Equipment in Anaesthesia and Critical Care

A complete guide for the FRCA

Daniel Aston
BSc, MBBS, MRCP, FRCA

Angus Rivers
BSc, MBBS, FRCA

Asela Dharmadasa
MA, BM BCh, FRCA

Scion

© **Scion Publishing Limited, 2014**

First published 2014

All rights reserved. No part of this book may be reproduced or transmitted, in any form
or by any means, without permission.

A CIP catalogue record for this book is available from the British Library.

ISBN 978 1 907904 05 9

Scion Publishing Limited

The Old Hayloft, Vantage Business Park, Bloxham Road, Banbury OX16 9UX, UK

www.scionpublishing.com

Important Note from the Publisher

The information contained within this book was obtained by Scion Publishing Ltd from
sources believed by us to be reliable. However, while every effort has been made to
ensure its accuracy, no responsibility for loss or injury whatsoever occasioned to any
person acting or refraining from action as a result of information contained herein can
be accepted by the authors or publishers.

Readers are reminded that medicine is a constantly evolving science and while the
authors and publishers have ensured that all dosages, applications and practices are
based on current indications, there may be specific practices which differ between
communities. You should always follow the guidelines laid down by the manufacturers of
specific products and the relevant authorities in the country in which you are practising.

Although every effort has been made to ensure that all owners of copyright material
have been acknowledged in this publication, we would be pleased to acknowledge in
subsequent reprints or editions any omissions brought to our attention.

Registered names, trademarks, etc. used in this book, even when not marked as such, are
not to be considered unprotected by law.

Cover design by Andrew Magee Design Ltd., Kidlington Oxfordshire, UK
Illustrations by Underlined, Marlow, Buckinghamshire, UK
Typeset by Phoenix Photosetting, Chatham, Kent, UK
Printed and bound by Charlesworth Press, Wakefield, UK

Contents

Preface

The Fellowship of the Royal College of Anaesthetists (FRCA) examination demands an in-depth knowledge of the mechanics, physics and clinical application of equipment used in anaesthesia and critical care.

Whilst working towards this exam ourselves, we struggled to find a textbook on equipment that distilled the required information into a clear and concise format that was easy to learn from. We have therefore spent considerable time researching equipment and liaising with manufacturers and trainees to produce a book specifically targeted at candidates sitting the primary and final FRCA exams. Our hope is that you will find it engaging, comprehensive and to the point.

For the sake of clarity, a standardized format is used throughout; each major piece of equipment is given a single section that includes photographs and simple line diagrams that can be reproduced in a viva or written exam. Each section is subdivided into an *overview*, a list of *uses* for the equipment, a description of *how it works*, an opinion on its relative *advantages* and *disadvantages*, and a list of *safety* considerations. Where relevant, we have also included chapter introductions that provide a framework to help understand and classify the equipment featured within it. A point to note is that the comments on the relative advantages and disadvantages of pieces of equipment may differ from those expressed by the manufacturer, but the views expressed are based on evidence, our experience or the opinions of other senior anaesthetists with whom we have worked.

A set of pertinent multiple choice, short answer and viva questions are provided to test your knowledge of each chapter.

Inevitably, many descriptions of equipment require an explanation of the physical variables used or measured. Where possible we have used the SI unit for these. However, in some areas of practice the unit in common use is not SI (e.g. the measurement of blood pressure) and in these cases we have used the more familiar term.

You will see that some words and phrases are written in blue. This highlighting indicates that a more detailed description of the subject can be found elsewhere in the book.

Thank you for using our book, we hope you find it useful and wish you the very best of luck with the exam.

Dan, Angus & Asela

August 2013

Acknowledgements

This book would not have been possible without the many people who helped us along the way.

For taking the time to proof-read some of our work and for inspiring us with suggestions and constructive criticism, we would like to thank:

Doug Barker, Alistair Blake, Ed Costar, Pascale Gruber, Stefan Gurney, James Ip, Rohit Juneja, Daniel Krahne, Helen Laycock, Geoff Lockwood, Shahan Nizar, Jeremy Radcliffe, Neville Robinson, Martin Rooms, Aarti Shah, Olivia Shields, Adam Shonfeld and Peter Williamson.

We are also most grateful to the significant number of individuals, hospitals, companies, museums and other sources who have generously supplied us with or allowed us to take photographs of their equipment. They are credited within the text.

For converting our hand drawn pictures into the high quality diagrams that appear in these pages, we owe our thanks to Elliot Banks.

Finally, there are three people who have been our principle source of inspiration and encouragement; our warmest and most heartfelt gratitude is reserved for Lindsay, Malin and Aneesha, to whom this book is dedicated.

Abbreviations

AC	alternating current
ACT	activated clotting time
AF	atrial fibrillation
APL	adjustable pressure limiting
APTT	activated partial thromboplastin time
AV	atrioventricular
BIPAP	bi-phasic positive airway pressure
BIS	bispectral index
COETT	cuffed oral endotracheal tube
CPAP	continuous positive airway pressure
CPB	cardiopulmonary bypass
CPU	central processing unit
CSA	compressed spectral array
CSE	combined spinal epidural
CSF	cerebrospinal fluid
CT	computed tomography
CVP	central venous pressure
CVVHD	continuous venovenous haemodialysis
CVVHDF	continuous venovenous haemodiafiltration
CVVHF	continuous venovenous haemofiltration
DC	direct current
DLT	double lumen tube
ECG	electrocardiograph
ECMO	extracorporeal membrane oxygenation
EEG	electroencephalograph
EMG	electromyography
ETT	endotracheal tube
EVD	external ventricular drain
EVLW	extravascular lung water
FFP	fresh frozen plasma
FGF	fresh gas flow
FiO_2	inspired fraction of oxygen
FRC	functional residual capacity
GEDV	global end diastolic volume
HFJV	high frequency jet ventilation
HFOV	high frequency oscillatory ventilation
HME	heat and moisture exchange
HMEF	heat and moisture exchange filter
IABP	intra-aortic balloon pump
ICD	implantable cardioverter defibrillator

ICP	intracranial pressure
ID	internal diameter
IPPV	intermittent positive pressure ventilation
ITTV	intrathoracic thermal volume
LMA	laryngeal mask airway
LOR	loss of resistance
MLT	microlaryngeal tube
MRI	magnetic resonance imaging
MV	minute ventilation
NG	nasogastric
NICE	National Institute for Health and Care Excellence
NIPPV	non-invasive positive pressure ventilation
NIST	non-interchangeable screw thread
NJ	nasojejunal
OD	outer diameter
PAC	pulmonary artery catheter
PCA	patient-controlled analgesia
PCWP	pulmonary capillary wedge pressure
PDPH	post-dural puncture headache
PEEP	positive end expiratory pressure
PEG	percutaneous endoscopic gastrostomy
PICC	peripherally inserted central catheter
PIP	peak inspiratory pressure
PPV	positive pressure ventilation
PRVC	pressure-regulated volume control
PT	prothrombin time
PTV	pulmonary thermal volume
PVC	polyvinylchloride
RIL	rigid indirect laryngoscope
RMS	root mean square
RRT	renal replacement therapy
RUL	right upper lobe
SIMV	synchronized intermittent mandatory ventilation
SVP	saturated vapour pressure
SVT	supraventricular tachycardia
TCI	target controlled infusion
TIVA	total intravenous anaesthesia
TPN	total parenteral nutrition
VAD	ventricular assist device
VF	ventricular fibrillation
VIC	vaporizer-in-circuit
VIE	vacuum insulated evaporator
VOC	vaporizer-out-of-circuit
VT	ventricular tachycardia

Chapter 1
Medical gases

Vacuum insulated evaporator

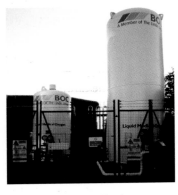

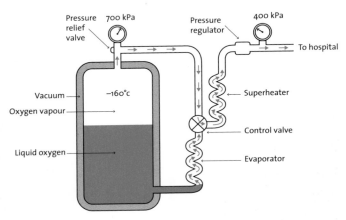

Fig. 1.1.1: The main and backup vacuum insulated evaporators outside a hospital.

Fig. 1.1.2: A schematic diagram of a vacuum insulated evaporator.

Overview

The vacuum insulated evaporator (VIE) is a storage tank for liquid oxygen with a vacuum insulated wall designed to keep the contents below −160°C. The wall consists of an inner stainless steel shell and an outer carbon steel shell. It may rest on a weighing tripod.

Uses

VIEs provide the piped oxygen supply in most hospitals.

How it works

General principles
Liquid oxygen is produced by fractional distillation of air, off-site. It is delivered to the hospital on a regular basis and stored in the VIE. Oxygen has a critical temperature of −119°C, meaning that above this temperature it must exist as a gas; the VIE is therefore kept between −160°C and −180°C.

The VIE is not actively cooled. Instead, as suggested by the name, it relies on insulation and evaporation to maintain the low temperature. Insulation is provided by the vacuum wall, which minimizes conduction and convection of heat into the chamber. The small amount of heat which does enter the VIE causes some of the liquid oxygen to evaporate. Evaporation uses energy in the form of heat (the latent heat of vaporization) and therefore the VIE remains cool.

Low and high use situations
The pressure in the VIE is approximately 700 kPa (7 Bar, the saturated vapour pressure of oxygen at −160°C). If left unvented (say all the oxygen taps in the hospital were turned off), the pressure in the VIE would rise as oxygen slowly evaporated. To prevent an explosion in this situation, a pressure relief valve vents unused oxygen into the atmosphere.

If instead demand is high, the rapid vaporization of large quantities of oxygen causes a drop in temperature, resulting in the reduction of vapour pressure and therefore reduced supply. In this circumstance, a valve is electronically opened, allowing liquid oxygen to enter an evaporator coil exposed to ambient temperature. This pipe is also known as a superheater, though the

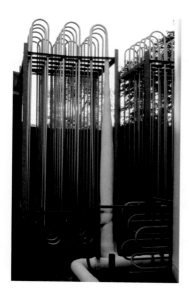

Fig. 1.1.3: Superheater coils. The pipes leading from the VIE are covered in frost because of the extreme cold.

only heat required is that from the air surrounding it – the large temperature difference causes rapid warming and vaporization.

Oxygen leaving the VIE is extremely cold and exceeds pipeline pressure. Before entering the hospital pipeline, it is therefore passed through another superheater that brings it to ambient temperature, and a pressure regulator that reduces its pressure to 400 kPa (4 Bar).

Measuring the contents

The amount of oxygen remaining in the VIE can be calculated from its mass. Traditionally this is done by weighing it using a tripod weighing scale – the VIE pivots on two legs, with the third resting on the scale. The VIE's empty (tare) weight is known and subtracted from the measured value to give the weight of oxygen inside.

Alternatively, the oxygen contents may be calculated from the difference between the vapour pressure at the top of the VIE and the pressure at the bottom of the liquid oxygen. Using these pressures, it is possible to calculate the height of the fluid column and, by knowing the VIE's cross-sectional area, the volume of liquid oxygen remaining.

⊕ Advantages

- Storing liquid oxygen is highly efficient in terms of space. It expands to 860 times its volume as it vaporizes to 20°C.
- Compared with a cylinder at room temperature, liquid oxygen is stored at a much lower pressure (700 instead of 13 700 kPa).
- The VIE does not require power to store oxygen in a liquid state.
- Oxygen is therefore cheaper both to deliver and to store as a liquid.

⊖ Disadvantages

- Initial equipment costs are much higher than a cylinder manifold.
- A backup cylinder manifold and/or second VIE is required in case of interruption to the oxygen supply.
- If demand is not fairly continuous a significant amount of oxygen will be unused and vented.

ⓘ Safety

- The VIE must be kept outside the building because of the fire risk.

1.2 Cylinder manifolds

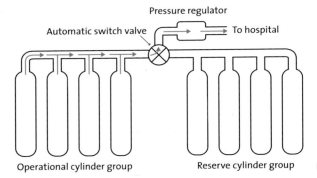

Fig. 1.2.1: A cylinder manifold.

Overview

A manifold is a pipe with several openings, in this case connected to cylinders supplying pipeline oxygen, nitrous oxide or Entonox.

Uses

Manifolds are used to supply piped nitrous oxide and Entonox, and they may also be used as a primary oxygen supply in small hospitals, or as a backup supply for larger hospitals.

How it works

The manifold usually connects two groups (occasionally there may be more) of high capacity cylinders (size J or L). Each cylinder is connected to the manifold and then to the pipeline. Pressure regulators reduce the pressure to that of a standard pipeline. All the cylinders in a group are utilized simultaneously until their pressure falls below a certain level, at which point an automatic valve switches to draw gas from the other group of cylinders. At this point an alarm indicates the need to change the cylinders in the empty group.

A cylinder manifold is typically designed with each cylinder group able to supply a typical day's demand, hence one group of cylinders is changed each day.

⊕ Advantages

- Simple and cheap.
- Provides an effective backup supply.
- The alarm system means it should never run empty, providing there are full cylinders available to swap in.

⊖ Disadvantages

- Limited capacity when compared with a VIE.

ⓘ Safety

- Medical gases are a potential fire and explosion risk so the manifold is kept in a well-ventilated building separate from the main hospital.
- The main cylinder store should be in a separate room.

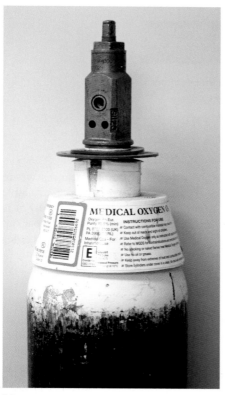 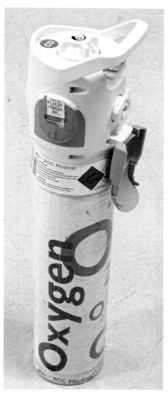

(a)　　　　　　　　　　　　　　　(b)

Fig. 1.3.1: (a) A size E oxygen cylinder. Note the disc around the valve block and the label information. This cylinder is ready to connect to the pin-index system on the anaesthetic machine. (b) A size CD oxygen cylinder. This size cylinder commonly has both a Schrader valve and a connection for standard oxygen tubing.

Overview

Medical gases are supplied in cylinders that are usually made of chromium molybdenum (chromoly) steel, or aluminium. They are available in a range of sizes; those most commonly encountered in anaesthetics are size E on anaesthetic machines and size CD, which is often used during the transfer of patients. A full size E oxygen cylinder yields 680 litres of oxygen, while a size CD oxygen cylinder releases 460 litres. Larger cylinders (e.g. size J) are used in cylinder manifolds. *Table 1.3.1* shows some commonly encountered cylinder sizes and their volumes.

Several pieces of important information are found on gas cylinders. There is a label that notes the name of the gas and its chemical formula, the cylinder size letter, a batch number, the maximum safe operating pressure, the expiry date, and notes on storage, handling and hazards. A plastic disc denotes the date that the cylinder was last subjected to testing, and the valve block is engraved with the testing pressure. The cylinder itself is also engraved with the test pressure and the dates of testing, along with the tare (empty) weight of the cylinder and the cylinder serial number.

Cylinders are colour coded for easy identification. In the UK, oxygen cylinders have a black body and a white shoulder. *Figure 1.3.2* shows the colours of commonly encountered gas cylinders.

Table 1.3.1: Properties of commonly encountered oxygen cylinder sizes.

Cylinder size	Cylinder oxygen volume at 137 Bar at 15°C (litres)	Cylinder water capacity (litres)	Approximate tare weight (kg)
CD	460	2.0	3.0
E	680	4.7	5.4
J	6800	47.0	69.0

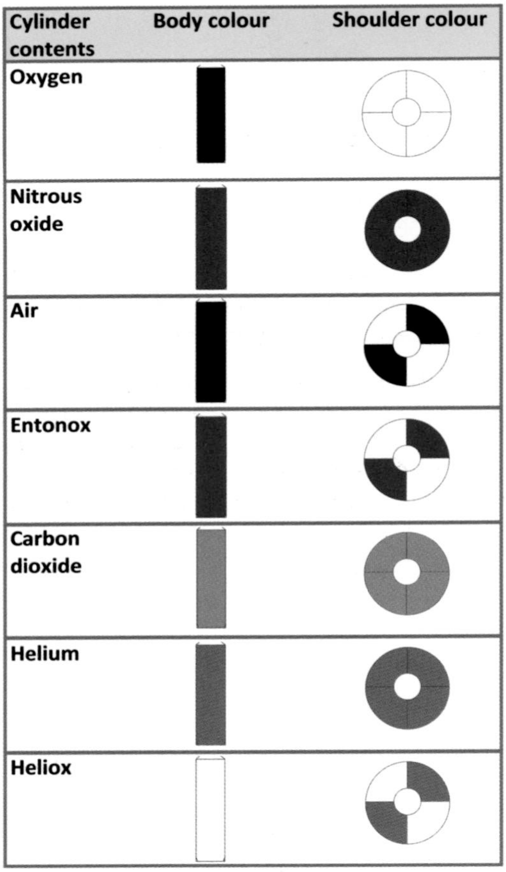

Cylinder contents	Body colour	Shoulder colour
Oxygen		
Nitrous oxide		
Air		
Entonox		
Carbon dioxide		
Helium		
Heliox		

Fig. 1.3.2: UK gas cylinder colour coding.

Uses

Cylinders are used in circumstances where a piped gas supply is either not available (e.g. in ambulances or small hospitals) or is inconvenient. They are also used as a backup to the piped supply on anaesthetic machines and where the gas is required infrequently or in small quantities (e.g. nitric oxide or heliox).

How it works

Size E or J cylinders containing oxygen or air have a gauge pressure of 13 700 kPa (137 Bar, 2000 psi) when they are full at 15°C. Size CD cylinders can be filled to a maximum pressure of 23 000 kPa (230 Bar). The pressure displayed on the Bourdon gauge is proportional to the volume of gas remaining in the cylinder (provided the temperature is constant), in accordance with Boyle's law.

It is impossible to compress a gas into a liquid, no matter what pressure is applied, if the temperature of the gas is above its critical temperature. The critical temperature of oxygen is −119°C and so it remains in its gaseous phase in cylinders at 15°C and obeys Boyle's law. However, other gases behave differently under pressure because they have different critical temperatures. The critical temperature of nitrous oxide is 36.5°C so it is possible to compress it into a liquid in a cylinder at 15°C.

A full nitrous oxide cylinder therefore contains nitrous oxide liquid and vapour in equilibrium. The Bourdon gauge on the cylinder measures the vapour pressure and gives no information about the amount of liquid remaining. The gauge will read 4400 kPa at 15°C (or 5150 kPa at 20°C), and this pressure will only begin to fall when the cylinder is very nearly empty (i.e. when all the liquid nitrous oxide is used up). Because of this, the only way to estimate how much nitrous oxide remains in a cylinder is to weigh it.

Gas can be released from cylinders in several ways, including a variable valve and tap that is calibrated in litres per minute and can be connected to standard oxygen tubing. These taps are usually found on size CD cylinders. Schrader valves, the pin index system and connection of cylinders to the anaesthetic machine are discussed in *Section 5.2*.

⊕ Advantages

- Smaller cylinders are portable.
- A variety of connectors exist.
- Can be refilled and reused.

⊖ Disadvantages

- Heavy to transport.
- Not all connectors are present on all cylinders.
- The amount of gas is limited by the volume of the cylinder, and there is no alarm when it runs out.

ⓘ Safety

All cylinders are tested once in every 5–10 years. Tests include endoscopic examination, pressurization tests (up to 25 000 kPa), and tensile tests; the latter involve destroying 1% of cylinders in order to perform impact, stretching, flattening and other tests of strength.

The filling ratio, defined as the weight of the liquid in a full cylinder divided by the weight of water that would completely fill the cylinder, is 0.75 at 15.5°C in the UK. This is so that if the temperature rises, the liquid can vaporize without the risk of large pressure increases and explosions. In countries with warmer climates, a lower filling ratio of 0.67 is often used instead of 0.75. A filling ratio of 0.75 is not exactly the same as the cylinder being 75% filled, due to the difference between the properties of water and the contents of the cylinder (e.g. density).

1.4 Compressed air supply

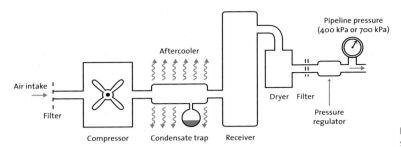

Fig. 1.4.1: The compressed air supply system.

Overview

Two pressures of medical grade air are used in hospitals, and these are usually provided using an air compressor. Smaller hospitals may use cylinder banks.

Uses

Air at 400 kPa (4 Bar) is piped for use in anaesthetic machines and ventilators. A second supply at 700 kPa (7 Bar) is used to power surgical equipment.

How it works

The air intake for a hospital is usually in an outside location and must be at a safe distance from exhaust fumes and other sources of pollution. The intake incorporates a filtering system. Two compressors are used, each capable of meeting expected demand, thus ensuring continued supply should one of them fail. The compressors are designed to minimize contamination of the air with oil. Compression causes the air to heat because of the 3rd gas law; aftercoolers are therefore employed. As the air cools, water condenses and is captured in condensate traps.

Compressed air may be stored in a receiver before being further dried, filtered and pressure regulated. It then enters the pipeline.

⊕ Advantages

- An on-site air compressor is far more cost-effective for a large hospital than a cylinder bank.

⊖ Disadvantages

- There is a higher initial cost than a cylinder bank in order to provide a safe, clean air supply.

⊘ Safety

- Risk of contamination at the air intake, which must be carefully situated and regularly inspected.
- Risk of oil mist contamination from the compressor.
- The two different pressure pipelines have non-interchangeable Schrader valves which prevents the connection of high pressure air to the anaesthetic machine.

1.5 Oxygen concentrator

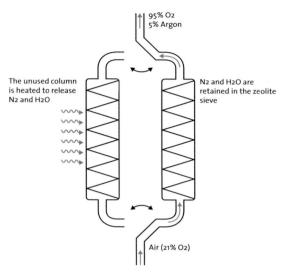

95% O2
5% Argon

The unused column is heated to release N2 and H2O

N2 and H2O are retained in the zeolite sieve

Air (21% O2)

Fig. 1.5.1: An oxygen concentrator.

Overview

Oxygen concentrators produce concentrated oxygen from air (which consists of 78% nitrogen, 21% oxygen, 1% argon, and a variable amount of water vapour). Nitrogen and water vapour are removed, leaving up to 95% oxygen and 5% argon.

Uses

Oxygen concentrators are commonly used to supply oxygen to individuals in the home. Larger concentrators may be used as a backup to the primary hospital oxygen supply or as a main oxygen supply in remote hospitals where deliveries of oxygen are unreliable.

How it works

Materials called zeolites, a family of aluminosilicates, form a lattice structure that acts as a molecular sieve, filtering specific molecules whilst allowing others to pass through. Oxygen concentrators contain two or more zeolite columns, used sequentially. Pressurized air is passed through the column and nitrogen and water vapour are retained by the sieve, leaving a high concentration of oxygen. When a zeolite column is not in use, it can be heated and the unwanted nitrogen and water released into the atmosphere.

The maximum achievable concentration of oxygen is around 95%. Argon, which makes up 1% of the atmosphere, is concentrated by the same factor as oxygen, yielding approximately 5% once all the nitrogen has been removed.

Personal oxygen concentrators may supply up to 10 l.min^{-1} oxygen, although they are normally used at much lower rates.

⊕ Advantages

- They are a cheap and reliable method of supplying home oxygen.
- Concentrators avoid or reduce the need for commercial deliveries of oxygen.

⊖ Disadvantages

- If used at low flows on an anaesthetic circle system, argon accumulates, eventually producing a hypoxic mixture.
- The system will stop producing oxygen if the power supply fails.

⊘ Safety

- As with all high concentrations of oxygen, explosions are a hazard and home users are therefore required to give up smoking before long-term oxygen therapy is prescribed.

1.6 Piped medical gas supply

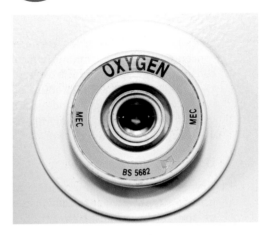

Fig. 1.6.1: A Schrader oxygen outlet.

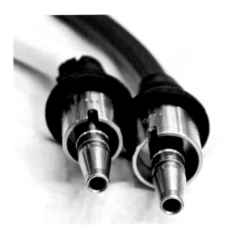

Fig. 1.6.2: Oxygen and nitrous oxide Schrader probes. The hoses are colour coded and the probes labelled with the gas name. The different diameter index collar physically prevents cross-connection.

Overview

The medical gas supply includes pipelines linking VIEs, cylinder banks and air compressors to wall outlets in wards and theatre suites. Indexed connectors prevent cross-connection.

Uses

Gases supplied include oxygen, air, nitrous oxide and Entonox.

How it works

The vast majority of hospitals have a piped oxygen supply, and most anaesthetic facilities also have piped air and nitrous oxide. Piped Entonox is used on many labour wards. Gases are supplied at 400 kPa (4 Bar), with the exception of air which is supplied at 400 kPa for therapeutic use and 700 kPa to power surgical equipment.

The pipeline is made of a special high quality copper to prevent corrosion or contamination and terminates in self-closing wall outlets called Schrader sockets. Schrader probes click into the sockets and connect via anti-kink hoses to anaesthetic machines, wall flowmeters, ventilators and other equipment.

⊕ Advantages

- Convenience.
- Central safeguarded supply ensures gas delivery.

⊖ Disadvantages

- High initial setup and ongoing maintenance costs.
- Leaks pose a fire hazard, and may be difficult to locate.

ⓘ Safety

A number of design features prevent the potentially fatal connection of the wrong gas type (for instance, nitrous oxide cross-connected with oxygen).

- *Clear labelling* – both Schrader sockets and connecting hoses are labelled with the gas name.
- *Colour coding* – both Schrader sockets and connecting hoses are colour-coded (oxygen is white, nitrous oxide is blue, air is black).
- *Index collar* connection, which is non-interchangeable – the hose terminates in a Schrader probe with an index collar of a specific diameter which will only fit into the appropriate socket.
- *NIST* – the hose connects to the anaesthetic machine by means of a Non-Interchangeable Screw Thread (NIST) which cannot be attached to the wrong connector (see *Section 5.2*).

The risks of fire or explosion due to a leaking oxygen or nitrous oxide pipeline are considerable and regular maintenance is required. Emergency shut-off valves allow isolation of particular areas.

1.7 Medical vacuum and suction

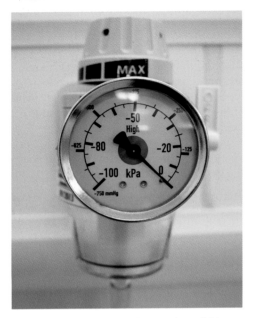

Fig. 1.7.1: A wall suction unit showing the variable pressure regulator and suction trap.

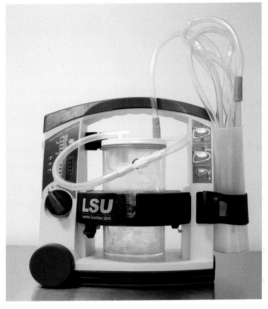

Fig. 1.7.2: The Laerdal suction unit (Laerdal Medical) is a battery operated portable suction unit.

Overview

Medical vacuum is used in suction devices throughout the hospital, usually from a central vacuum plant. It is recommended that one vacuum outlet is present in each anaesthetic room, with two in each operating theatre (including one dedicated to anaesthetic use). Portable vacuum units are also available.

Pressures are typically described in gauge pressure; negative pressures are therefore relative to atmospheric pressure. Gauge pressures of less than −101 kPa (−760 mmHg) cannot be achieved because a negative absolute pressure is impossible.

Uses

The immediate availability of functioning suction apparatus is mandatory for safe anaesthesia, and is used to clear secretions, vomitus and blood from the airway. Suction is also required for most surgical procedures and for a wide array of other uses such as bronchoscopy and cell salvage.

How it works

A medical vacuum system should be capable of creating a pressure of −53 kPa (−400 mmHg) with a flow of 40 l.min^{-1}. It is therefore a high-pressure, low-flow system (scavenging systems are low-pressure, high-flow).

The central medical vacuum system is based around a vacuum receiver vessel (essentially a large empty tank) which is maintained at the required sub-atmospheric pressure by at least two pumps, so that the supply continues even if one pump fails. The receiver and pumps are protected from contamination by an arrangement of secretion traps and filters. Pipelines then connect to vacuum outlets throughout the hospital.

In order to use suction, a pressure is selected using a variable pressure regulator attached to the wall outlet. Tubing transmits the negative pressure to a disposable collection bottle. Aspirated fluid passes into the collection bottle and the volume of liquid can be measured. A valve shuts off the suction once the liquid reaches the top of the bottle. In order to further protect the pipeline from contamination, a suction trap is integrated into the pressure regulator unit.

An alternative to centralized suction is portable suction which consists of a battery operated pump and integrated collection bottle. Devices powered by pressurized medical gas from a cylinder are also available.

Advantages

- Essential for safe anaesthesia.
- Centralized vacuum supplies are highly reliable.
- Collection systems are simple, cheap and disposable.

Disadvantages

- Disconnections and leaks in collection system are common, limiting suction pressure and flow.
- Battery life in portable units is limited.

1.8 Scavenging

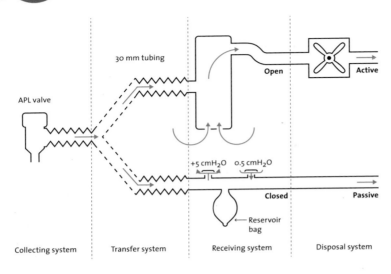

Fig. 1.8.1: Schematic diagram showing the components of active and passive scavenging systems.

Overview

The safe environmental levels of anaesthetic gases have not yet been determined. UK legislation, somewhat arbitrarily therefore, limits environmental concentrations to 100 parts per million (ppm) for nitrous oxide (N_2O) and 50 ppm for isoflurane, as time-weighted averages over 8 hours. Newer volatiles are not included in the legislation, but 20 ppm has been suggested as a limit for sevoflurane (being 100 times less than the concentration which has any clinical effect).

The USA takes an alternative approach and limits concentration to 25 ppm for N_2O and 2 ppm for volatile anaesthetics, these being levels that can be reasonably achieved.

Uses

Scavenging systems are designed to reduce environmental anaesthetic gas concentrations by collecting waste gases and venting them outside the building.

How it works

Scavenging systems may be divided into active or passive designs, depending on the disposal system used. Active systems use a pump to generate a negative pressure and require an open receiving system to prevent transfer of the negative pressure to the patient. Passive systems use the positive pressure generated by the patient's expiration to transmit gas to the atmosphere via a closed receiving system.

There are four components to a scavenging system:

Collecting system
This typically connects to the adjustable pressure limiting (APL) valve, using a 30 mm connection to avoid accidental cross-connection with the breathing system.

Transfer system
This is the corrugated plastic hose which connects the collecting system to the receiving system.

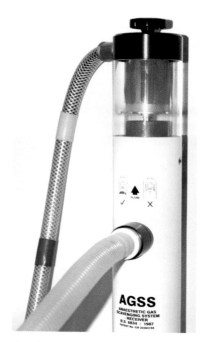

Fig. 1.8.2: An open receiving system (the opening is at the bottom of the device, not shown in the image). The 30 mm corrugated hose connects to the APL valve and the top hose connects to the active disposal system.

Receiving system

Open receiving systems consist of a reservoir with a mesh-covered opening that is usually mounted on the anaesthetic machine. The opening allows compensation for variations in expiratory flow without generating positive or negative pressures. Open receiving systems are used in active scavenging.

Closed receiving systems consist of a length of tubing with positive and negative pressure relief valves. The valves open at +5 cmH$_2$O and −0.5 cmH$_2$O respectively. In the absence of a relief valve, pressure may increase if the system is blocked or decrease if the opening is in a windy area. Many systems also incorporate a reservoir bag, which reduces valve opening by accommodating small variations in pressure and therefore increases efficiency of scavenging. The tubing in a passive system should be kept as short as possible to decrease the resistance.

Disposal system

Modern hospitals use active scavenging with a high-flow (over 100 l.min^{-1}), low-pressure vacuum system to draw exhaust gases from the receiving system and vent them to the atmosphere. This system is separate from the high-pressure, low-flow vacuum used for suction.

Passive systems consist of tubing that directly vents to the atmosphere through an external wall. They are affected by wind direction, and may lead to increased resistance to expiration.

Advantages
- Required to reduce theatre pollution to within legal limits.
- Systems are simple and effective.

Disadvantages
- Does not prevent environmental pollution (volatile anaesthetics are potent greenhouse gases).
- Positive or negative pressures may be transmitted to breathing system if the system is poorly designed or malfunctions.

Other notes
- Ventilation systems change the air in operating theatres at least 20 times per hour, which further reduces ambient anaesthetic gas concentrations.
- Cardiff aldasorber is a simple passive device used in resource-poor locations, consisting of a canister containing activated charcoal which absorbs volatile anaesthetic agents. When heated the agents are vented back into the atmosphere.

1.9 Delivery of supplemental oxygen

Hospital patients often have an increased oxygen demand and/or impaired oxygen delivery and so administration of supplemental oxygen is commonly required. Delivering supplemental oxygen may be achieved using devices that deliver oxygen to the nose only, or via masks covering the nose and mouth.

Minute ventilation in an adult is approximately $6\,l.min^{-1}$ at rest, and it would therefore appear at first glance that an inspired oxygen fraction (FiO_2) of 1.0, (i.e. 100% oxygen) could be achieved by administering over $6\,l.min^{-1}$ via a simple face mask. Unfortunately this is not the case, because inspiratory flow rates are non-uniform and peak at over $60\,l.min^{-1}$. Air is therefore entrained and dilutes the supplied oxygen.

Reservoir devices

In order to provide an FiO_2 of 1.0, a device must be able to match the patient's peak inspiratory flow. Whilst this could be achieved using a higher oxygen supply flow, it is more efficient to have a reservoir which fills with oxygen during expiration and is drawn upon during inspiration. This is the principle underlying all anaesthetic breathing systems, and the reservoir mask.

Variable performance devices

A further problem caused by non-uniformity of inspiratory flow is that it is not possible to set a specific FiO_2 when using simple face masks or nasal cannulae. In order to compensate for the difference between the flow delivered to the mask and the flow required by the patient, air will be entrained around the side of the device and through the expiration ports. Increasing the oxygen flow will see some increase in FiO_2, but the exact amount will depend on the volume of the mask (which acts as a reservoir), the patient's respiratory dynamics, and the seal of the mask. Such a system is called a variable performance device.

Fixed performance devices

In some conditions, such as in patients with chronic lung disease, delivering a fixed FiO_2 is desirable. This may, in theory, be achieved by supplying a specific oxygen/air mix at a flow greater than the patient's peak inspiratory flow. In practice, peak flows are highly variable and may exceed the delivered flow, reducing the FiO_2. Unlike a variable performance device, however, a fixed device can never deliver *more* than the specified FiO_2. The most common fixed performance device is the Venturi mask, though nasal high flow devices are also available.

1.10 Nasal cannulae

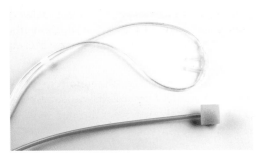

Fig. 1.10.1: Nasal cannulae and a nasal catheter, which supplies oxygen to one nostril only.

Overview

Nasal cannulae are variable performance devices that are effective and well tolerated in many patients with low supplemental oxygen requirements.

Uses

An alternative to an oxygen mask in those requiring low level supplemental oxygen.

How it works

The tubing is looped around the patient's ears and the prongs inserted into the nose. Gas flows of 1–4 l.min^{-1} are typically used because higher flows cause drying of the nasal mucosa leading to discomfort, epistaxis and impaired mucociliary clearance.

During use, the nasopharynx acts an oxygen reservoir. Even if the patient breathes through the mouth, oxygen will be entrained from the nasopharynx and a majority of studies have shown that mouth breathing results in either the same inspired oxygen concentration, or a higher concentration. This effect is unpredictable, however, and therefore nasal cannulae deliver a variable FiO$_2$.

Advantages

- Simple and cheap.
- Patients can speak, eat and drink.
- Good patient compliance.

Disadvantages

- Variable FiO$_2$.
- Drying of nasal mucosa limits FiO$_2$ unless humidified gas is supplied (see *Section 1.13*: nasal high flow).

Other notes

A nasal catheter is a single lumen catheter that is inserted into a single nostril. It has a sponge tip which holds it in place and it is usually also secured with tape to the patient's face. Once in place it is well tolerated. It may be used in situations such as carotid surgery, where traditional nasal cannulae would interfere with the surgical field.

1.11 Variable performance masks

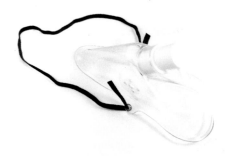

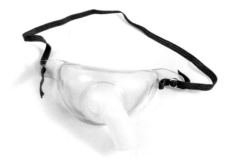

Fig. 1.11.1: A simple face mask, also commonly known as a Hudson mask.

Fig. 1.11.2: A tracheostomy mask.

Overview

The simple face mask, a variable performance device, is the most common means of delivering supplemental oxygen. Modifications include the reservoir mask and the tracheostomy mask.

Uses

Variable performance masks are used for delivery of oxygen in situations where the precise FiO_2 is unimportant. Reservoir masks are the simplest means of delivering high oxygen concentrations and are thus used in emergency situations.

How it works

Simple face masks do not form a tight seal against the patient's face and may have holes on each side to allow air entrainment to meet peak inspiratory flow and to vent expired gases. Plastic tubing connects to the oxygen supply.

An oxygen flow of up to $15\,l.min^{-1}$ may be used depending on the patient's requirements. It is important to realize that air is entrained with the supplied oxygen and the FiO_2 delivered is therefore imprecise.

Reservoir mask

This is a modification of a simple face mask and is also known as a non-rebreather mask. Oxygen is supplied into a reservoir bag which is connected to the mask via a simple flap valve. The side holes in the mask are covered by further flap valves which allow expiration, but reduce entrainment of air.

During inspiration, 100% oxygen is drawn from the reservoir bag. Some air will still be entrained around the mask, because it isn't fully sealed, so the FiO_2 remains variable at around 0.6–0.8. Expired gas is vented through the side holes and around the mask, with the valve and the oxygen flow preventing it entering the reservoir.

⊕ Advantages

- Simple, cheap and widely available.
- Easy to vary the oxygen delivered (though not from or to known fractions, c.f. Venturi masks (see *Section 1.12*)).
- Reservoir masks are the simplest means of delivering high concentrations of oxygen.

⊖ Disadvantages

- Variable performance device:
  - the precise FiO_2 is unknown
  - not suitable for performing calculations such as A/a gradients.
- Rebreathing of exhaled CO_2 from within the mask may occur.

1.12 Venturi mask

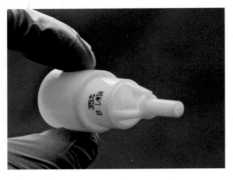

Fig. 1.12.1: A Venturi device.

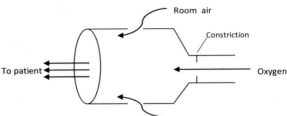

Fig. 1.12.2: Schematic of a Venturi device.

Overview

Venturi masks are fixed performance devices that utilize the Venturi effect to deliver a precise concentration of oxygen to the patient.

Uses

Venturi masks are used to deliver oxygen to patients when a specific and consistent concentration is needed. Unlike variable performance devices, the fixed performance of the Venturi mask allows interpretation of oxygen saturations and blood gases in the context of a known inspired fraction of oxygen (FiO_2). A 24% Venturi mask can be relied upon to deliver no more than 24% oxygen.

How it works

The colour-coded Venturi device (see *Table 1.12.1*) comprises a distal connection to standard oxygen tubing and a proximal nozzle that connects to a mask. Oxygen flows through a central constriction within the device and room air is entrained through surrounding apertures due to a combination of the Venturi effect and frictional drag of air. This dilutes the oxygen to the required concentration.

The Venturi effect is a consequence of the Bernoulli principle, which states that in order to maintain a constant flow, a fluid must increase its velocity as it flows through a constriction. This increase in kinetic energy occurs at the expense of its potential energy or, in other words, through a decrease in pressure. The energy in the system is therefore constant, in keeping with the first law of thermodynamics.

If the constriction in the tubing is opened to the outside environment, surrounding air will be entrained into the tubing due to the pressure drop generated as the velocity of gas flowing through the constriction increases. This is the Venturi effect. The relative contributions of the Venturi effect and of frictional drag to the volume of air entrained are difficult to quantify and subject to debate. The volume of air entrained compared with the flow of oxygen (the entrainment ratio) is determined by the

Table 1.12.1: UK colour coding for Venturi devices

Colour	Inspired oxygen concentration
Blue	24%
White	28%
Yellow	35%
Red	40%
Green	60%

size of the apertures around the nozzle. A Venturi mask delivering 60% oxygen will therefore have smaller apertures than a 24% mask, because the latter has to dilute the oxygen with more air to achieve the required concentration.

A Venturi mask is intended to deliver accurate concentrations of oxygen to the patient, provided that the oxygen flow is set above the recommended minimum rate, which is printed on the side of the device. The total flow delivered to the patient is the sum of the set oxygen flow through the Venturi device and the volume of air entrained through its apertures. For the delivered oxygen concentration to remain accurate, the total flow delivered must be greater than the patient's peak inspiratory flow. Oxygen flows above the minimum do not alter the final concentration of oxygen produced by the device because the oxygen flow and amount of air entrained are proportional.

Unfortunately, although the concentration produced by the Venturi is constant, in certain circumstances the patient's inspired oxygen concentration may be less. In their 2008 guideline *Emergency Oxygen Delivery in Adults,* the British Thoracic Society recommends that at respiratory rates of greater than 30 breaths per minute the oxygen flow through the Venturi should be increased above the minimum rate printed on the device. The table below is adapted from the guideline and demonstrates the total flow delivered to the patient (oxygen + entrained air), for a given oxygen flow. Interestingly, a Venturi that is intended to deliver 60% oxygen can only actually deliver a total diluted flow of $30\,l.min^{-1}$, even with an oxygen flow of $15\,l.min^{-1}$. Given that a patient *in extremis* may have a far greater peak inspiratory flow than this, they are likely to receive an oxygen concentration below 60%. At this extreme, the Venturi has changed from a fixed to a variable performance device.

Table 1.12.2: The total flow (oxygen + entrained air) delivered to the patient for a given oxygen flow setting.

Set oxygen flow ($l.min^{-1}$)	24% Venturi ($l.min^{-1}$)	28% Venturi ($l.min^{-1}$)	35% Venturi ($l.min^{-1}$)	40% Venturi ($l.min^{-1}$)	60% Venturi ($l.min^{-1}$)
15			84	82	30
12			67	50	24
10			56	41	
8		89	46		
6		67			
4	102	44			
2	51				

Adapted from the 2008 BTS guideline: *Emergency Oxygen Delivery in Adults.*

⊕ Advantages

- Simple and lightweight.
- Able to deliver a specific and consistent concentration of oxygen to the patient under most circumstances, provided that the set oxygen flow is above the minimum recommended by the manufacturer.
- The patient's respiratory rate and pattern do not alter the inspired concentration of oxygen.

⊖ Disadvantages

- Risk of hypoxia by under-delivering oxygen.

- High flows of oxygen can lead to drying of airways.
- Less accurate at higher inspired concentrations of oxygen.
- At low oxygen flows and very high inspiratory flows, the device stops behaving like a fixed performance oxygen delivery device and may behave like a variable performance device.

ⓘ Safety

- Humidifiers used with a Venturi mask create water droplets that may occlude the narrow oxygen inlet and alter the device's entrainment ratio.

1.13 Nasal high flow

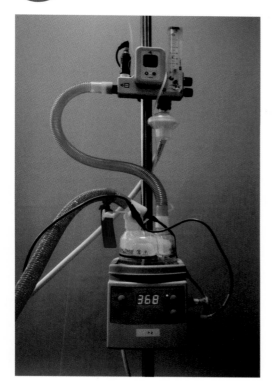

Fig. 1.13.1: An Optiflow system (Fisher & Paykel Healthcare) in use on an intensive care unit. It consists of a unit to alter oxygen concentration and flow, and a unit which warms and humidifies the gas before it is delivered to the patient via modified nasal cannulae.

Overview

Nasal high flow is a relatively new innovation. Warm, humidified oxygen and air mixtures can be supplied at flows of up to 60 l.min^{-1}. Its use is not widespread outside critical care and there are limited data on clinical outcomes.

Uses

A nasal high flow system may be used as an alternative to high flow face mask oxygen, particularly in post-surgical or critical care patients. It may also have a role in the management of patients requiring fixed oxygen concentrations or low level continuous positive airway pressure (CPAP).

How it works

Nasal high flow is an evolution of simple nasal cannulae (see *Section 1.10*). Gases are warmed and humidified prior to delivery to the patient, preventing drying of the nasal mucosa and overcoming the flow limitation of traditional cannulae. The device allows adjustment of inspired oxygen concentrations by mixing oxygen and air. This gas mixture may be delivered at flows of up to 60 l.min^{-1} and therefore, under normal conditions, nasal high flow acts as a fixed performance device.

An additional benefit is that nasal high flow devices have been shown to produce positive airway pressures of over 5 cmH$_2$O, thus permitting their use in place of low level CPAP (see *Section 4.1: Introduction to ventilators*).

⊕ Advantages

- Better tolerated in some patients than face masks.
- Fixed performance, permitting accurate delivery of up to 100% oxygen in most clinical situations.
- Gas is warmed and humidified.
- Low level positive airways pressure is possible.

⊖ Disadvantages

- Results of large scale clinical trials are still awaited.
- More expensive than standard oxygen delivery devices.
- Not yet available in all hospitals, and rarely outside of critical care.

Chapter 2
Airway equipment

2.1 Sealing face masks

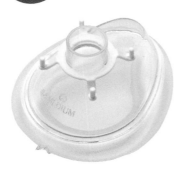

Fig. 2.1.1: Size 4 face mask (medium adult). Image courtesy of Timesco Healthcare Ltd.

Overview

Face masks have a soft seal that fits over the patient's nose and mouth. All masks in current use in the UK are disposable.

Uses

The seal permits non-invasive positive pressure ventilation, and allows effective administration of 100% oxygen.

How it works

The breathing system is usually attached to the mask via a catheter mount and 90° angle piece. This angle piece attaches to the mask via a standard 22 mm connector. The mask is designed to seal to the face using either an inflatable air cushion or a silicone seal. Paediatric masks may have a pleasant scent to improve patient acceptance.

A hooked connector may be used to attach a harness which straps around the patient's head. This has been superseded in anaesthetic practice by the laryngeal mask airway (see *Section 2.6*), but it is commonly used for non-invasive positive pressure ventilation (NIPPV).

⊕ Advantages

- A sealing face mask allows 100% oxygen to be delivered using an appropriate breathing system.
- A face mask is the simplest method of applying positive pressure ventilation and its use is an essential component when managing respiratory or airway emergencies. An appropriately sized mask should therefore be available for every anaesthetic.

⊖ Disadvantages

- Achieving a seal may prove difficult in some patients, particularly the edentulous.
- The volume within the mask is dead space. Paediatric masks are smaller and are often used without a catheter mount to offset this.
- Claustrophobia is a significant problem in some patients. This problem is improved by modern transparent masks.

ⓘ Safety

- Mask use can cause pressure injuries. Both skin breakdown and facial and trigeminal nerve injury have been reported, usually after prolonged NIPPV.

2.2 Magill forceps

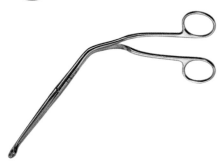

Fig. 2.2.1: Adult size Magill forceps. The curved design allows the anaesthetist's hand to be out of the line of vision. Image courtesy of Timesco Healthcare Ltd.

Overview

Magill forceps are shaped to enable manipulation of objects within the oropharynx without the operator's hand being in the line of sight.

Uses

Originally designed to aid placement of bougies (see *Section 2.7*) into the larynx, Magill forceps are commonly used to manipulate all manner of objects, including tracheal tubes, nasogastric tubes, throat packs, reinforced laryngeal mask airways and foreign bodies. They are essential for safe practice and should be immediately available during every anaesthetic.

How it works

The forceps are available in adult and paediatric sizes. The curved design allows the anaesthetist's hand to be out of the line of vision when used within the tight confines of the oropharynx.

⊕ Advantages

- Facilitates manipulation of objects within the oropharynx.
- Positions hand out of line of sight.

⊖ Disadvantages

- Potential to cause trauma.

⊘ Safety

Care should be taken to avoid damaging the cuff on the endotracheal tube, and to avoid oral trauma, particularly to the uvula.

2.3 Guedel airways

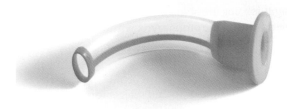

Fig. 2.3.1: A Guedel airway, size 3.

Overview

The terms 'oropharyngeal airway' and 'Guedel airway' are usually used interchangeably to describe the airway adjunct designed by American anesthesiologist, Arthur Guedel. There are, however, other oropharyngeal airways, such as the Berman airway (see *Section 2.10*: Fibreoptic endoscopes for intubation).

Uses

Used in unconscious patients to improve upper airway patency. In an anaesthetic setting, Guedel airways may be used prior to the insertion of, or after the removal of, a more definitive airway. They are also used in emergency situations by other health professionals who do not have advanced airway skills.

How it works

A Guedel airway maintains upper airway patency by keeping the mouth open and preventing the tongue falling backwards.

The airway is available in a range of sizes from neonate to adult. To determine the correct size, the airway is held up to the patient's face. The size that is most appropriate for the patient can be estimated in two ways: either the 'hard-to-hard' method, where the flange is placed at the level of the incisors and the tip at the angle of the mandible, or the 'soft-to-soft' method, from the angle of the mouth to the tragus of the ear. In adults, the Guedel is usually inserted upside down and then rotated 180 degrees once it has reached the back of the oropharynx. However, using this manoeuvre in young children may result in trauma to their soft palate, so the airway is usually inserted without inverting it in this age group. A tongue depressor or laryngoscope may be used to facilitate placement.

⊕ Advantages

- The airway is simple and easy to use and is available in all clinical areas.
- All healthcare professionals should be familiar with its use.

⊖ Disadvantages

- Guedel airways are poorly tolerated by semi-conscious patients and they may induce vomiting.
- Blind insertion of a Guedel may cause bleeding, especially from upper airway tumours.
- Incorrect sizing may cause obstruction:
  - too long, and it may push the epiglottis over the laryngeal inlet
  - too short, and it will not pass the base of the tongue.

2.4 Nasopharyngeal airways

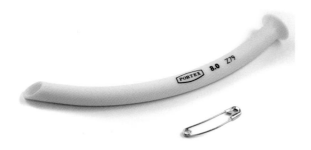

Fig. 2.4.1: A nasopharyngeal airway. The safety pin is passed through the proximal end to prevent it from fully entering the nostril.

Overview

The nasopharyngeal airway adjunct is used as an alternative to an oropharyngeal airway.

Uses

It is most commonly used in emergency situations, but may be used in anaesthetized patients who have poor mouth opening. It is also sometimes used to facilitate regular suctioning of the oropharynx using a suction catheter.

How it works

The airway is traditionally sized by matching its diameter with that of the patient's little finger. This should only be taken as an estimate – some airways will be too large for the patient's nostril, others may be too short and not successfully pass the base of the tongue, leading to obstruction.

A safety pin is often inserted through the flange to prevent loss of the airway into the nose; some modern designs have a larger flange and therefore do not need this.

The airway is lubricated with aqueous gel and inserted gently into a nostril. It is passed directly posteriorly through the nose and along the posterior pharyngeal wall. If significant resistance is encountered, an alternative size or technique should be used. When ideally positioned, the airway tip sits just above the epiglottis providing a clear passage behind the base of the tongue.

Advantages

- Tolerated in semi-conscious patients.
- Suctioning can take place through the nasopharyngeal tube.

Disadvantages

- Contra-indicated when there is deranged coagulation.

Safety

The potential risk of intracranial placement of the airway in cases of basal skull fracture must be balanced with the need to maintain an airway.

2.5 Bite blocks

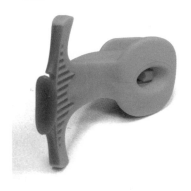

Fig. 2.5.1: A Breathesafe Bite Block.

Overview

A roll of gauze between the molars has traditionally been improvised by anaesthetists for the purpose of preventing patients obstructing their airway by biting the endotracheal tube. However, they are not always effective and the gauze may itself cause an airway obstruction. The use of midline devices such as a Guedel airway is also not an ideal solution because there are numerous reports of incisors being broken by patients biting down against its hard plastic coating. Newer purpose-designed bite blocks such as the Breathesafe Bite Block (OGM Ltd) have proved to be an effective solution.

Uses

These devices prevent patients from biting down and obstructing airway devices during emergence from anaesthesia and sedation. The Breathesafe Bite Block may also aid emergency reintubation or the insertion of a laryngeal airway by keeping the mouth open whilst situated in a lateral position within the mouth.

How it works

The Breathesafe Bite Block is a single use, sterile device with a soft, moulded plastic block that is positioned between the upper and lower molars on one side of the mouth. The block is continuous, with a rigid plastic handle and anti-swallowing T-shaped flange. The soft but strong core of the bite block is capable of resisting compression forces of up to 1500 N, which is in excess of the maximum bite force that can be generated by humans. It is capable of maintaining an inter-incisor distance of over 7.5 mm.

⊕ Advantages

- Reduces the risk of dental damage when compared to the use of Guedel airways for this purpose.
- Positioned laterally between the incisors, allowing instrumentation of the airway.

⊖ Disadvantages

- The T-shaped handle and anti-swallow flange may hinder conventional bag mask ventilation.

2.6 Laryngeal mask airways

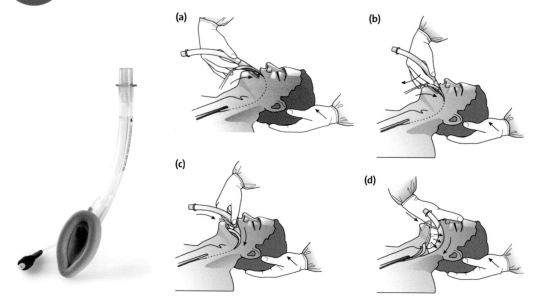

Fig. 2.6.1: The LMA Classic.

Fig. 2.6.2: The manufacturer's recommended method of insertion. Images courtesy of Teleflex Incorporated. © 2013 Teleflex Incorporated. All rights reserved.

Overview

The original laryngeal mask airway (LMA Classic, Teleflex Inc.) was introduced in 1988 by the British anaesthetist, Dr Archie Brain. It is a reusable device and may be steam autoclaved 40 times. The success of the LMA Classic led to the introduction of many other sealing supraglottic airways, including a number of single use designs. A selection of these is described here.

Uses

LMAs are most commonly used for airway management in fasted patients who do not suffer from significant gastro-oesophageal reflux. They may also be used as an emergency airway where a practitioner skilled in intubation is not available (e.g. some paramedic crews), or as an emergency airway in 'can't intubate, can't ventilate' situations.

Table 2.6.1: Sizing an LMA.

LMA size	Patient weight (kg)
1	<5
1½	5–10
2	10–20
2½	20–30
3	30–50
4	50–70
5	70–100
6	>100

How it works

Insertion of an LMA requires the patient's airway reflexes to be absent and is therefore only possible if they are anaesthetized or unconscious. LMAs are available in a broad range of sizes (*Table 2.6.1*). These sizes do not correspond to any particular dimension and are a guide only; in many instances it is possible to use a size higher or lower and achieve a similar, or superior, result.

Some sealing supraglottic airways have a design feature to prevent the epiglottis from obstructing the airway; in the LMA Classic, this is the two flexible 'aperture bars' (visible in *Fig. 2.6.1*). The utility of these features has been questioned.

Technique for inserting LMA

The technique for insertion as described by Dr Brain may be examined in the FRCA and is as follows.

- Prepare the LMA by fully deflating the cuff, apply water-soluble gel to the back of the cuff (not to the front as it may cause laryngospasm).
- Hold the LMA like a pen, with the index finger placed anteriorly at the junction of the cuff and tube (*Fig. 2.6.2a*).
- Push the mask backwards along the hard palate. As the mask moves downwards, the index finger maintains pressure backwards against the posterior pharyngeal wall to avoid collision with the epiglottis (*Figs 2.6.2b & c*).
- Insert the index finger fully into the mouth to complete insertion, stopping when resistance is felt (*Fig. 2.6.2d*).
- Inflate the cuff without holding the tube or connecting the breathing system. When correctly positioned, the LMA will be seen to rise slightly in the mouth.
- The manufacturers recommend using a bite block with the LMA Classic.

Other methods are routinely used in clinical practice.

Advantages

Advantages common to all sealing supraglottic airways
- Neuromuscular blocking drugs are not required.
- Insertion requires less skill than intubation.
- There is minimal haemodynamic response to insertion and removal (cf. endotracheal intubation).
- Emergence is smooth, which is particularly useful in head and neck surgery.

Specific advantages of the LMA Classic
- It has a proven track record during widespread use – there are over 2500 publications relating to the LMA Classic, far more than any other supraglottic airway.
- The LMA Classic (or alternatively the iLMA, see below) form part of the difficult airway algorithm.
- Aperture bars may prevent the epiglottis blocking the airway.

Disadvantages

Disadvantages common to all sealing supraglottic airways
- Achieving an adequate seal is not possible in a small proportion of patients.
- There is a risk of aspiration of gastric contents – it is not a 'definitive airway'.
- They may cause laryngospasm.

Specific disadvantages of the LMA Classic
- It seals to a relatively low airway pressure of around 20 cmH$_2$O.
- It has no integrated bite block so it may be bitten flat during emergence.
- Its position is less stable in edentulous patients.
- The aperture bars may impede fibreoptic intubation through the LMA.

⚠ Safety

The LMA Classic is a reusable device, but sterilization may not inactivate prions. Concerns regarding the transmission of variant Creutzfeldt–Jakob disease, as well as economic considerations, have led to many hospitals phasing out reusable airway equipment in favour of single use devices.

Other notes

Propofol, introduced in 1986, inhibits airway reflexes to a much greater degree than thiopentone and is therefore ideal for anaesthetizing patients having an LMA inserted. Propofol and the LMA were therefore responsible for each other's success.

Other sealing supraglottic airways

Single use LMAs

A number of companies manufacture single use LMAs using similar designs to the LMA Classic. They are factory sterilized using ethylene oxide, and discarded following use.

Whilst they share similar advantages and disadvantages to the reusable design, there are minor design differences (such as alternatives to aperture bars), and few comparative studies, so it should not necessarily be assumed that performance will be equal to the LMA Classic.

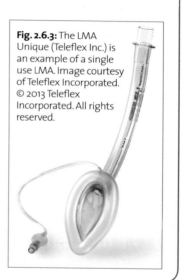

Fig. 2.6.3: The LMA Unique (Teleflex Inc.) is an example of a single use LMA. Image courtesy of Teleflex Incorporated. © 2013 Teleflex Incorporated. All rights reserved.

LMA Proseal (Teleflex Inc.)

This is a reusable LMA designed to overcome problems encountered with the LMA Classic. The inflatable cuff extends onto the reverse of the device in order to improve the seal, particularly around the oesophagus. Unlike the LMA Classic, there is a gastric drain tube that opens at the tip. This is designed to channel fluid away or permit the passage of an orogastric tube; it also reduces the likelihood of inflation of the stomach during prolonged ventilation. The LMA Proseal has an integrated bite block and a preformed metal introducer is available to aid insertion.

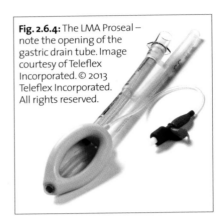

Uses
- Obese patients, laparascopic surgery, positive pressure ventilation (i.e. in those likely to have high airway pressures).

Advantages
- Seals to around 30 cmH$_2$O.
- Gastric drain tube.
- Integrated bite block.
- May seal where other LMAs have failed.

Disadvantages
- Bulky.
- A different technique is required for insertion (rarely practiced).

LMA Supreme (Teleflex Inc.)

The LMA Supreme was recently designed by Archie Brain and attempts to overcome some of the shortcomings of his LMA Classic. It is a single use device similar, but not identical, to the LMA Proseal. Unlike the LMA Proseal, it is pre-curved to facilitate insertion and has its gastric tube integrated with the airway tube. The cuff does not extend onto the reverse of the device, but is designed to provide an improved oesophageal seal. The LMA Supreme tends to seal to a slightly lower airway pressure than the LMA Proseal, at approximately 25 cmH$_2$O.

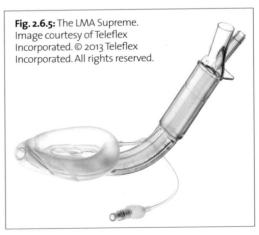

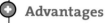

Advantages
- Gastric drain tube.
- Integral bite block.
- Single use.
- Can be inserted without placing one's hand in the patient's mouth.

Disadvantages
- Relatively new, therefore little evidence base.

i-gel (Intersurgical Ltd)

The i-gel has a non-inflatable cuff made of an anatomically shaped elastomer gel which further moulds to the airway shape when it warms to body temperature. It seals to around 25 cmH$_2$O. A thin coating of lubricant should be applied to all sides of the device before insertion.

Advantages
- Integrated gastric drain tube.
- Integrated bite block.
- Simple insertion without inserting hand into patient's mouth.
- No cuff to inflate.
- Improved stability in edentulous patients.

Disadvantages
- Bulky – oral surgery is impossible.
- Lower pharyngeal and oesophageal seal pressures compared with the LMA Proseal.

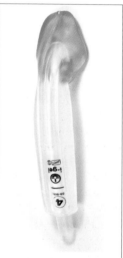

Fig. 2.6.6: The i-gel has an elastomer gel seal instead of an inflatable cuff.

Flexible LMAs

The LMA Flexible (Teleflex Inc.) and similar designs differ from the single use LMAs due to the wire-reinforced airway tube, which facilitates positioning away from the surgical field whilst maintaining a good seal.

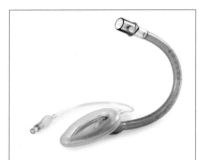

Uses
- Dental, ophthalmic and head and neck surgery.

Advantages
- Less likely to become dislodged during surgery to the head and neck than a non-flexible device.
- Compared with an endotracheal tube, the large cuff may reduce tracheal soiling in tonsillectomy and dental surgery.

Fig. 2.6.7: The LMA Flexible. Image courtesy of Teleflex Incorporated. © 2013 Teleflex Incorporated. All rights reserved.

Disadvantages
- Insertion may prove more difficult than the non-flexible designs.
- The coil reinforcement remains deformed once bitten, and may therefore cause airway obstruction if the patient bites down.
- It carries a higher risk of becoming dislodged during surgery than a reinforced endotracheal tube.

Intubating LMA (Teleflex Inc.)

The intubating LMA is designed to facilitate endotracheal intubation. It is rigid and anatomically curved, with a lumen wide enough to accept a reinforced size 8.0 endotracheal tube, and short enough to ensure passage of the endotracheal tube cuff beyond the vocal cords.

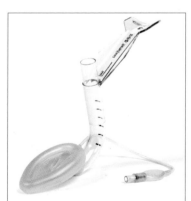

Uses
- Achieving and maintaining control of the airway in anticipated or unexpected difficult airways.

Advantages
- Can be used blindly or to facilitate fibreoptic intubation.
- Allows ventilation between intubation attempts.
- All sizes (3, 4 and 5) will accept an 8.0 mm endotracheal tube (whereas a size 4 LMA Classic will accept a 6.5 mm tube).

Fig. 2.6.8: The LMA Fastrach has a short, wide lumen to permit passage of an endotracheal tube. Image courtesy of Teleflex Incorporated. © 2013 Teleflex Incorporated. All rights reserved.

- Reusable and single use designs available.

Disadvantages
- Blind intubation can lead to pharyngeal trauma and the deterioration of an already difficult airway.

CobraPLA (perilaryngeal airway, Pulmodyne Ltd.)

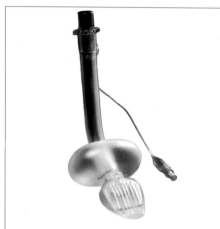

Fig. 2.6.9: The CobraPLA (Pulmodyne Ltd.).

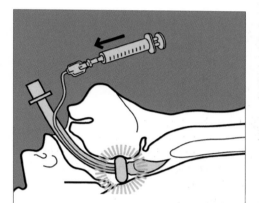

Fig. 2.6.10: The CobraPLA creates a seal in the hypopharynx rather than at the laryngeal inlet. Images courtesy of Pulmodyne Ltd.

The CobraPLA was designed as an alternative to a laryngeal mask. The 'cobra head' abuts the laryngeal inlet holding the epiglottis out of the airway, but the device seals using a cuff in the hypopharynx.

Uses
- Controlled or spontaneous ventilation.

Advantages
- Insertion time and success are similar to the LMA Classic.
- Airway pressures of up to 30 cmH$_2$O are possible.

Disadvantages
- There may be an increased risk of pulmonary aspiration; one prospective study was halted after two cases.

Oesophageal/tracheal tubes

These are often called Combitubes after the Covidien/
Nellcor version. The device has two cuffs and is designed
for blind insertion. It usually enters the oesophagus where
the distal cuff is inflated. The proximal cuff then acts as
a pharyngeal seal, and ventilation takes place through
the side holes between the cuffs. If the device enters the
trachea, the other lumen is used as a normal tracheal tube.

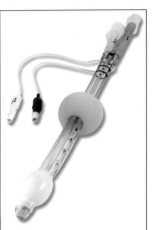

Uses
- Resuscitation, usually in pre-hospital settings.

Advantages
- Blind insertion.
- Ventilation theoretically possible wherever the tube is
  placed.
- Protection from aspiration.

Disadvantages
- Identifying which lumen to ventilate is critical.
- It is unsuitable in patients with oesophageal pathology.
- Tracheal suctioning is not possible.
- It has been largely superseded by LMAs.

Fig. 2.6.11: Combitube
(Covidien Corporation) – an
example of an oesophageal/
tracheal tube. Image
reproduced with permission
from Nellcor Puritan Bennett
LLC, Boulder, Colorado, doing
business as Covidien.

2.7 Bougies, stylets and airway exchange catheters

Bougies

The original Portex bougie (Portex, Smiths Medical) was 60 cm long with a 5 mm diameter and an angled 'Coude' tip. It was reusable and made of beige resin over fibreglass, which allowed it to retain some of its shape when bent. Newer designs are available from a variety of manufacturers and are often single use. When in use, the tip is angled anteriorly and can be used to identify tracheal rings that may be felt as ridges on insertion, in contrast to the smooth oesophagus. Adult (15 Fr) and paediatric (10 Fr) bougies are available.

The endotracheal tube (ETT) may be railroaded following bougie placement or pre-loaded.

Uses
- To facilitate tracheal intubation.
- For airway exchange (ETT or tracheostomy).
- During emergency surgical cricothyroidotomy.

Advantages
- The narrow diameter allows superior visualization of the airway anatomy in comparison to an ETT.
- Angled tip to identify tracheal rings.
- Some shape retention, so can be curved to shape.

Disadvantages
- Size 4.0 ETT minimum (paediatric bougie).

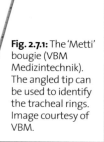

Fig. 2.7.1: The 'Metti' bougie (VBM Medizintechnik). The angled tip can be used to identify the tracheal rings. Image courtesy of VBM.

Guides

A guide is a bougie with a straight tip. It is used only for airway exchange so its ability to retain shape is much less important and the angled tip is unnecessary because the tube being exchanged is already in the trachea.

Uses
- Airway exchange.

Advantages
- Sizes available down to 1.7 mm outer diameter, thus allowing use with paediatric tubes.
- No resistance from straight tip on inserting or removing endotracheal tube.

Stylets

Stylets are placed within an ETT prior to intubation and used to hold the tube in a particular shape. They are made of polyethylene with an aluminium core. The proximal end is curved over to prevent the stylet migrating distally. The tip of the stylet must remain proximal to the tip of the tube to prevent airway trauma.

Uses
- To add rigidity and shape to ETTs.

Advantages
- Available for all sizes of tube.
- Retains its shape fully and stiffens the ETT.

Disadvantages
- Potential for airway trauma.

Fig. 2.7.2: A Mallinckrodt intubating stylet (Covidien Corporation). Image reproduced with permission from Nellcor Puritan Bennett LLC, Boulder, Colorado, doing business as Covidien.

Airway exchange catheter

The airway exchange catheter is used as an alternative to a guide for airway exchange, but has an adaptor for connection to a standard 15 mm connector or a jet ventilator. It thus allows oxygenation or ventilation during airway exchange. Distal side ports reduce the chance of obstruction.

Uses
- Airway exchange.

Advantages
- Ability to oxygenate or jet ventilate through the catheter.
- Available to fit within ETTs greater than 4.0 mm internal diameter.
- It is possible to extubate onto an airway exchange catheter permitting oxygenation and easy reintubation if required.

Disadvantages
- More prone to kinking than a bougie or guide.
- Does not retain its shape.

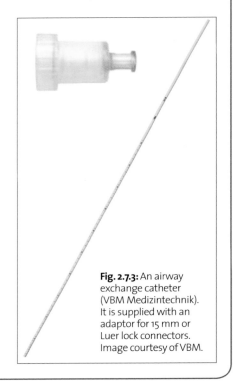

Fig. 2.7.3: An airway exchange catheter (VBM Medizintechnik). It is supplied with an adaptor for 15 mm or Luer lock connectors. Image courtesy of VBM.

Intubation catheter for fibreoptic intubation

A modification of the airway exchange catheter with an increased internal diameter designed to fit over a standard 4 mm paediatric bronchoscope. It is 56 cm long, which allows the flexible tip of the bronchoscope to remain free. It can then be guided visually through a standard (non-intubating) LMA (see *Section 2.6*) and into the larynx. The catheter is left in place whilst the bronchoscope and LMA are removed. An ETT is then railroaded in place.

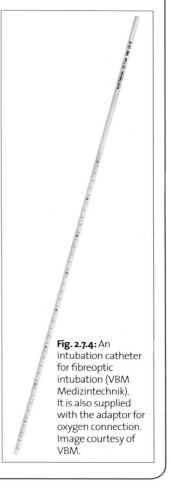

Fig. 2.7.4: An intubation catheter for fibreoptic intubation (VBM Medizintechnik). It is also supplied with the adaptor for oxygen connection. Image courtesy of VBM.

Uses
- Intubation through an LMA.

Advantages
- Allows fibreoptic intubation through a standard LMA using a larger ETT than would usually be possible. (A size 4 LMA will only accept a 6.5 mm tube.)
- Ability to oxygenate or ventilate through catheter.

Disadvantages
- The 56 cm length is barely long enough for changing a tube through an LMA.
- The thin-walled design kinks easily when railroading the ETT.

Laryngoscope blades

Macintosh

The most commonly used blade in the UK is the English profile Macintosh. American and German profiles are also available.

The curved blade is designed with a large reverse-Z shaped flange to sweep the tongue to the left of the mouth. The tip is placed in the vallecula, indirectly lifting the epiglottis via pressure on the hyoepiglottic ligament.

The light source pierces the blade towards the tip so as not to interfere with the view.

Left-handed Macintosh blades are available for use in patients with right-sided facial deformities. Despite the name, they are not specifically designed for use by left handed operators.

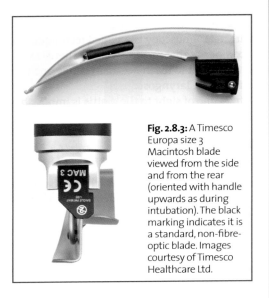

Fig. 2.8.3: A Timesco Europa size 3 Macintosh blade viewed from the side and from the rear (oriented with handle upwards as during intubation). The black marking indicates it is a standard, non-fibre-optic blade. Images courtesy of Timesco Healthcare Ltd.

Sizing: neonate (0), infant (1), child (2), adult (3), large adult (4).

Miller

Again available in English, American and German designs, the Miller is the most commonly used straight blade. It is also manufactured in neonate to adult sizes, though the adult designs are rarely used.

The small flange does not permit a tongue sweep; instead the blade is directed along the right side of the mouth and the tip re-angled once it has passed the base of the tongue. In contrast to the standard curved blade technique, the tip of a straight blade is placed over the epiglottis (instead of in the vallecula), lifting it directly. Straight blades are particularly useful in neonates and infants because of the relatively large epiglottis.

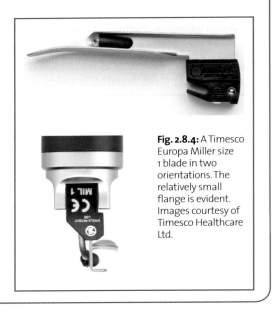

Fig. 2.8.4: A Timesco Europa Miller size 1 blade in two orientations. The relatively small flange is evident. Images courtesy of Timesco Healthcare Ltd.

McCoy

The McCoy is a modification of a Macintosh blade. Its design allows the tip to be flexed (using the lever alongside the handle) in order to lift the epiglottis without the degree of force that would be required using a standard blade. It makes some difficult intubations easier and is commonly found on difficult airway trolleys.

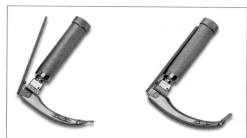

Fig. 2.8.5: A McCoy-bladed laryngoscope. Pulling the lever flexes the tip to lift the epiglottis. Images courtesy of Penlon.

Polio Macintosh

A modification of the Macintosh design with the blade mounting on the handle at 135° rather than 90°. This allowed it to be used in polio patients being ventilated in an iron lung which would otherwise obstruct the handle. It now finds occasional use in patients with restricted neck mobility or large breasts, sometimes in conjunction with a stubby handle.

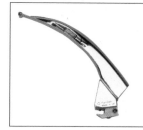

Fig. 2.8.6: A Polio Macintosh blade, which mounts at 135° rather than 90°. Image courtesy of Penlon.

2.9 Rigid indirect laryngoscopes

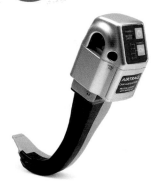
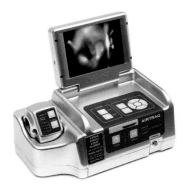

Fig. 2.9.1: An Airtraq laryngoscope with optional camera attachment. The image is wirelessly transmitted to the monitor. Image courtesy of Airtraq.

Overview

Rigid indirect laryngoscopes (RILs) allow visualization of the larynx by a means other than direct line of sight, using a combination of mirrors, prisms, fibreoptics or video cameras.

Uses

RILs may be used for any intubation, but are especially useful for difficult intubations, where the larynx is anterior, neck extension is limited or there are upper airway abnormalities. RILs are also now finding a use in awake intubation following local anaesthesia to the airway.

How it works

Many RILs have appeared on the market in recent years, largely as a result of new camera, display or lighting technologies. Their chief advantage over direct laryngoscopes is their ability to help the anaesthetist see around corners in the upper airway and thus obtain a view of the glottis. RILs may be categorized either by the method used to produce the image (video, fibreoptic or mirror/prism) or by the means used to deliver the tube.

- *Non-guided:* the tube is steered into position by the anaesthetist, usually on a curved stylet [e.g. Glidescope (Verathon Inc.), McGrath (Aircraft Medical), C-MAC (Karl Storz)].
- *Tube-guided:* the laryngoscope incorporates a channel to deliver the tube [e.g. Airtraq (Airtraq), Bullard (Gyrus Medical)].
- *Optical stylet:* the tube is preloaded over the stylet [e.g. Bonfils (Karl Storz), Clarus Shikani and Levitan (Timesco)]. Stylets are covered with fibreoptic endoscopes in *Section 2.10*.

Curved stylets and tube channels are methods that attempt to circumvent one of the main drawbacks of non-guided RILs, which is the difficulty in getting the tube to the glottis despite an excellent view produced by the device.

Laryngoscopic technique varies between devices but, with the exception of optical stylets, most are introduced along the midline of the mouth, over the tongue. As the device is advanced, the anaesthetist looks at the screen rather than at the tip of the scope until the larynx is visualized.

⊕ Advantages

- RILs convert some difficult intubations into easy intubations.
- The reduced lifting force during laryngoscopy (because the oral and pharyngeal axes do not need to be aligned) minimizes the haemodynamic response.

- Cervical spine movement may be minimized.
- Airway trauma may be reduced because of improved vision (fewer blind attempts).
- It is easier to teach than direct laryngoscopy since trainee and trainer can usually both see the same image.

Disadvantages

- It is often possible to obtain an excellent view but then find it difficult to pass the tube.
- Better mouth opening is required than for flexible fibreoptic intubation.
- Cost.
- Blood and secretions may significantly impair the view.

Other notes

- The following tips may improve success.
- Vertically lifting the device once in position lifts the epiglottis and often improves exposure of the glottis (at the expense of increasing neck movement).
- Positioning the tip beyond the epiglottis may improve the view in some patients.
- Withdrawing the scope slightly whilst keeping the larynx in view may aid passage of the tube. This is because the wide angle lens that features on most RILs makes the glottis appear further away than it really is.

Glidescope (Verathon Inc.)

The Glidescope is a non-guided video laryngoscope with a camera on the end of a reusable video baton (paediatric and adult sizes). This is placed inside a disposable shaped clear plastic surround called the 'Stat' by the manufacturers (available in sizes 0–4). The large screen is usually mounted on a dedicated trolley.

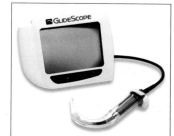

Fig. 2.9.2: The Glidescope AVL reusable, with disposable surround. Image courtesy of Verathon.

Advantages

- It is simple and quick to setup.
- Image quality is excellent and the display is large.
- A heater at the lens limits fogging.
- Stylets are available from Verathon shaped to match the Glidescope.

Disadvantages

- It is an unguided device.
- A stylet is required to facilitate tube placement.
- Portability is limited.

McGrath MAC (Aircraft Medical)

The McGrath MAC is a non-guided video laryngoscope with handle-mounted screen and is fully self-contained. A disposable plastic blade mounts over the non-disposable camera and has the same shape as a standard Macintosh blade. The device can therefore be used for both direct and indirect laryngoscopy, the operator choosing the technique that provides the best intubating conditions.

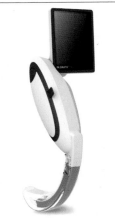

Advantages
- The device is compact and easily portable.
- Both direct and indirect laryngoscopy can be carried out.
- The low profile permits use where mouth opening is limited.

Disadvantages
- The device is unguided.
- It may be less useful in patients with very anterior larynxes or unstable cervical spines than designs with greater curvature.
- Small screen.

Fig. 2.9.3: The McGrath MAC is a self-contained video laryngoscope. Image courtesy of Aircraft Medical Limited, ©2010.

Airtraq (Airtraq)

The Airtraq is a disposable device with an LED light source at the tip and prisms and mirrors to direct the image to an eyepiece at the proximal end.

It is a guided device, incorporating a tube channel. Each Airtraq is supplied with batteries *in situ* so is ready for immediate use when removed from the packaging. Four sizes are available, from neonate to adult with additional designs for nasal intubation and double lumen tubes.

An eyepiece-mounted camera which communicates wirelessly with a monitor is also available and improves the ergonomics and view when using the Airtraq, at the expense of portability.

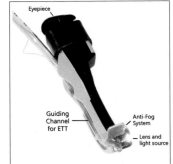

Fig. 2.9.4: A 'Regular' size Airtraq. An ETT is within the channel and the scope switched on ready for intubation. Image courtesy of Airtraq.

Advantages
- The device is self-contained and disposable, so is ideal for difficult airway trolleys and transfer bags.
- Heating at the lens limits fogging.
- The tube guide directs the tube or bougie through the larynx.

Disadvantages
- Using the eyepiece can be ergonomically awkward.
- The ETT may be difficult to feed unless well lubricated.
- Setting up camera and screen is less simple than the Glidescope.

2.10 Fibreoptic endoscopes for intubation

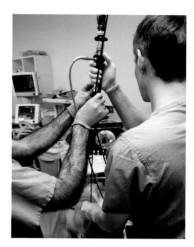

Fig. 2.10.1: Awake fibreoptic intubation.

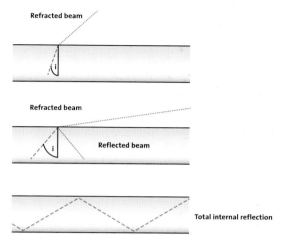

Refracted beam

Refracted beam

Reflected beam

Total internal reflection

Fig. 2.10.2: As the angle of incidence (i) increases to approach the critical angle, the refracted beam gets closer to the surface of the glass. At angles above the critical angle, the entire beam is reflected. This is total internal reflection.

Overview

Fibreoptic endoscopes rely on total internal reflection to transmit light to, and an image back from, the tip of a flexible insertion cord. The tip may be angled in order to steer the scope into position. The image may be viewed on an eyepiece or transmitted onto a screen.

Uses

- Awake or asleep intubation, particularly in patients with a difficult airway.
- To check the position of ETTs (particularly double lumen tubes; see *Sections 2.11* and *2.12*).
- For placement of bronchial blockers (see *Section 2.13*).
- To guide percutaneous tracheostomy (see *Section 2.15*).
- Suctioning and pulmonary toilet.
- Diagnosis of upper airway pathology.

How it works

Total internal reflection

Refraction (change of direction) of light occurs at the boundary of two materials with different refractive indices. A familiar example of refraction occurs when looking at a half-submerged object. Water and air have different refractive indices causing the object to appear to kink at the water's surface.

Under certain conditions, refraction is so great that the whole beam is bent back into the original material; this is called *total internal reflection*. The angle of incidence above which total internal reflection occurs is termed the *critical angle* (*Figure 2.10.2*).

Fibreoptic devices have bundles of around 15 000 glass fibres, each about 20 μm in diameter. Each glass fibre is covered in glass of a different refractive index, causing total internal reflection to occur and light to be transmitted along the bundle.

Components of a fibreoptic bronchoscope

The main body of the scope consists of an eyepiece and control section. It contains:

- the eyepiece (which may be used directly, or be attached to a camera)
- a connection for the light source
- a control lever permitting movement of the tip in a vertical plane with respect to the eyepiece
- a suction port (which may also be used for insufflation of oxygen, or administration of local anaesthetic).

The insertion cord is the flexible cord which is passed into the airway. It contains:

- the fibreoptic *light bundle*, which transmits light to the tip
- the fibreoptic *image bundle*, which transmits the image from the tip to the eyepiece
- a suction channel
- wires from the control lever which permit movement of the tip.

The light bundle may contain glass fibres in any alignment because it is simply transmitting white light to the tip. On the other hand, the 15 000 fibres in the image bundle are in effect each transmitting a pixel of image to the eyepiece. They must therefore be precisely aligned at each end in order for the image to be correctly displayed.

Fibreoptic intubation

A fibreoptic endoscope is particularly useful in patients with abnormal oropharyngeal anatomy (such as in cervical spine instability, or oropharyngeal tumours) which make visualization of the glottis difficult using a direct vision laryngoscope. It is less clearly indicated in patients with glottic or subglottic causes of difficult intubation, but may still be used.

Awake fibreoptic intubation, under local anaesthesia may be useful in a number of situations. It is particularly indicated in patients in whom both intubation *and* ventilation are predicted to be difficult because it permits control of the airway prior to the administration of general anaesthesia.

Preparation of the scope involves checking the control mechanism, focusing the eyepiece and attaching the light source and camera (if used). When a camera is used, it must be independently focused (on the image from the eyepiece) and the white balance adjusted. It is important to note that the eyepiece must be focused before the camera is attached, because it is impossible to adjust for a poorly focused eyepiece using the camera.

An ETT (see *Section 2.11*) is positioned proximally on the insertion cord, to be railroaded into position once the scope is passed through the glottis. The tip may be steered in a vertical plane relative to the eyepiece, using the control lever. Movement in other directions is achieved by rotating the entire scope.

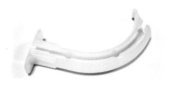

Fig. 2.10.3: A Berman intubating airway facilitates oral fibreoptic intubation.

Nasal fibreoptic intubation is generally simpler, as the nose naturally directs the scope down the posterior pharynx. In situations where oral intubation is preferred, an airway adjunct such as the Berman intubating airway may be used to facilitate passage of the scope and tube past the tongue. Such airways are designed with a slit in the side to allow them to be removed following successful passage of the bronchoscope through the cords. Railroading of the ETT maythen take place.

⊕ Advantages

- A fibreoptic scope permits visualization of the airway beyond the glottis.
- It may facilitate intubation, particularly in patients with difficult oropharyngeal anatomy.
- Once the insertion cord is correctly positioned, the ETT is railroaded into position (cf. some rigid indirect laryngoscopes in *Section 2.9*).
- Permits pulmonary suction under direct vision.

⊖ Disadvantages

- Fibreoptic bronchoscopy and intubation are skilled techniques.
- Blood or secretions in the airway will obscure the view.
- Passing an endoscope may cause complete airway obstruction in patients with a critically narrowed airway ('cork-in-a-bottle').
- The equipment is expensive and fragile.
- Decontamination is required after each use (see *Section 12.5*).

Other notes

The decontamination of fibreoptic scopes following use is commonly examined and is covered in *Section 12.5*: Decontamination of equipment.

Optical stylets

Optical stylets rely on fibreoptics to transmit an image along a rigid (or malleable) steel tube.

Some, for instance the Clarus Levitan (Timesco), are designed for use in conjunction with a conventional laryngoscope. In this circumstance they function as a normal stylet but allow the user to look through the eyepiece if necessary.

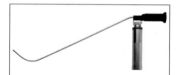

Fig. 2.10.4: Clarus Shikani SOS optical stylet. Image courtesy of Timesco Healthcare Ltd.

Others, for instance the Clarus Shikani SOS (Timesco), are designed as an alternative to a flexible fibreoptic bronchoscope and are used alone. The Clarus Shikani SOS is particularly marketed as an effective 'Plan B' in the event of an unanticipated difficult airway.

The Bonfils stylet (Karl Storz) is a further alternative, designed for a retro-molar approach.

The light source may be either a special LED light, or a standard laryngoscope handle, as shown in the image.

⊕ Advantages

- The familiar direct laryngoscopy technique is used, with the possibility of an alternative view in case of difficulty.

⊖ Disadvantages

- The rigid scope cannot be steered around obstructions.

Ambu aScope (Ambu)

The Ambu aScope is a disposable alternative to a fibreoptic bronchoscope. It uses a camera and an LED light source at the tip with the image transmitted electronically to the monitor. It is therefore not a fibreoptic scope; nevertheless, in use, it is similar being flexible and having a steerable tip and injection port.

Advantages
- Inexpensive.
- Decontamination facilities are not required.
- Reduced risk of transmission of infection.

Disadvantages
- There is no suction port.
- The insertion cord has a large diameter (5.4 mm) and is less flexible.
- Image quality is inferior to a good fibreoptic bronchoscope.

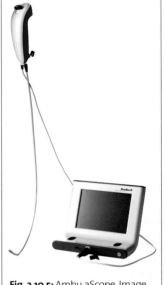

Fig. 2.10.5: Ambu aScope. Image courtesy of Ambu Ltd.

2.11 Endotracheal tubes

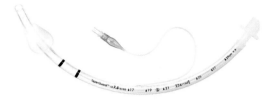

Fig. 2.11.1: A Mallinckrodt Taperguard size 7.5 cuffed oral endotracheal tube (Covidien). The cuff shape is intended to prevent micro-aspiration. Image reproduced with permission from Nellcor Puritan Bennett LLC, Boulder, Colorado, doing business as Covidien.

Overview

The cuffed oral endotracheal tube (COETT) is the most commonly used ETT and is covered first. Other types of ETT are then compared.

Uses

COETTs are used to secure the airway, allowing spontaneous or controlled ventilation while reducing the risk of aspiration. They are used in anaesthesia, resuscitation and critical care situations.

How it works

Modern tubes are single use and made of clear polyvinyl chloride (PVC), whereas the original designs used sterilizable rubber. The internal diameter (ID) in millimetres is used to define the size of the tube; for instance an 8.0 mm tube might be used for an average adult male. The outer diameter (OD) is also marked. Larger tubes are more likely to cause trauma on insertion but have less resistance to gas flow, though in adult practice this is usually insignificant. Larger tubes are, however, less likely to become blocked by secretions and may be used where ventilation is expected for long periods in intensive care.

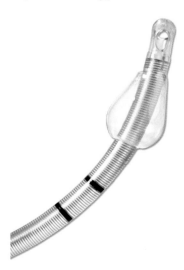

Fig. 2.11.2: A Murphy eye in a Mallinckrodt reinforced ETT (Covidien). Image reproduced with permission from Nellcor Puritan Bennett LLC, Boulder, Colorado, doing business as Covidien.

The distal end of the tube has a left-facing bevel to improve the view at laryngoscopy, during which the tube is inserted from the right-hand side. The cuff is positioned just distal to the glottis which, in an adult, leaves the tip of the tube a few centimetres proximal to the carina. There is often a mark which should remain visible just proximal to the glottis to aid positioning. Many tubes incorporate a 'Murphy eye', a side hole at the tip which allows continued ventilation if the end abuts the tracheal wall. It also allows ventilation of an aberrant right upper lobe, which occasionally originates from the trachea several centimetres above the carina. This is known as a tracheal bronchus and has an incidence of 0.1–2%.

The tube has a gentle curve that approximates the curve of the oropharynx and improves manipulation during intubation. Distance from the tip is marked in centimetres along the tube's length; tubes are often cut prior to insertion to reduce kinking under the weight of the breathing system. In situations in which facial swelling may occur, such as burns and intensive care, the tube should be left uncut. There is a standard 15 mm connection for the breathing system at the proximal end. A radio-opaque line runs the length of the tube to allow identification by X-ray.

The cuff

The cuff creates a seal in the trachea to allow higher ventilation pressures and to prevent aspiration. It is connected to a pilot balloon which incorporates a valve for injecting air. The cuff should be inflated to the lowest pressure at which there is no longer an air leak, which should be in the range of 20–30 cmH$_2$O.

Modern cuffs are usually low-pressure, high-volume designs which spread lower pressures over a larger area of trachea. Older cuffs were high-pressure, low-volume and risked tracheal ischaemia and necrosis if used for long periods. Low-pressure, high-volume cuffs are, however, less effective at preventing aspiration because wrinkles form, which over time allow the passage of fluids.

In order to compensate for this new cuff designs are being introduced. These include the Mallinckrodt Taperguard (*Fig. 2.11.1*), which is stated to reduce micro-aspiration by 90% and the Kimvent Microcuff (*Fig. 2.11.5*). Other tube designs feature a suction lumen which ends just above the cuff to prevent pooling of secretions (*Fig. 2.15.1*).

⊕ Advantages

- The gold standard 'definitive' airway.
- Helps prevent aspiration.
- Allows some leeway in sizing of the tube (cf. uncuffed).
- Allows high ventilation pressures.

⊖ Disadvantages

- Requires advanced airway skills to insert when compared with supraglottic airway devices.
- Risk of pressure necrosis both at the level of the cuff, and in the oropharynx if used for long periods.
- Risk of micro-aspiration through cuff wrinkles, which may lead to ventilator-associated pneumonia.
- Risk of endobronchial intubation (the tube is in too far).
- Risk of cuff herniation proximally through the glottis (the tube is not in far enough).

Other notes

Uncuffed tubes were traditionally favoured in paediatrics, however, new paediatric COETTs are becoming popular as the low-pressure, high-volume cuff has reduced the risk of tracheal ischaemia.

Sizing endotracheal tubes

ETT sizing is patient-specific. The ETT should always pass easily through the glottis, but be large enough to prevent a leak and to minimize resistance to airflow. The appropriate size cuffed tube (*Table 2.11.1*) will be one size smaller than the uncuffed equivalent in a particular patient.

Table 2.11.1: Typical tube sizes. A size smaller or larger may be required and should be immediately available at time of intubation.

Age	Internal diameter	Length to teeth
Term–neonate	3 mm (uncuffed)	9 cm
1 year old	4 mm (uncuffed)	10 cm
Child >1 year	Age/4 + 4 mm (uncuffed)	Age/2 + 12 cm
Adult	>7.0 mm	18–22 cm

Uncuffed tube

Uncuffed tubes are often used in paediatrics because of concerns of necrosis caused by cuff pressure at the level of the cricoid cartilage, the narrowest point of the paediatric airway.

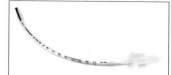

Fig. 2.11.3: An uncuffed endotracheal tube. Image courtesy of Timesco Healthcare Ltd.

Uses
- Paediatrics (neonate to puberty).
- Adult sizes are available but are used infrequently.

Advantages
- Uncuffed tubes provide the widest possible lumen for a given external diameter, thus reducing resistance.
- The risk of pressure necrosis caused by a cuff is avoided.
- The lack of cuff reduces risk of trauma at glottis during insertion (or nose during nasal intubation).

Disadvantages
- Must be correctly sized to prevent a leak.
- Unable to compensate for changes in airway diameter (caused by oedema) occurring during long term ventilation.
- High ventilation pressures not achievable due to leak.

Cole tube

The Cole is a shouldered, uncuffed tube.

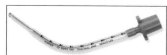

Fig. 2.11.4: A Portex Cole neonatal tube.

Uses
- Neonates (though less commonly than standard uncuffed tubes).

Advantages
- The tube is tapered so that it has a wider diameter proximally than distally. This decreases kinking and reduces resistance to gas flow.

Disadvantages
- The shoulder causes turbulence and may actually increase resistance to airflow.
- Tracheal injury may result if tube inserted too far.

Microcuff tube

The Kimberly Clark Microcuff tube has been specifically designed for paediatrics. This contrasts with existing paediatric cuffed tubes which are smaller versions of the standard adult tube.

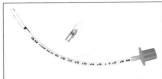

Fig. 2.11.5: A Kimvent Microcuff paediatric tube.

It has a modified short tip, which reduces the risk of endobronchial intubation, and a polyurethane cuff. The cuff is made of thinner (10 µm) material compared to standard 70 µm PVC cuffs and therefore inflates and seals at lower pressures (average 11 cmH$_2$O), reducing the risk of mucosal ischaemia. When inflated it has a smooth surface, unlike PVC cuffs which can wrinkle and therefore increase the risk of aspiration. The cuff is short and designed to sit below the vulnerable subglottic region.

Uses
- Paediatrics.
- Adult versions may be used in place of cuffed tubes to reduce micro-aspiration risk.

Advantages
- Specifically designed for paediatrics.
- Very low pressure, smooth cuff.

Disadvantages
- Expensive.
- Smaller internal diameter than an uncuffed tube which may lead to increased blockage by secretions.

South RAE (Ring, Adair and Elwyn) tube

Anatomically shaped tubes introduced by Ring, Adair and Elwyn, designed to position the tube and breathing circuit out of the surgical field. They are available cuffed or uncuffed, and the uncuffed versions have a double Murphy eye. In most individuals, the tube is correctly positioned when the thick black line is at the lower lip.

Uses
- Head and neck surgery, ophthalmic surgery.

Advantages
- Improves surgical access.
- Reduces surgical interference with the tube.

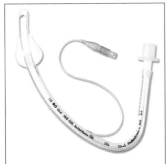

Fig. 2.11.6: A Mallinckrodt South RAE tube. Image reproduced with permission from Nellcor Puritan Bennett LLC, Boulder, Colorado, doing business as Covidien.

Disadvantages

- The preformed shape may not fit all individuals and increases the risk of endobronchial intubation or cuff prolapse.

North RAE/Nasal tube

Anatomically curved shape. May be cuffed or uncuffed. To insert under direct vision, laryngoscopy is performed and the tube is gently inserted through the nostril, directed towards the glottis. Final placement with Magill's forceps is often required. Following insertion, the right-angle curve (indicated by the thick black line) is designed to sit at the external nares and the tube is taped in place along the nose.

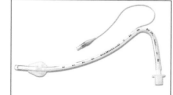

Fig. 2.11.7: A Mallinckrodt North RAE tube. Image reproduced with permission from Nellcor Puritan Bennett LLC, Boulder, Colorado, doing business as Covidien.

Uses

- Maxillofacial or dental surgery.
- As an alternative to tracheostomy for respiratory wean.

Advantages

- Permits unimpeded surgical access to the oral cavity.
- Better tolerated in semi-conscious or awake patients.
- The patient cannot bite the tube.
- The tube is easily stabilized.

Disadvantages

- Risk of epistaxis.
- Contraindicated in basal skull fracture.

Other notes

Oral north-facing tubes are available. Nasal intubation is also possible using a standard or reinforced ETT.

Reinforced tube

Reinforced tubes are made of PVC, with a spiral metal reinforcement which allows the tube to bend without kinking. Often used in situations where the tube must be positioned away from the surgical field.

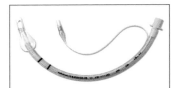

Fig. 2.11.8: A Mallinckrodt reinforced ETT. Image reproduced with permission from Nellcor Puritan Bennett LLC, Boulder, Colorado, doing business as Covidien.

Uses
- Neurosurgery, maxillofacial surgery, shoulder surgery.
- Prone positioning.
- With some fibreoptic or indirect laryngoscopy techniques.

Advantages
- Bends without kinking.

Disadvantages
- Cannot be cut to size.
- Remains deformed if bitten by the patient, causing obstruction (a bite block can prevent this).

Laser tube

Laser tubes are designed to resist laser damage, usually by means of a metal exterior. The cuff is often filled with saline or foam to allow early detection of perforation.

A low cost, less effective alternative to a laser tube is a standard tube wrapped in a special laser-resistant foil tape.

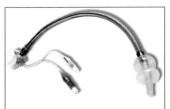

Fig. 2.11.9: A Mallinckrodt laser dual cuffed tube. The second cuff maintains a seal if the first is perforated Image reproduced with permission from Nellcor Puritan Bennett LLC, Boulder, Colorado, doing business as Covidien.

Uses
- Laser airway surgery (laser tubes are not required for laser surgery away from the airway).

Advantages
- Resists melting and combustion.
- The matt surface defocuses reflected beams to protect healthy tissue.
- Some tubes incorporate a double cuff to maintain the seal if first cuff is perforated.

Disadvantages
- Stiff, abrasive, potential for mucosal trauma.
- Will burn if exposed to high energy laser for around 10 seconds.
- Although it is defocused, the reflected laser beam may still cause damage.

Microlaryngeal tube (MLT)

These are 4.0–6.0 mm ID ETTs with a longer length than normal for a tube of that diameter so that they can be used in adults. The cuff has a high volume to provide an effective seal despite the narrow tube.

Uses

- Microlaryngeal surgery (for alternatives see *Section 2.14*: Airway devices for jet ventilation).
- For adults with a pathologically narrow larynx or trachea (oedema, masses, etc.).

Advantages

- Permit surgical access during microlaryngeal procedures.
- Standard anaesthetic techniques and breathing systems may be used (cf. jet ventilation).
- The cuff protects the airway.

Disadvantages

- The narrow lumen may become blocked by secretions.
- The high resistance caused by the long, narrow lumen precludes spontaneous ventilation.
- Surgical access is poorer than during jet ventilation.

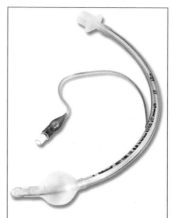

Fig. 2.11.10: A 6.0 mm Mallinckrodt microlaryngeal tube. Image reproduced with permission from Nellcor Puritan Bennett LLC, Boulder, Colorado, doing business as Covidien.

2.12 Double lumen endobronchial tubes

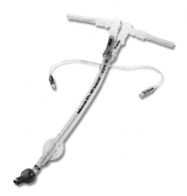

Fig. 2.12.1: A left-sided Mallinckrodt endobronchial tube, based on the Robertshaw design. As with most double lumen tubes, the bronchial cuffs, lumens and pilot balloons are coloured blue for easy recognition. Available in 28, 32, 35, 37, 39 and 41 Fr sizes. Image reproduced with permission from Nellcor Puritan Bennett LLC, Boulder, Colorado, doing business as Covidien.

Overview

Double lumen tubes (DLTs) are specialized tubes which allow isolation of a lung and single lung ventilation. Alternative, infrequently used techniques include positioning a single lumen tube beyond the carina or using a bronchial blocker (see *Section 2.13*).

Uses

DLTs are most commonly used to facilitate thoracic surgery, but may also be used on intensive care. There are a number of absolute and relative indications for one lung ventilation; note that the majority of surgery is possible, though more difficult, using two lung ventilation.

Absolute indications

- To protect the good lung from contralateral pathology:
  - massive haemorrhage
  - pus (i.e. empyema or abscess).
- To allow ventilation in the presence of a major air leak:
  - bronchopleural fistulae
  - tracheobronchial trauma
  - surgery to the major airways (e.g. bronchial sleeve resection).
- Whole lung lavage (as a treatment for pulmonary alveolar proteinosis).

Relative indications

- To facilitate surgery:
  - video assisted thoracoscopy (VATS); this is often stated to be an absolute indication, but in some circumstances can be carried out with a single lumen tube.
  - pneumonectomy
  - lobectomy
  - thoracic aortic aneurysm
  - oesophagectomy
  - spinal surgery.
- Split lung ventilation on intensive care (in a patient with a single diseased lung, ventilation of each lung at different pressures may be useful).

How it works

DLTs have a tracheal lumen and a bronchial lumen, each with an inflatable cuff. The tube has two curves, a bronchial curve at the tip and an oropharyngeal curve more proximally.

There have been a number of different designs of DLT. Some earlier designs such as the Carlens tube had a carinal hook to aid bronchial placement, however, this also made intubation of the glottis more difficult. The majority of DLTs in current use are based on the Robertshaw design, which was originally manufactured in red rubber. Re-useable red rubber tubes are still available

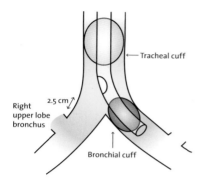

Tracheal cuff

Right
upper lobe
bronchus

2.5 cm

Bronchial cuff

Fig. 2.12.2: A correctly positioned DLT.

(P3 Medical), however, disposable clear PVC versions are more common. Many tubes are supplied with a stylet that makes the tube more rigid and easier to manipulate.

In order to understand how a DLT should function, consider a correctly positioned left-sided tube. The bronchial cuff is in the left main bronchus and the tracheal cuff is positioned in the trachea. With both cuffs inflated, ventilating the bronchial lumen will ventilate only the left lung, whereas ventilating the tracheal lumen will ventilate only the right lung. Whilst the chest is open, if either lumen is left open to air, its lung will collapse, facilitating surgical access.

Left- and right-sided tubes are available, but left-sided tubes are preferred even for right-side surgery because the right main bronchus is shorter (≈ 2.5 cm long) than the left. Therefore the bronchial cuff of a right-sided DLT may easily obstruct the origin of the right upper lobe (RUL). A Murphy eye with a shaped or slotted bronchial cuff is present on right-sided DLTs in order to ventilate the RUL, but the fine positioning required means it is easily dislodged.

Achieving correct tube positioning may be challenging and there are a number of approaches. The following is the classic insertion technique.

Insertion of a DLT

- Select an appropriate size tube (35 Fr or 37 Fr for women, 39 Fr or 41 Fr for men).
- Ensure that you have the connection to the breathing system and that the stylet is appropriately curved; exaggerating the bronchial curve is often helpful.
- Perform direct laryngoscopy and intubate the larynx with the bronchial curve angled anteriorly.
- As soon as the tip passes through the cords, remove the stylet and rotate 90° towards the desired bronchus (i.e. to the left for a left-sided DLT). Airway trauma can result if the stylet is not removed.
- Continue advancing until resistance is felt.
- Connect the breathing system and inflate the tracheal cuff. At this point, a correctly positioned DLT should function like a standard single lumen tube and ventilate both lungs.

Checking position

- Clamp tracheal lumen, open tracheal cap. There should be a 'whoosh' as the lung empties and air escapes through the tracheal lumen.
- Ventilate the bronchial lumen – a leak will be felt through the tracheal lumen. Inflate the bronchial cuff (this requires only around 2 ml of air). The leak through the tracheal lumen will stop once the cuff is correctly inflated. Check you are ventilating only the appropriate lung (left for a left-sided DLT).
- Swap the clamp to the bronchial lumen and open the cap. Check that you are ventilating only the opposite side.

Possible incorrect positions

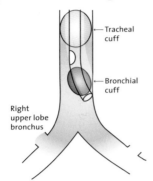

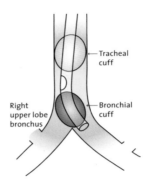

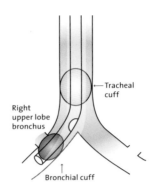

Fig. 2.12.3: Bronchial lumen in trachea – lung isolation not possible. Remedy: insert tube further, or choose a larger size.

Fig. 2.12.4: Bronchial cuff herniates proximally so cuff covers the other bronchus. Unable to ventilate lung via tracheal lumen. Remedy: insert tube further.

Fig. 2.12.5: Upper lobe occlusion (most common with right-sided tubes). Remedy: manipulate tube position so that Murphy's eye is correctly placed.

Alternatively it is possible to insert the bronchial lumen into the wrong bronchus. Remedy: re-site the DLT.

Bronchoscopy

Ideally, tube position should be confirmed by bronchoscopy. A narrow diameter (e.g. 2.8 mm) bronchoscope is required.

- Examine the tracheal lumen. The carina should be visible beyond the end of the tube. A rim of bronchial cuff should be visible in the appropriate bronchus.
- Examine the bronchial lumen. The upper lobe bronchus should be visible beyond the end of the tube.

⊕ Advantages

- Isolates lung from contralateral pathology.
- Permits independent suctioning of each lung.
- Permits independent ventilation of each lung.
- Allows CPAP to be applied to the non-ventilated lung.

⊖ Disadvantages

- DLTs are bulky and may be challenging to insert.
- Prone to moving during patient positioning or surgery (though less so than bronchial blockers).
- Too large for children under around 8 years old (28 Fr DLT is smallest available).
- May need to change from or to a single lumen tube before or after surgery.

Other notes

Some degree of hypoxia during one lung ventilation is expected owing to the large shunt. If the degree of desaturation is unacceptable, a number of manoeuvres may improve the situation.

- Recheck tube position and ventilation. Use bronchoscopy if available.
- Suction down each lumen.
- Improve oxygenation via the ventilated lung:
  - 100% oxygen
  - apply PEEP (though this may worsen shunt)
  - increase tidal volume.
- Improve oxygenation via the non-ventilated lung:
  - insufflate oxygen
  - CPAP (a special circuit is available)
  - surgical clamping of the pulmonary artery (obliterates shunt).
- Revert to two lung ventilation.

2.13 Bronchial blockers

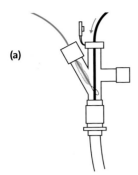 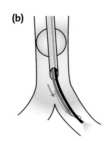 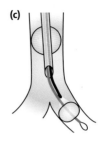

(a)   (b)   (c)

Fig. 2.13.1: Insertion of a bronchial blocker.
(a) The tip of a fibreoptic bronchoscope is placed through the loop bronchial blocker within a special multiport adapter.
(b) The bronchoscope is positioned in the bronchus and the blocker is advanced off the end of the bronchoscope.
(c) Cuff inflation takes place under bronchoscopic vision, and the wire loop is then removed.

Overview

A bronchial blocker is a balloon-tipped catheter used to isolate a lung or lobe. Purpose-designed catheters are available, such as the Cook Arndt bronchial blocker (Cook Medical). These are used in combination with a special endotracheal tube (ETT), or ETT adapter (*Fig. 2.13.1*) for ease of placement. Fogarty embolectomy catheters with a 3 mm balloon or Foley catheters have also been used.

Uses

Used to isolate a lung, or portion of lung in situations in which a double lumen endobronchial tube (DLT) (see *Section 2.12*) is contra-indicated or difficult to insert.

How it works

Bronchial blockers are usually inserted using a fibreoptic bronchoscope. The wire loop protruding from the blocker lumen is hooked over the bronchoscope within the multiport adapter in the arrangement shown in *Fig. 2.13.1a*. This may take place prior to attachment of the adaptor to the ETT. The bronchoscope is then passed into the bronchus to be blocked, the blocker advanced off the end of the bronchoscope, and the bronchoscope retracted proximal to the still deflated balloon. The balloon is then inflated under bronchoscopic vision. Once the position is acceptable, the wire loop is removed. The lung slowly deflates through the long, narrow lumen.

⊕ Advantages

- Permits lung isolation in children too small for a DLT, or in adults in whom a DLT is difficult to insert.
- No ETT change is required at the end of the case.
- Permits isolation of a single lobe.
- Less airway trauma compared to a DLT.

⊖ Disadvantages

- Bronchial blockers are difficult to position and prone to dislodging.
- The lung is slow to deflate owing to the narrow lumen of the blocker.
- It is not possible to suction the deflated lung unit.
- Once the wire loop has been removed, it cannot be replaced for repositioning.

2.14 Airway devices for jet ventilation

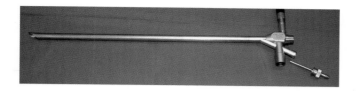

Fig. 2.14.1: A Storz rigid bronchoscope with jet cannula (Karl Storz). Image courtesy of Andrew Sutherland, www.surgicalexam.com.

Overview

Jet ventilation permits positive pressure ventilation in the absence of a sealed airway, using a high pressure oxygen source such as a Sanders injector, or a high frequency jet ventilator (see *Section 4.9*). The high pressure also allows ventilation to take place through a narrow lumen, providing there is a patent airway for expiration around the device. Jet ventilation can be manual or automated, low frequency or high frequency; it should not, however, be confused with high frequency oscillatory ventilation, which is a technique used in neonatal and adult intensive care patients (see *Section 4.10*).

Uses

- Anaesthesia for airway surgery.
- Emergency ventilation.

How they work

Devices for jet ventilation are divided into supraglottic and infraglottic.

- Supraglottic ventilation is carried out using a jetting needle attached to the surgical laryngoscope.
- Infraglottic ventilation may be *transglottic*, using a specialized catheter placed at laryngoscopy (e.g. a Hunsaker tube), or *percutaneous,* via a jet ventilation catheter placed under local or general anaesthesia (e.g. a Ravussin needle). Percutaneous devices are covered under cricothyroidotomy devices (see *Section 2.16*).

In all cases a high pressure source is required to overcome the resistance offered by the 2–3 mm lumen, and to provide a sufficient flow for lung expansion despite the lack of an airway seal. Passive expiration cannot take place through the narrow jet lumen and must therefore occur around it, usually through the patient's own patent airway.

Since jet ventilators cannot deliver an anaesthetic gas mixture, anaesthesia is usually maintained intravenously.

ⓘ Safety

Barotrauma is a significant risk with all techniques and therefore care must be taken to allow full expiration between jets. For the same reason, significant lung disease is a relative contraindication.

Supraglottic jet ventilation via a surgical laryngoscope

A surgical laryngoscope is fitted with a metal cannula for supraglottic jet ventilation. This is also called a jetting needle or nozzle and may be built in, or attached prior to use. A 14–16 G cannula is suitable for adults, allowing the delivery of a jet pressure of around 30–50 cmH$_2$O. A 19 G cannula may be used for children and allows a jet of approximately 15 cmH$_2$O.

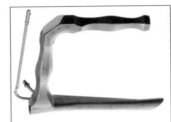

Fig. 2.14.2: A surgical laryngoscope. A jet needle adapter, which may clip on or replace the suction port permits attachment of a jet ventilator. Image courtesy of Teleflex Inc. ©2013 Teleflex Inc. All rights reserved.

Air entrainment

As the oxygen jet emerges from the cannula, air is entrained in a process called jet mixing. The Venturi effect (see *Section 1.12: Venturi masks*) is widely, and probably incorrectly, quoted as the cause. For the Venturi effect to be the cause, the jet must create a sub-atmospheric pressure as it leaves the cannula and thus entrain surrounding air. Experimental evidence suggests that a negative pressure occurs only under specific conditions and that most of the entrainment occurs because of the frictional drag of the jet on the surrounding air.

Uses
- Laryngeal surgery, including laser.

Advantages
- There is a tubeless surgical field.
- There is no extraneous flammable material in the airway.

Disadvantages
- Air entrainment leads to a variable FiO$_2$.
- Poor alignment of the laryngoscope may lead to impaired ventilation.
- Significant movement of the vocal cords during ventilation. This may make surgery difficult.
- Debris is carried into the airway by the jet and may cause obstruction.
- Capnography is not possible (see *Section 6.9*).
- Gastric distension may occur.

Transglottic jet ventilation via a Hunsaker tube

The Hunsaker tube is a 33 cm long plastic tube with a 3 mm OD which is placed through the larynx at laryngoscopy by the anaesthetist. There is a basket at the tip to stabilize the tube in the trachea and to ensure therefore that the jet is not directed into the tracheal wall. There is a main lumen for jet ventilation and a narrower secondary lumen for capnography. Both lumens have a Luer lock connector at the proximal end (see *Section 8.7*).

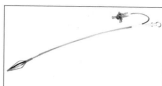

Fig. 2.14.3: A Medtronic Xomed Hunsaker jet ventilation catheter.

Uses
- Laryngeal surgery, including laser.

Advantages
- Good surgical access.
- Suitable for use with lasers.
- Surgical debris is likely to be carried outwards.
- Less vocal cord movement occurs than with other techniques.
- Capnography is possible.
- There is less air entrainment and therefore the inspired oxygen concentration is more predictable.

Disadvantages
- The tube may impede surgical access.
- There is an increased risk of barotrauma because the jet emerges below the glottis.
- Use is controversial in glottic and subglottic stenosis because of the reduced expiratory flow which may result in gas trapping.
- May be technically difficult to insert.

Other notes

The Benjet and Laserjet tubes are alternative, similar devices.

Ventilation via a rigid bronchoscope

Rigid bronchosopes (*Fig. 2.14.1*) are available in sizes from neonate to adult. The bronchoscope consists of a stainless steel tube which is positioned in the trachea or bronchus. An optical telescope or other instruments can be passed through the lumen.

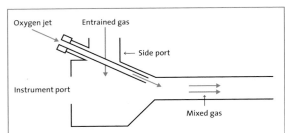

Fig. 2.14.4: Jet ventilation through a rigid bronchoscope. The jet is delivered down a jet cannula placed within the angled port (see also *Fig. 2.14.1*). Air is entrained via the 15 mm side port.

The proximal end of the bronchoscope has a 15 mm side port for connection to a breathing system, and an angled port through which a cannula can be inserted for jet ventilation. The distal end of the bronchoscope has side openings to allow ventilation of the contralateral lung.

Spontaneous, or low pressure manual ventilation, via the 15 mm side port may be used in patients undergoing upper airway procedures, particularly in children or during foreign body removal. A standard Mapleson or circle breathing system is used (see *Sections 3.5* and *3.7*). During low pressure manual ventilation, the proximal end of the bronchoscope must be occluded during inspiration.

Jet ventilation is used more commonly in adults; this must incorporate pauses because otherwise the surgeon receives a jet in the eye whilst operating. Manual jet ventilation is therefore most commonly used.

Jet mixing occurs as the jet enters the bronchoscope, with air being entrained via the side port, reducing the FiO_2 by a variable amount. An oxygen source may therefore be connected to the side port to raise the delivered oxygen concentration. Although the jet is delivered transglottically, air entrainment occurs above the glottis and thus many characteristics are shared with supraglottic devices.

Uses
- Major airway stenting or foreign body removal.
- Emergency ventilation of a critically narrowed airway.

Advantages
- Improved surgical access compared with a flexible bronchoscope.
- May allow emergency ventilation in upper airway obstruction.

Disadvantages
- Jetting cannot be carried out whilst the surgeon is looking down the scope.
- Air entrainment leads to a variable FiO_2.
- Poor alignment of the bronchoscope may lead to impaired ventilation.

2.15 Tracheostomy tubes

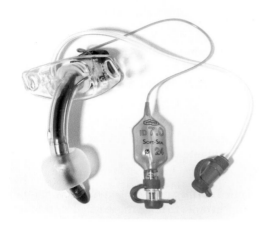

Fig. 2.15.1: Portex Blue Line Ultra Suctionaid cuffed tracheostomy tube with obturator (purple) *in situ* (Smiths Medical). The Suctionaid port permits suctioning directly above the cuff to reduce the risk of microaspiration.

Overview

Tracheostomy tubes are curved tubes inserted through an opening created in the patient's neck which passes into the upper trachea. They are therefore infraglottic airways.

Uses

Upper airway obstruction
- Tracheostomies are indicated in upper airway obstruction which cannot be bypassed by an oral endotracheal tube.
- They may be used prior to, or following, head and neck surgery.
- They are an option in 'can't intubate, can't ventilate' situations.

Respiratory wean
- Tracheostomies are well tolerated by non-sedated patients, thus facilitating long-term support of ventilation during respiratory wean.
- They permit suctioning of the airway in patients unable to clear secretions.

Severe sleep apnoea
- In patients unresponsive to continuous positive airways pressure (CPAP).

How it works

The tracheostomy tube may initially be inserted surgically or using a percutaneous technique. Most commonly, this is performed under general anaesthesia, however, tracheostomy under local anaesthesia may be carried out in patients in whom there is a risk of complete airway obstruction under general anaesthesia.

A typical tracheostomy tube is made up of three parts, an outer tube, an inner tube and an obturator.

Outer tube

This consists of a curved plastic tube with a proximal flange that is sutured or tied in position on the neck. The tube has a proximal 15 mm connection for a breathing system. Some devices have an adjustable flange, allowing accommodation of abnormal anatomy such as a large neck, or a distal tracheal obstruction.

Adult tubes of ID 6.0–10.0 mm are available. Larger sizes are preferable where possible because of the reduced chance of mucus plugging. The outer tube may be cuffed or uncuffed.

Inner tube

The inner tube is a simple plastic sleeve that slides inside the outer tube and may easily be replaced if it becomes plugged with mucus. Paediatric tubes are often of a single lumen design (without an inner tube) because of their narrow diameter; this necessitates more frequent tube changes to prevent mucus plugging.

Obturator

This is a plastic insert with a bullet-shaped tip which protrudes from the tracheostomy tube to facilitate tube insertion. It must be removed in order to ventilate.

Speech with a tracheostomy

In some patients, deflating the cuff or using an uncuffed tracheostomy tube will allow enough airflow around the tube to permit speech and coughing. In order to force the exhaled air through the vocal cords rather than the tube, the tracheostomy may be covered by hand or a one-way speaking valve such as a Passy-Muir.

To improve speech quality, a fenestrated tracheostomy tube may be used. Both the outer and inner tube must be fenestrated, though the inner tube may be changed back to a plain tube for suctioning or for short term ventilation.

Advantages

- Tracheostomies are better tolerated than oral or nasal intubation, allowing sedation to be weaned.
- Oral hygiene is improved.
- A tracheostomy may be the only airway option in patients with upper airway lesions.
- Dead space and airway resistance are reduced.
- Facilitation of pulmonary suctioning.

Disadvantages

Immediate complications:
- airway loss
- haemorrhage
- pneumothorax.

Early complications:
- dislodged tracheostomy tube; within the first few days, it may be difficult to reinsert a tracheostomy which becomes dislodged and there is a risk of creating a false passage
- secretions may block the tube causing airway obstruction
- local infection.

Late complications:
- tracheal stenosis
- tracheomalacia.

Safety

The National Tracheostomy Safety Project (www.tracheostomy.org.uk) issues guidance on the safe management of tracheostomies, and emergency algorithms for use in airway emergencies in patients with tracheostomies or laryngectomies.

Uncuffed tracheostomy tube

Uses

- In patients who can protect their own airway and manage their secretions by coughing.
- In paediatrics (avoidance of pressure necrosis of the trachea and to maximize the internal diameter).

Disadvantages

- Unless the tube is a close fit, positive pressure ventilation will not be possible because of the air leak around the tube.

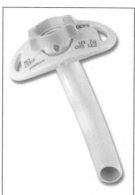

Fig. 2.15.2: Shiley uncuffed fenestrated tracheostomy tube (Covidien). Image reproduced with permission from Nellcor Puritan Bennett LLC, Boulder, Colorado, doing business as Covidien.

Fenestrated tracheostomy tube

Uses

- Fenestrations are used to allow exhalation through the glottis as part of the weaning process, and in particular to permit speech.

Disadvantages

- Positive pressure ventilation will result in air leak and should be avoided where possible.
- There is a risk of surgical emphysema in patients with newly formed tracheostomies.
- Granuloma formation may occur around the fenestrations.

Other notes

A non-fenestrated inner tube should be reinserted for suctioning.

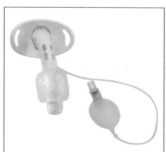

Fig. 2.15.3: Shiley cuffed fenestrated tracheostomy tube (Covidien). Image reproduced with permission from Nellcor Puritan Bennett LLC, Boulder, Colorado, doing business as Covidien.

Adjustable flange tracheostomy tube

Uses
- The adjustable flange allows the distance before the angle to be adjusted to take into account factors such as obesity or a neck mass.

Disadvantages
- The adjustment clamp is bulky and may therefore be unsuitable for long-term use. A variety of longer fixed length tubes is therefore available.

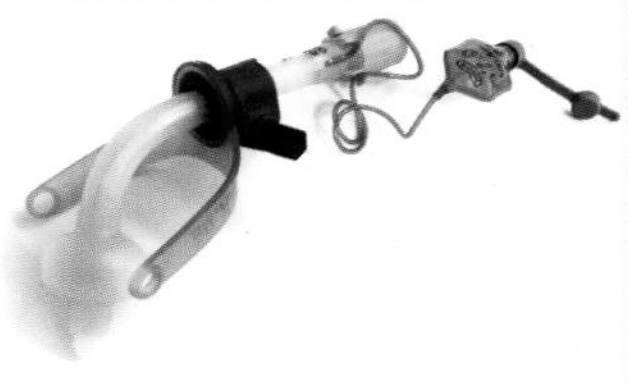

Fig. 2.15.4: A Portex blue line cuffed adjustable flange tracheostomy tube (Smiths Medical).

Other notes

Some patients, for example, those with a tracheal stenosis, may need a tracheostomy tube with extra length *after* the angle. This may be accomplished with a flexible adjustable length tube, or a longer fixed design. Custom tracheostomy tubes are also available.

Mini-tracheostomy

This is a cannula with a 4 mm ID. It may be inserted percutaneously, or exchanged for an existing tracheostomy tube. The patient breathes normally around the tube while the tube accepts a size 10 Fr suction catheter for tracheobronchial toilet.

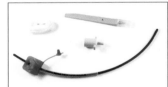

Uses
- Tracheobronchial suctioning.

Fig. 2.15.5: A Portex Mini-Trach II kit (Smiths Medical).

Other notes

Mini-tracheostomy kits are sometimes found on emergency airway trolleys. They are, however, unsuitable for this purpose because the ID is too narrow for effective ventilation and because the tube lacks a cuff.

Laryngectomy tube (Montandon)

A laryngectomy tube is a J-shaped tube with an extended proximal limb designed for use in place of a standard tracheostomy tube during laryngectomy. It keeps the breathing system away from the surgical site, facilitating surgical access.

Uses

- Laryngectomy and other major head and neck surgery in patients with a tracheostomy.

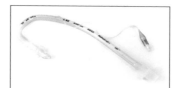

Fig. 2.15.6: A Mallinckrodt J-shaped laryngectomy tube, also known as a Montandon tube (Covidien).

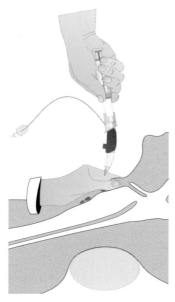

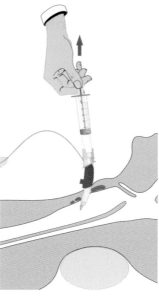

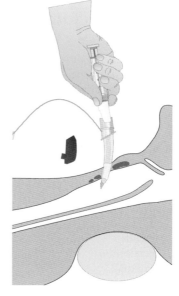

(a) The neck is extended and the larynx fixed by the operator's hand prior to insertion.

(b) Insertion takes place in the midline through the cricothyroid membrane until air is aspirated.

(c) The red spacer designed to prevent over-insertion and damage to the posterior tracheal wall is removed.

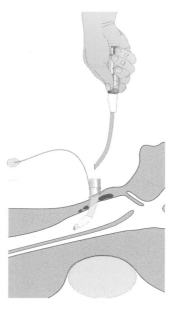

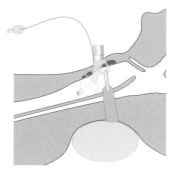

(d) The cannula is advanced off the needle.

(e) The cuff is inflated and the tube secured.

Fig. 2.16.1: The insertion and final positioning of VBM's Quicktrach II. Images courtesy of VBM.

Overview

Cricothyroidotomy devices are designed for insertion through the cricothyroid membrane. They may be classified by internal diameter (ID) as:

- ID <4 mm: small cannula devices, designed for oxygenation.
- ID >4 mm: large bore devices, designed for ventilation.

Surgical cricothyroidotomy is an alternative technique in which a standard 6 mm or larger cuffed endotracheal or tracheostomy tube is inserted through a surgical incision.

Uses

- *Elective prophylactic cricothyroidotomy* in an anticipated difficult airway.
- *Emergency cricothyroidotomy* in a 'can't intubate, can't ventilate' scenario.

How it works

Insertion

The cricothyroid membrane connects the thyroid cartilage to the cricoid cartilage, a distance of approximately 10 mm in the adult. Prior to cricothyroidotomy, the neck should be fully extended and the larynx fixed with one hand. The needle puncture should be in the midline.

Cricothyroidotomy devices use either a cannula-over-needle or Seldinger design. In either case, a syringe is attached to the needle and aspiration of air confirms placement in the larynx. Once the needle tip is in the larynx, the cannula is fed off the needle and/or the wire inserted, depending on the technique.

Oxygenation and ventilation

As a result of the Hagen–Poiseuille equation (see *Fig. 6.3.3*), gas flow drops dramatically as ID decreases. Whilst a 4 mm device permits expiration in around 4 seconds, expiration through a 2 mm (14 G) cannula takes 30 seconds.

Small cannula devices

Small cannula devices such as a Ravussin needle are chiefly useful for temporary oxygenation, rather than true ventilation. The high resistance caused by the narrow bore means that the best chance of good ventilation involves a high pressure oxygen delivery system (see Jet ventilators). Expiration must take place through the patient's own patent upper airway. Even in this situation, CO_2 build up will occur. Some authorities quote 45 minutes as the time until CO_2 levels will be significantly increased.

As an alternative in emergency situations, many small cannula devices have a 15 mm connector for a standard breathing system in addition to the Luer lock connector (see *Section 8.7*) for jet ventilation. Use of a standard breathing system should permit short-term oxygenation, but there will be no meaningful CO_2 removal.

Small cannula devices may also be used prophylactically prior to induction of general anaesthesia in patients with anticipated difficult airways. They are easily inserted under local anaesthesia and are relatively atraumatic. The anaesthetist then has a back-up means of oxygenating the patient should intubation prove difficult or impossible.

Large bore devices

Conventional ventilation using a breathing system is possible through large bore devices (>4 mm ID) providing that they have a cuff. During ventilation, an uncuffed 4 mm tube will usually result in a large leak through the patient's upper airway. Whilst this may sometimes be successfully managed by inserting throat packs, it is preferable to use a cuffed device such as a Quicktrach II or Melker.

Surgical cricothyroidotomy

Surgical cricothyroidotomy may be carried out with a blade and a 6 mm cuffed endotracheal tube, equipment which should always be available in anaesthetic or critical care settings. The use of artery forceps or a tracheal hook facilitates insertion and is recommended.

Other notes

The Royal College of Anaesthetists 4th National Audit Project (NAP4) found the failure rate for cannula cricothyroidotomy to be 65%, with surgical techniques being more successful. It is unclear whether cannula techniques are inherently inferior, or whether there were patient or operator factors which accounted for this difference.

Ravussin needle (VBM)

The Ravussin needle is a 13 G cannula-over-needle device designed for jet ventilation. The needle and cannula are curved to reduce the chance of posterior tracheal wall damage and kinking, and there are side holes at the end of the cannula to keep it from obstructing if it abuts the tracheal wall. In addition to the Luer lock connection for a jet ventilator, there is also a 15 mm connection for a breathing system that should permit oxygenation if a jet ventilator is not available.

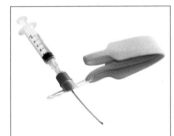

Fig. 2.16.2: A Ravussin needle. Image courtesy of VBM.

 Advantages

- Simple and quick to insert.
- Relatively atraumatic.
- Useful prophylactically prior to an expected difficult intubation.

Disadvantages

- Requires a patent upper airway for ventilation.
- Requires jet ventilation, with its attendant risks.
- The cannula may kink.

Quicktrach II (VBM)

This is a cannula-over-needle device with a 4 mm ID. It is supplied preassembled and does not require a skin incision. Quicktrach II is a cuffed device, whereas Quicktrach I is uncuffed.

The needle is designed to cut to 2 mm and dilate to 4 mm. The red stopper prevents the needle from being inserted too deep and therefore reduced the risk of damage to the posterior tracheal wall.

The procedure may be completed in around 30 seconds in skilled hands following the steps in *Fig. 2.16.1*.

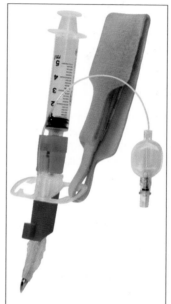

 Advantages
- Simple and quick to insert.
- Skin incision not required, though it may aid placement.
- Ventilation may take place using a standard breathing system.
- The cuff permits positive pressure ventilation and protects against aspiration.

Fig. 2.16.3: VBM Quicktrach II. Image courtesy of VBM.

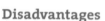 **Disadvantages**
- Greater trauma and associated risk of bleeding than a Ravussin needle.

Melker cricothyroidotomy set (Cook)

This is an example of a device which uses the Seldinger technique. A percutaneous needle is inserted (a Ravussin cannula which is already *in situ* may also be used). The wire is then threaded and a skin incision made with a scalpel. The dilator, with the pre-loaded cricothyroidotomy cannula is railroaded into position.

It is available in 4 and 6 mm ID uncuffed and 5 mm ID cuffed versions. The procedure takes around 40 seconds in skilled hands.

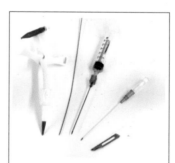

Advantages
- Uses the familiar Seldinger technique.
- Ventilation may take place using a standard breathing system.
- The cuff permits positive pressure ventilation and protects against aspiration.

Fig. 2.16.4: A Cook Melker cricothyroidotomy set incorporating a needle and saline-filled syringe, wire, blade, dilator and uncuffed Melker tube.

Disadvantages
- The multistep technique is more complex than cannula-over-needle, and increases the time required for insertion.

Surgicric I (VBM)

This is an example of a surgical cricothyroidotomy kit which includes a scalpel, tracheal hook and 7.0 mm cuffed tracheal tube with an adjustable flange, allowing the tube to be secured in an appropriate position once inserted.

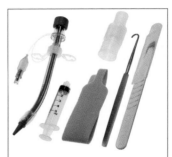

Advantages
- All the required equipment is in the pack.
- Ventilation may take place using a standard breathing system.
- Surgical cricothyroidotomy may have higher success rates than needle.

Fig. 2.16.5: VBM Surgicric I. Image courtesy of VBM.

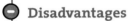
Disadvantages
- Anaesthetists may feel more confident using non-surgical, needle-based techniques.

2.17 Retrograde intubation set

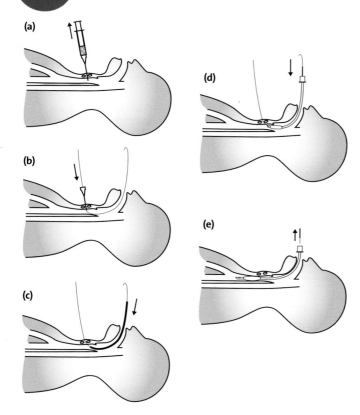

(a)

(b)

(c)

(d)

(e)

Fig. 2.17.1: Technique for retrograde intubation (adapted from Cook Medical instructions).

(a) Cricothyroid puncture.

(b) Retrograde passage of the wire.

(c) Antegrade passage of the intubation catheter over the wire

(d) Intubation over the catheter.

(e) Removal of catheter and wire together.

Overview

Retrograde intubation involves a wire being passed cephalad through the cricothyroid membrane, to exit the mouth or nose. The wire may then be used to guide placement of an ETT.

Uses

It may be used in patients in whom antegrade oral or nasal intubation is difficult or dangerous. Examples of patients include those with oropharyngeal masses or where upper airway haemorrhage obscures the view.

Retrograde intubation takes several minutes and is therefore not suitable for critical emergency situations.

How it works

A kit is available from Cook Medical containing a cannula for cricothyroid puncture, a J-tipped guide wire and a retrograde intubation catheter (a hollow airway exchange catheter). Alternatively these components can be sourced separately.

Under suitable anaesthesia, the cricothyroid membrane is punctured as for a needle cricothyroidotomy, however, the cannula is directed in a cephalic direction. The guide wire is passed through the cannula to exit either the nose or the mouth. The retrograde intubation catheter is then threaded over the guide wire in an antegrade direction and passed through the glottis. The wire is held tight and an ETT is railroaded over the catheter. The wire and catheter are then removed and the ETT secured.

Advantages

- Permits intubation in patients with distorted upper airway anatomy.
- Bag-mask ventilation may continue throughout most of the procedure.
- Oxygenation may take place down the airway exchange catheter once sited.

Disadvantages

- Retrograde intubation is a multistep procedure that takes several minutes and is therefore only suitable for patients in whom oxygenation can be maintained.
- Potential for pneumothorax and haemorrhage.

Chapter 3
Breathing systems

3.1 Introduction to breathing systems

Classification

A breathing system is a device that conducts gases such as oxygen and anaesthetic agents to the patient and conducts waste gases such as CO_2 away.

Classically, breathing systems are classified as open, semi-open, semi-closed and closed. Semi-closed systems are further divided into rebreathing systems with CO_2 absorption, rebreathing systems without CO_2 absorption and non-rebreathing systems. This classification is confusing, and systems are classified differently by different authors.

More simply, systems can be classified in two groups:

- systems with CO_2 washout (includes open and semi-open systems)
- systems with CO_2 absorption (includes closed and semi-closed systems).

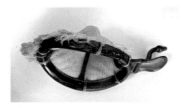

Fig. 3.1.1: A Schimmelbusch mask – an historical example of an open breathing system.

Examples of *open systems* include the use of chloroform dripped onto gauze (for example, a Schimmelbusch mask, *Fig. 3.1.1*), or the delivery of the fresh gas into an anaesthetist's cupped hands for inhalational induction in paediatrics. *Semi-open systems* include those in the Mapleson classification; they rely on their gas dynamics to ensure that CO_2 is washed out and not rebreathed.

The circle system incorporates a soda lime canister for CO_2 absorption. It usually functions as a semi-closed system. When the fresh gas flow is greater than the patient's gas uptake, some gas is vented via the adjustable pressure limiting (APL) valve, and the circle behaves as a *semi-closed* system. It is possible to use a circle as a fully *closed* system. To do this, the APL valve is closed and the fresh gas flow is set equal to the uptake by the patient so that the overall volume of gas in the system is constant. It is difficult to estimate the patient's oxygen uptake accurately and therefore fully closed systems are rarely used in practice.

Efficiency

The efficiency of a breathing system is defined by the lowest fresh gas flow that prevents the patient rebreathing CO_2. Low fresh gas flows are desirable to reduce the amount of expensive (and polluting) volatile anaesthetic that is used. In an inefficient open system, most anaesthetic will be vented into the atmosphere, whereas in a closed system, only the amount taken up by the patient is required.

An ideal breathing system

Examiners sometimes ask the characteristics of the mythical 'ideal' breathing system. Some suggestions are that it should:

- be simple and portable
- be safe to use in all age groups
- reliably deliver the intended gas mixture
- be efficient in both spontaneous and controlled ventilation
- protect patients from barotrauma
- permit scavenging of waste gases
- offer low resistance to gas flow
- conserve heat and moisture.

Unfortunately, no system fits all criteria and a compromise is therefore made depending on the situation.

3.2 Bag valve mask

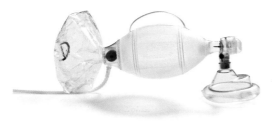

Fig. 3.2.1: The Ambu SPUR II (single patient use resuscitator). Image courtesy of Ambu.

Overview

The bag valve mask was first brought to market in 1956 by Ambu; these systems are therefore Ambu bags. The primary benefit of bag valve masks over other breathing systems is their self-inflating bag, which enables them to be used without a pressurized gas supply.

Uses

Bag valve masks are used for emergency ventilation, with or without a pressurized gas supply. The bag and valve may also be used to ventilate via an ETT (see *Section 2.11*) or laryngeal mask airway (see *Section 2.6*).

How it works

The self-inflating bag is usually made of clear silicone and returns to its original shape when squeezed. Some designs may be collapsed in on themselves for storage.

Between the bag and the mask is a one-way 'non-rebreathing' valve which vents expired gases. There are a number of designs by different manufacturers (Ambu use their proprietary Ambu-E valve). Most valve designs permit both spontaneous and controlled ventilation. The device may be used with room air, or with supplementary oxygen. Most have an oxygen reservoir to maximize the concentration of inspired oxygen.

Advantages

- May be used to deliver room air without a pressurized gas supply.
- Self-contained and widely available.

Disadvantages

- There is little tactile feedback during ventilation.
- There is no visual indication of spontaneous ventilation.
- Although positive end expiratory pressure (PEEP) valves are available from the manufacturer, the device is less suitable for applying PEEP than Mapleson breathing systems (see *Section 3.5*).
- All expired gas is vented, thus making the system expensive to use with anaesthetic gases. For this reason, it is rarely used (though see the Triservice apparatus in *Section 5.11*).

3.3 Adjustable pressure limiting valve

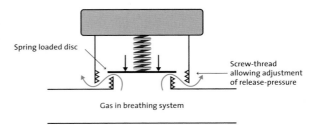

Spring loaded disc

Screw-thread allowing adjustment of release-pressure

Gas in breathing system

Fig. 3.3.2: Diagram of the APL valve. The pressure exerted by the spring-loaded disc can be varied by screwing the valve top.

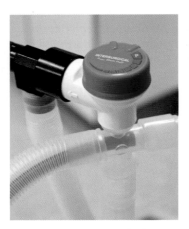

Fig. 3.3.1: An APL valve attached to a Bain system and scavenging (black 30 mm connector).

Overview

The APL valve is a spring-loaded pressure release valve in which the release pressure can be varied to suit the situation.

Uses

APL valves are an essential component of most breathing systems (except the Mapleson E or F) allowing control of the pressure within the breathing system and therefore the airway.

How it works

The valve consists of a lightweight disc which is held against the base by a spring, closing the valve. The pressure exerted by the spring may be adjusted by screwing the valve cap. When the pressure beneath the disc (i.e. the pressure in the breathing system) exceeds the pressure exerted by the spring, the valve will open, allowing gas to escape.

When the valve cap is fully unscrewed, the pressure exerted by the spring is less than 1 cmH$_2$O and gas vents easily. In order to protect against barotrauma, modern valves are designed so that the valve will open at pressures above 60 cmH$_2$O even when the cap is screwed down and the valve fully 'closed'.

Modern valves are designed so that all exhaust gases exit through a 30 mm port, allowing a scavenging system to be connected.

⊕ Advantages

- Permits control of the airway pressure during positive pressure ventilation.
- Permits application of PEEP.
- Facilitates scavenging.

⊖ Disadvantages

- Water vapour may condense on the disc, causing it to stick. Discs are made of a hydrophobic material to reduce the likelihood of this.
- Valves introduce greater resistance and are less suitable for small children. This is the reason the APL valve is absent from the Mapleson E and F systems.
- Barotrauma may result from inadvertent closure of the APL valve.
- Adds bulk to the breathing system.

3.4 Reservoir bag

Overview

The reservoir bag is an essential component of most breathing systems because it improves efficiency and permits manual ventilation. Bags are available in both rubber and latex-free versions. The standard adult size is 2 litres, with paediatric sizes down to 0.5 litres. Larger sizes are occasionally used for inhalational induction in adults.

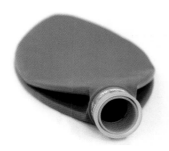

Fig. 3.4.1: A 2 litre reservoir bag.

Uses

A component of most anaesthetic breathing systems.

How it works

The reservoir bag has a number of useful properties.

- It acts as a reservoir for oxygen and anaesthetic gases, which enter the bag from the fresh gas flow during expiration and are drawn upon during inspiration, thus allowing lower fresh gas flows to be used.
- Manual ventilation is achieved by squeezing the bag.
- It acts as a visual indicator of spontaneous ventilation.
- In the event of a valve becoming stuck or being left unintentionally closed, pressure will build up in the breathing system. The reservoir bag will then distend, limiting the pressure to around 60 cmH$_2$O and thus reducing barotrauma. According to the law of Laplace, the pressure will fall as the bag's radius increases – an effect that can be demonstrated using the pressure gauge on an anaesthetic machine.

The law of Laplace

$$P = \frac{2T}{r}$$

where P = pressure, T = tension in the wall of a sphere, r = radius.

The bag contains a plastic cage at the opening which prevents apposition of the two sides of the bag. Without the cage, the apposition of the bag can occlude the flow of gas, particularly during spontaneous inspiration.

Open-ended bags are used for the Mapleson F paediatric breathing system, which has no valves. The anaesthetist partially occludes the open-ended tail of the bag in order to maintain and adjust positive pressure in the system.

Advantages

- An essential component of anaesthetic breathing systems.
- Permits tactile feedback.

Disadvantages

- It is relatively easy to tear the bag.
- It is not self-inflating and must therefore be used with a pressurized gas supply.

3.5 The Mapleson classification

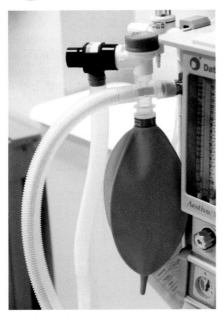

Fig. 3.5.1: The Bain system which is derived from, and functionally similar to, Ayre's T-piece. The bag and APL valve are at the machine end and a narrow inner tube carries fresh gas flow to the patient end.

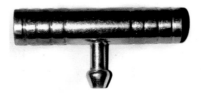

Fig. 3.5.2: An early version of Ayre's T-piece. Tubing would be attached to complete the system. Image courtesy of the Anaesthesia Museum, Sheffield Teaching Hospitals NHS Foundation Trust.

Overview

In 1954, Mapleson performed mathematical modelling of the semi-open breathing systems available to him. He classified them into five breathing systems (A–E) and a sixth (F) was added later. Systems are classified according to the relative positions of three components: the fresh gas flow (FGF), the APL valve and a gas reservoir. Variable lengths of corrugated tubing connect the components.

Mapleson systems are semi-open and rely on sufficient fresh gas flow to wash out exhaled gas and prevent rebreathing.

Uses

In comparison with a circle system, Mapleson breathing systems are inefficient (meaning that higher FGFs are required to prevent rebreathing) and are therefore expensive to use with volatile anaesthetics. They are therefore not used for anaesthetic delivery to adult patients in theatre – circle systems are used instead.

Mapleson systems continue to be used in the anaesthetic room (D and, occasionally, A), for transfers or management of critically ill patients outside of theatre (C), and for paediatric patients (F and, occasionally, E).

How it works

When Mapleson performed his mathematical modelling of how each breathing system worked, he used a number of simplifications and assumptions.

- Gases move en block. In other words, they maintain their identity as fresh gas flow, dead space gas, alveolar gas, etc., and do not mix.
- The reservoir bag continues to fill up, without offering any resistance until it is full.
- The expiratory (APL) valve opens as soon as the reservoir bag is full and the pressure inside the breathing system is greater than atmospheric pressure.
- The valve remains open throughout the expiratory phase, without offering any resistance to gas flow, and closes at the start of the next inspiration.

The efficiency of a breathing system is defined by the lowest FGF required to prevent rebreathing of CO_2. High flows waste anaesthetic gases, therefore the use of efficient systems has become more important due to the use of volatile agents that are currently expensive, such as sevoflurane and desflurane.

The limbs of the breathing system are named relative to the patient. Therefore the afferent limb carries gas towards the patient, whereas the efferent limb carries gas away. The reservoir may be on the afferent or efferent limb of the system, and may consist of a reservoir bag, reservoir tubing, or both.

Afferent reservoir systems

Mapleson A, B and C are afferent reservoir systems – the reservoir bag is situated on the afferent limb. They do not have an efferent limb as the APL valve is at the patient end (except in the Lack system, which is nevertheless functionally identical). Afferent reservoir systems are *efficient during spontaneous ventilation* providing the APL valve is separated from the FGF by more than the patient's tidal volume, which is the case in the Mapleson A. These systems are all *inefficient during controlled ventilation*, requiring a FGF over 3 times the minute ventilation (MV).

Efferent reservoir systems

Mapleson D, E and F are efferent reservoir systems derived from Ayre's T-piece. Without a reservoir, a T-piece requires an FGF of greater than the patient's peak inspiratory flow rate (which may exceed $60\,l.min^{-1}$) in order to prevent air entrainment. A reservoir or tubing and/or a bag, is therefore situated on the expiratory limb to reduce FGF requirements. Providing the reservoir's volume is greater than the patient's tidal volume, the system will be *efficient for controlled ventilation*. The mechanics are complicated but there will almost always be some rebreathing, which must be offset by increasing the ventilatory rate. Normocapnia may then be achieved with a FGF of around 0.7 times MV. Efferent reservoir systems are *inefficent during spontaneous ventilation*, requiring FGF of 1.5–2 times MV.

⊕ Advantages

Mapleson systems remain in use because they:

- are simple and cheap
- do not require CO_2 absorption
- are easily portable (particularly C, E and F)
- have some specific advantages in paediatric anaesthesia (F).

⊖ Disadvantages

- Compared with a circle system, all Mapleson systems are inefficient.

Magill system (Mapleson A)

Fresh gas flow enters at the machine end, just proximal to the reservoir bag, which is connected by approximately 1.6 m of tubing to the APL valve at the patient end. The volume of this tubing must exceed one tidal volume to ensure efficient spontaneous ventilation.

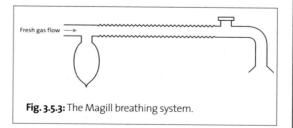

Fig. 3.5.3: The Magill breathing system.

Spontaneous ventilation (efficient)
- During inspiration, the APL valve closes and the patient inspires fresh gas from the tubing.
- During expiration, the expiratory gas initially enters the reservoir tubing until the bag fills and the pressure opens the APL valve allowing gas to escape.
- During the expiratory pause, fresh gas displaces the remaining expired gas out of the APL valve.
- At flows equalling MV, no rebreathing occurs.
- The system can be made more efficient because gas from anatomical dead space is expired first and therefore vented from the APL valve last. If this dead space gas, which does not contain CO_2, is rebreathed, flows of 0.7 times the patient's MV may be used (this is equivalent to alveolar MV and approximately 70 ml.kg^{-1}.min^{-1}).

Controlled ventilation (inefficient)
- Venting of FGF occurs during positive pressure inspiration and exhaled gas is not vented until the APL valve reopens (a higher APL valve opening pressure has to be set than during spontaneous ventilation).
- Rebreathing of expired gas therefore occurs unless FGF exceeds 3 times MV.

Advantages
- Efficient for spontaneous ventilation.

Disadvantages
- Inefficient for controlled ventilation.
- The APL valve at the patient end adds bulk and drags on breathing circuit connections, particularly if connected to scavenging.
- Not suitable for paediatrics.

Lack system (Coaxial Mapleson A)

The Lack system is a modification of the Magill system, designed to eliminate the problem of having the APL valve at the patient end. It consists of a 30 mm outer tube for inspiration, and a 14 mm inner tube for expiration. This wider bore tubing is required in order to reduce resistance to expiration.

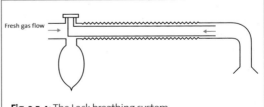

Fig. 3.5.4: The Lack breathing system.

The Lack system has similar characteristics to the Magill system, being efficient for spontaneous ventilation and inefficient for controlled ventilation.

Advantages
- Efficient for spontaneous ventilation.
- Bulky components are all at the machine end.

Disadvantages
- Inefficient for controlled ventilation.
- If the inner tube develops a leak, the entire system becomes dead space and CO_2 rapidly builds up.

Other notes
A parallel Lack circuit also exists, with separate inspiratory and expiratory limbs. In use it has similar characteristics to the coaxial version and avoids the problem of the inner tube leaking.

Mapleson B

This circuit is not in common usage. The FGF and APL valve are at the patient end of the tubing, which causes complete mixing of fresh and expired gas. It is therefore inefficient for both spontaneous and controlled ventilation.

Fresh gas flows of 2–3 times MV are required (this is slightly more efficient than Mapleson A for controlled ventilation, but significantly worse during spontaneous ventilation).

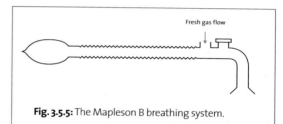

Fig. 3.5.5: The Mapleson B breathing system.

Mapleson C

This system is similar to a Mapleson B system, but without the reservoir tubing. The bag, FGF and APL valve are all at the patient end. It is inefficient for both spontaneous and controlled ventilation and requires FGFs of 2–3 times minute volume ($15\,l.min^{-1}$ is therefore appropriate).

It is used in resuscitation situations as an alternative to a self-inflating bag. In these situations, volatile anaesthetics are not used and therefore efficiency is less important than portability.

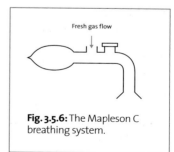

Fig. 3.5.6: The Mapleson C breathing system.

Advantages
- Simple and lightweight.
- Useful for resuscitation, allowing PEEP to be applied and giving a visual and tactile indication of ventilation.

Disadvantages
- Inefficient, CO_2 accumulates over time.
- APL valve adds bulk at the patient end.

Other notes
This system is commonly called a Waters circuit, although Ralph Waters' design incorporated a soda lime canister for CO_2 absorption. Waters' design is no longer in use because the canister adds bulk and there is a risk of the patient inhaling dust from the soda lime.

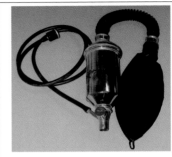

Fig. 3.5.7: A true Waters circuit, which incorporated a soda lime canister. Image courtesy of the Anaesthesia Museum, Sheffield Teaching Hospitals NHS Foundation Trust.

Bain system (Coaxial Mapleson D)

In a Mapleson D system, the FGF enters at the patient end, with the APL valve and bag being located at the machine end. Most Mapleson D systems in use are the coaxial Bain modification, in which fresh gas flows down a narrow (6 mm) inner tube and exhaled gas passes down the 22 mm outer tube. This is the reverse arrangement to the co-axial Mapleson A.

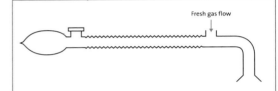

Fig. 3.5.8: The Mapleson D breathing system. The fresh gas flow enters at the patient end.

Spontaneous ventilation
(inefficient)
- During inspiration, fresh gas is supplemented by gas from the outer tubing.
- During expiration, exhaled gases pass back down the outer tubing to the bag, and mix with fresh gas, until the bag is full and the APL valve opens to allow venting.

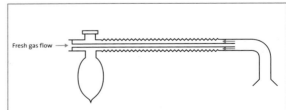

Fig. 3.5.9: The Bain system is functionally identical to the Mapleson D, but the fresh gas is delivered to the patient end co-axially down a narrow inner tube.

- Mixed gas from the tubing and bag will be used for the next inspiration.
- FGFs of 3 times the patient's MV are required to prevent rebreathing completely, however, flows of 1.5–2 times MV are usually sufficient to reduce it to an acceptable level.

Controlled ventilation (efficient)
- During expiration, expired gas is mixed with fresh gas.
- During the expiratory pause, fresh gas washes expired gas from the outer reservoir tubing.
- During inspiration the patient inspires fresh gas from the outer tube.
- Some rebreathing will usually occur, however, with an increased ventilatory rate, flows of 0.7 times MV are possible.

Advantages
- Compact system with all the major components at the machine end, facilitating scavenging.
- Low dead space because the APL valve is at the machine end.
- May be used with a Penlon Nuffield 200 ventilator (see *Section 4.5*).

Disadvantages
- Inefficient for spontaneous ventilation.
- If the inner tube becomes disconnected or breaks, the entire system becomes dead space.

Other notes
- When used with the Penlon Nuffield 200 ventilator, the bag is removed and the ventilator attached in its place. The APL valve is fully closed. It can be seen that following the effective removal of these two components, the system is now a T-piece.

Ayre's T-piece (Mapleson E)

A Mapleson E system consists of a T-shaped rigid tube, with connections for the FGF, the patient, and a variable length of reservoir tubing.

It is a valveless, bagless breathing system. Whilst intermittent positive pressure ventilation (IPPV) is possible by intermittently occluding the expiratory limb, this affords little control and there is the risk of high pressures occurring. Mapleson E systems have been superseded in clinical use by the Mapleson F system.

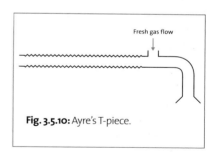

Fresh gas flow

Fig. 3.5.10: Ayre's T-piece.

Spontaneous ventilation (inefficient)
- During the expiratory pause, fresh gas enters the reservoir tubing. The volume of this tubing should exceed the expected tidal volume because it will supply the fresh gas during inspiration.
- During inspiration, fresh gas is drawn from the reservoir (as well as the FGF).
- During expiration, exhaled gas is vented down the reservoir tubing.
- FGF of 2–3 times MV are required.

If the volume of the reservoir tubing is too large, rebreathing may occur, whereas if it is too small, air may be entrained.

Advantages
- There is minimal dead space.
- It is a valveless system. There is therefore minimal resistance to breathing, and the high pressures that would be encountered in the event of valve failure, are avoided.
- It is suitable for paediatric patients (up to 25 kg).

Disadvantages
- Application of PEEP is not possible. This is particularly important in anaesthetized paediatric patients who are dependent on positive airways pressure to maintain functional residual capacity (FRC).
- Positive pressure ventilation is difficult and potentially hazardous.
- Scavenging is difficult.

Jackson–Rees modification (Mapleson F)

The Jackson–Rees modification of Ayre's T-piece incorporates an open-ended bag attached to the end of the reservoir tubing. Partially occluding the 'tail' of the bag permits positive pressure ventilation or the application of PEEP. The bag also gives a visual indication of ventilation.

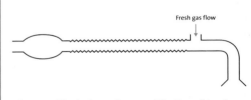

Fig. 3.5.11: The Jackson–Rees modification of Ayre's T-piece.

Gas dynamics during spontaneous or controlled ventilation are similar to Mapleson E systems. FGF of 2–3 times MV is required.

Advantages
- As for Mapleson E.
- Positive pressure ventilation and PEEP are possible.
- More suitable for inhalational induction than a circle system.
- This is the standard breathing system for paediatric patients (up to 25 kg) although a small calibre circle system may also be used.

Disadvantages
- Scavenging is difficult.
- The system is inefficient, requiring high FGFs.
- Partially occluding the tail, whilst at the same time squeezing the bag is a moderately skilled technique.

3.6 Humphrey ADE block

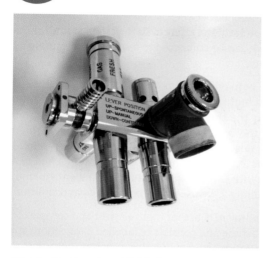

Fig. 3.6.1: The Humphrey ADE block.

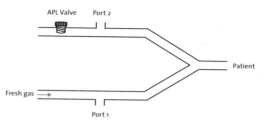

Fig. 3.6.2: A simplified schematic of the Humphrey ADE block.

Overview

The Humphrey ADE block was designed and introduced into anaesthetic practice by David Humphrey in 1983. Its design allows the anaesthetist to switch between Mapleson A, D and E systems quickly and easily, without the need to disconnect from the fresh gas flow or change the breathing tubing that goes to and from the patient; this is achieved in part simply by switching a lever on the block. The system can be used in the Mapleson A configuration to improve efficiency during spontaneous breathing and the Mapleson D mode to improve efficiency during positive pressure ventilation. The Mapleson E configuration allows the Humphrey ADE block to be used in children as well as adults. Independent studies have shown that the Humphrey ADE block mechanics are more efficient than conventional Mapleson breathing systems. For example, a conventional Mapleson A system, during spontaneous ventilation, allows fresh gas flows as low as 70 ml.kg^{-1}.min^{-1} before carbon dioxide is rebreathed. The Humphrey ADE block, when in the Mapleson A configuration, allows considerably lower fresh gas flows of 50 ml.kg^{-1}.min^{-1} before carbon dioxide is rebreathed.

Uses

A block that connects to the common gas outlet of an anaesthetic machine and allows the efficiency of the breathing system to be maintained when switching between spontaneous and controlled ventilation. It can be used in adults and children.

How it works

Although the Mapleson A, D and E breathing systems are functionally very different, they only differ physically by the relative positions of the reservoir bag (*Section 3.4*) and APL valve (*Section*

Table 3.6.3 The relative location of the fresh gas flow, reservoir bag and APL valve in conventional Mapleson circuits.

Circuit	Location within breathing circuit		
	Fresh gas flow	**Reservoir bag / ventilator**	**APL valve**
Mapleson A	Afferent limb	Afferent limb	Efferent limb
Mapleson D	Afferent limb	Efferent limb	Efferent limb
Mapleson E	Afferent limb	None	None

3.3) relative to the patient. For example, the main difference between Mapleson A and D breathing systems is that the reservoir bag changes its position from the afferent to the efferent limb of the breathing system. Equally, a Mapleson A or D circuit can be converted to a Mapleson E simply by removing the APL valve and reservoir bag altogether.

The Humphrey ADE block exploits the relative ease with which it is possible to transition between these three breathing circuits. *Figure 3.6.2* shows a highly simplified schematic of the principles of how a Humphrey ADE block works. It combines the three Mapleson circuits by the addition of ports into the afferent and efferent limbs of the breathing system. A rotary lever is then capable of isolating one or both ports and the APL valve, depending on its position. The reservoir bag is attached to port 1, whilst port 2 can either be left open to the atmosphere or attached to a ventilator. Smooth bore tubing of 15 mm diameter (with external corrugations to prevent kinking) is used to reduce resistance. This allows identical tubing to be used with both adults and children.

In reality of course, the inner workings of the Humphrey ADE are far more elegant and complex. A Humphrey block is mounted on the anaesthetic machine and consists of labelled connections for a reservoir bag, a ventilator, inspiratory and expiratory limbs of a breathing system, a 60 cmH$_2$O pressure relief safety valve, an APL valve and a lever to select spontaneous or controlled ventilation.

When the lever is up (spontaneous and manual bag ventilation)

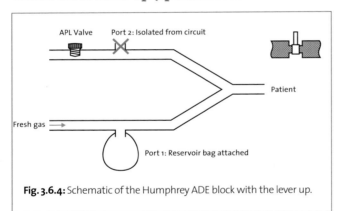

APL Valve   Port 2: Isolated from circuit

Patient

Fresh gas →

Port 1: Reservoir bag attached

Fig. 3.6.4: Schematic of the Humphrey ADE block with the lever up.

Port 2 is disconnected from the system, but the FGF and APL valve remain connected. The system therefore acts as a Mapleson A. In fact, due to its design and the use of low resistance tubing, studies have shown it to be more efficient than a standard Mapleson A circuit during spontaneous ventilation, requiring FGFs as low as 50 ml.kg^{-1}.min^{-1}.

Bag ventilation is also possible with the lever in this position. Waste gases can be scavenged through the exhaust valve.

When the lever is down (controlled ventilation or T-piece)

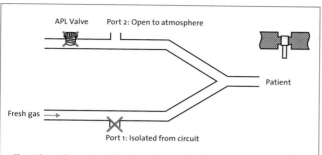

APL Valve   Port 2: Open to atmosphere

Patient

Fresh gas

Port 1: Isolated from circuit

Fig. 3.6.5: Schematic of the Humphrey ADE block with the lever down and used as a T-piece.

Port 1 and the APL valve are disconnected from the system whilst port 2 remains connected. If port 2 is left open to the atmosphere, it behaves as a Mapleson E (T-piece) system. If a ventilator is attached to port 2, the system then operates as a Mapleson D, although, because the APL valve is redundant, it is not strictly a Mapleson D.

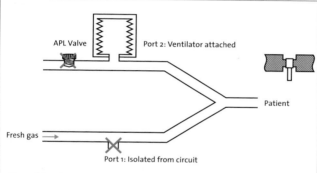

APL Valve   Port 2: Ventilator attached

Patient

Fresh gas

Port 1: Isolated from circuit

Fig. 3.6.6: Schematic of the Humphrey ADE block with the lever down and attached to a positive pressure ventilator.

⊕ Advantages

- Versatile: may be used in adults and children.
- Switches instantly between three different breathing system configurations.
- More efficient than standard Mapleson systems; significantly lower gas flows are needed in any given configuration to prevent CO_2 rebreathing, compared to conventional Mapleson circuits.
- Smooth bore 15 mm tubing reduces turbulence and resistance to breathing. Therefore the resistance to breathing is not much different to a similar length of corrugated 22 mm internal diameter tubing.

⊖ Disadvantages

- Not immediately intuitive to use.
- Heavy block may dislodge easily from common gas outlet.

3.7 The circle system

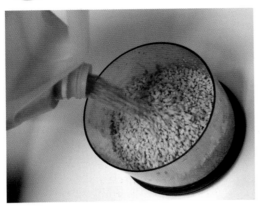

Fig. 3.7.1: Soda lime.

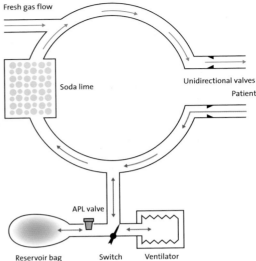

Fig. 3.7.2: Schematic of a circle system.

Overview

The circle system (*Fig. 3.7.2*) is a highly efficient breathing system that conserves anaesthetic gases, heat and moisture. By actively removing carbon dioxide from exhaled gas, the circle system allows re-breathing of anaesthetic gases. In theory, the fresh gas flow (FGF) that is added to the circle system need only match the oxygen consumption of the patient and any anaesthetic losses through leaks, absorption or metabolism; i.e. it can operate as a closed breathing system. However, in practice the circle system is almost always used as a semi-closed system, because the FGF is usually greater than the patient's gas uptake (see *Section 3.1*).

Uses

This breathing system is particularly useful for long cases because it efficiently conserves anaesthetic gases, heat and moisture. It is the main alternative to the Mapleson systems for conveying gas to and from the patient in theatre, and often in the anaesthetic room.

How it works

A circle system comprises:

- a fresh gas inlet
- a reservoir bag (see *Section 3.4*)
- two one-way valves (one in each of the inspiratory and expiratory limbs)
- a Y-piece connector from the one-way valves to the patient (not shown in *Fig. 3.7.2*)
- an APL valve (see *Section 3.3*)
- a soda lime canister that absorbs carbon dioxide
- lengths of corrugated (kink-resistant) tubing to connect the components to one other and the patient.

Volatile anaesthetic agents may be added to the gas mixture in two ways. A vaporizer (see *Chapter 5*) may be included in the circuit itself, so that gas flows through it on its way round the circle.

This configuration is known as vaporizer-in-circuit (VIC). More commonly, the vaporizer is located outside the circuit (VOC) and fresh gas flows through it before entering the circle.

Fresh gas flow and the reservoir bag are usually found in the inspiratory limb of the circuit to reduce the resistance to inspiration. The APL valve is ideally located in the expiratory limb of the circuit so that only CO_2-containing gas is expelled through it. While in theory it could be placed in the inspiratory limb, fresh gas would be wasted in this configuration as it may be vented before it reached the patient.

The soda lime canister is situated after the APL valve and removes carbon dioxide through an exothermic reaction. Soda lime comprises sodium hydroxide, calcium hydroxide and potassium hydroxide. Sodium and potassium hydroxide are recycled through a series of reactions that aim to permanently neutralize and trap gaseous carbon dioxide as solid calcium carbonate (chalk). By-products of these reactions are heat and water, which maintain the temperature and humidity of the circuit.

Table 3.7.3 The chemical reaction between soda lime and CO_2

CO_2	+	H_2O	→	H_2CO_3				
H_2CO_3	+	2NaOH (or 2KOH)	→	Na_2CO_3 (or K_2CO_3)	+	$2H_2O$	+	HEAT
Na_2CO_3 (or K_2CO_3)	+	$Ca(OH)_2$	→	2NaOH (or 2KOH)	+	$CaCO_3$		

Baralyme is popular in the USA and contains barium hydroxide and calcium hydroxide. It also traps carbon dioxide as insoluble barium carbonate through a similar series of reactions.

The monitoring of the FiO_2 and inspired anaesthetic concentration within the circle system is mandatory. Expired gas has a lower oxygen concentration than the inspired gas because of oxygen uptake (VO_2) by the patient. When the flow of fresh gas into the circle is high, this is of no consequence because the incoming oxygen is more than enough to compensate for the deficit in the recycled gas. Under these circumstances, the FiO_2 within the circle system approximates the FiO_2 in the FGF entering the circle. However, when low flows are used, the recycled expired gas dilutes the fresh gas and the FiO_2 falls. The VO_2 stays constant and because of this, the partial pressure of oxygen (PO_2) in the next expiration is even lower than it was in the first. The fresh gas is therefore diluted further. The end result is that over the course of a low flow anaesthetic, the FiO_2 may drift down to dangerous levels unless a high oxygen concentration is set at the flowmeters.

The concentration of anaesthetic in a low flow circle will also drift downwards due to the same process in addition to losses due to absorption (by the patient and materials within the circuit), leaks and metabolism. However, the rate of fall will slow over time because uptake of anaesthetic by the patient reduces as equilibrium is approached. The concentration of anaesthetic in a high flow system approximates that set by the anaesthetist on the vaporizer.

VIC systems are rarely used but do have a role in the field and for veterinary anaesthesia. They must be low resistance and therefore the plenum vaporizer is not suitable. Draw-over vaporizers are more appropriate, but their output is difficult to calibrate and maintain. Output and performance depend on the minute volume of the patient, the fresh gas flow and ambient temperature (for which they cannot readily compensate). Accidental spillage of the vaporizer contents into the circuit can lead to dangerous surges in volatile concentration. Because of this, an inefficient draw-over VIC may be safer than an efficient one, especially if potent anaesthetic agents are being used.

⊕ Advantages

- The circle system conserves anaesthetic gases, heat and moisture.
- Low flow anaesthesia is possible provided concentrations are monitored.
- There is a low dead space. The Y-piece tubing between the patient and the inspiratory and expiratory valves creates mechanical dead space, but this is no greater than in non-rebreathing circuits.
- The soda lime canister is distant from the patient's airway, reducing the risk of soda lime dust inhalation.
- Reduced atmospheric pollution because anaesthetic gases can be recycled.

⊖ Disadvantages

- Changes made at the vaporizer dial take a long time to equilibrate with the circle system, especially at low flows.
- The circle system apparatus is bulkier than Mapleson breathing systems.
- Complexity of connections mean that leaks and disconnections are more difficult to identify quickly.
- The extra valves, tubing and soda lime canister increase the resistance.
- At low flows, recycled expired gases progressively dilute the fresh gas flow risking hypoxia and awareness.
- Soda lime may degrade sevoflurane into harmful substances such as compound A. Animal models have demonstrated that compound A can produce hepatic and renal toxicity. As it is only produced in very low concentrations in circle systems, its clinical significance is debated.
- Anaesthetic agents (in particular desflurane and enflurane) have been reported to produce clinically significant levels of carbon monoxide when passed over desiccated (dry) Baralyme and to a lesser extent soda lime.

Chapter 4
Ventilators

4.1 Introduction to ventilators

Overview

Most physicians understand the basic role of a ventilator – it moves gas in and out of the lungs to maintain oxygenation and remove carbon dioxide. However, ventilators are complicated and are a common source of confusion. It is easy to lose sight of the basic concepts of mechanical ventilation when trying to understand the growing number of trade names and acronyms which relate to advanced modes of ventilation: CMV, IPPV, PSV-PRO, SIMV/PS, Autoflow, PRVC, BIPAP, BiPAP, Adaptive Pressure Ventilation, Volume A/C, to name but a few.

What manufacturers won't tell you is that many of these ventilator modes are actually very similar to one another and, in spite of what the manufacturers and some senior clinicians insist, the evidence for one mode being better than another is limited.

Having multiple ventilator modes with different trade names may also be a threat to patient safety; lack of familiarity or confusion concerning the operation of any medical device is dangerous. For many years professional associations and regulatory bodies such as the AAGBI and MHRA have tried, unsuccessfully so far, to convince manufacturers to reach a consensus and standardize the names of their ventilator modes.

This section begins by introducing four basic modes of positive pressure ventilation (PPV), and shows how these can be combined or modified to create advanced modes of ventilation. It then goes on to discuss the interpretation of ventilator graphics and ends with a description of how ventilators may be classified, based on their internal mechanics.

Negative versus positive pressure ventilation

Ventilators can be either negative pressure or positive pressure generators. A negative pressure ventilator reduces intrathoracic pressure so that it becomes sub-atmospheric. Gas flows into the lungs down this pressure gradient and therefore these ventilators mimic normal respiratory physiology. Positive pressure ventilators drive gas into the lungs by creating a pressure within a breathing system that is above atmospheric pressure.

The first commercially successful negative pressure ventilator, the 'iron lung', was developed in the late 1920s. It was an air-tight cylindrical drum with a port so that the head and neck could remain free. Powerful pumps intermittently generated a negative pressure by drawing air out of the sealed chamber. The intermittent negative pressure leads to chest wall expansion and air being drawn into the patient's lungs. The iron lung was popular in the management of respiratory failure secondary to poliomyelitis, but it is rarely used in modern practice.

PPV is now the mainstay of mechanical ventilation, and from here on in, the term 'ventilation' refers to PPV, which can be delivered to the patient 'invasively' through, for example, an endotracheal tube or 'non-invasively' via a tight-fitting face mask.

Basic ventilator modes

The two most fundamental variables in ventilation are:

- *respiratory rate* (breaths per minute) and
- *tidal volume* (ml per breath).

The product of the respiratory rate and tidal volume is the *minute volume*, defined as the total volume delivered to the lungs in one minute. The main differences between modes of ventilation are therefore how the respiratory rate is determined and how the desired tidal volume is delivered.

The respiratory rate may be set by either the:

- *ventilator* (mandatory breaths) or the
- *patient* (triggered breaths).

These triggering options help define control, support and spontaneous breathing modes of ventilation:

- *control mode*: the ventilator delivers a mandatory breath and does all the work of breathing
- *support mode*: the patient triggers the ventilator to deliver a breath; although some respiratory effort is made by the patient, the ventilator does most of the work
- *spontaneous breathing mode*: the patient triggers all breaths and makes all the respiratory effort but the ventilator may provide continuous positive airway pressure (CPAP) and/or supplementary oxygen.

A tidal volume breath may be delivered as a:

- fixed volume (e.g. 500 ml) or a
- fixed pressure (e.g. 15 cmH$_2$O).

The way that the tidal volume is delivered (fixed volume or fixed pressure) and the way that the respiratory rate is set (patient or ventilator), generate four variables which can be combined in different ways to produce four different basic ventilator modes. These ventilator modes are described in more detail in *Tables 4.1.1* and *4.1.2* but in summary they are:

- Volume Control (VC)
- Pressure Control (PC)
- Volume Support (VS)
- Pressure Support (PS)

These basic ventilator modes form the fundamental building blocks of all other modes. Microprocessor controlled ventilators are able to modify or combine these basic modes to create highly sophisticated settings, which are discussed later in this chapter.

In VC and VS, the set volume is delivered regardless of the compliance of the lungs. The flow during inspiration is relatively high and constant until the desired tidal volume is reached, at which point the ventilator cycles into passive expiration. If the patient has severe lung disease and poorly compliant lungs, this type of ventilation can generate high airway pressures, risking barotrauma.

In PC and PS modes, the ventilator generates a set positive pressure which drives air into the lungs until the pressure in the lungs equals the driving pressure. At this point there is no pressure gradient for gas to flow and the ventilator will cycle into expiration. Like physiological inspiration, flow is high at the start of inspiration, then slows as the pressure gradient between the ventilator and the lungs falls. The advantage of this mode is that the risks of barotrauma are reduced because the pressure is limited. The main disadvantage is that the delivered tidal volume is unpredictable. For example, the reduction in compliance that occurs due to abdominal insufflation during laparoscopy will result in a reduced tidal volume for a given airway pressure. Changes in compliance may result in the tidal volume being too low, reducing ventilation, or too high, risking volutrauma.

Choice of support or control modes
This is a compromise between the level of control over minute ventilation and how well a patient tolerates the ventilator mode (see *Table 4.1.1*). The first ventilators were developed for theatre use and involved deeply anaesthetized patients. Control modes were therefore used. Patients being

Table. 4.1.1: The basic building blocks of ventilator modes.

Tidal volume delivered as a set:	Respiratory rate set by the:	Flow of air into patient	Generic name of ventilator mode	Synonyms & trade names	Degree of control over minute volume	Patient tolerance of ventilation
Volume	Ventilator	Constant (high flow)	Volume Controlled Ventilation (VCV)	CMV, IPPV	High	Low
Pressure	Ventilator	Decreasing (dependent on lung compliance)	Pressure Controlled Ventilation (PCV)	PC	↑	↑
Volume	Patient	Constant (high flow)	Volume Support Ventilation (VSV)	VS	↓	
Pressure	Patient	Deceasing (dependent on lung compliance)	Pressure Support Ventilation (PSV)	ASB, PS, SM, PSV	Low	High

Note that most modern ventilator modes providing positive inspiratory pressure are a *variation* or *combination* of these basic ventilator modes.

Key to trade names:

CMV: controlled mandatory ventilation or control mode ventilation
IPPV: intermittent positive pressure ventilation (Draeger)
PC+: pressure control (Draeger)
VS: volume support (Maquet, Puritan-Bennett)
ASB: assisted spontaneous breathing (Draeger)
PS: pressure support (Maquet)
SM: spontaneous mode (Hamilton)
PSV: pressure support ventilation (Viasys)

ventilated longer-term on intensive care, however, develop muscle atrophy caused by lack of use, which makes weaning from the ventilator difficult. PS ventilation modes were therefore developed to permit weaning from ventilation. These modes of ventilation allow the patient's respiratory muscles to be trained; the patient must trigger breaths and the support from the ventilator is progressively reduced as the patient improves clinically. In support modes, some control over the minute volume is conceded, but patient comfort and tolerance of these modes is high as breaths are synchronized with ventilator support. Patients may therefore be ventilated with light, or no, sedation.

Ventilator graphics

Graphs associated with different ventilator modes may seem daunting at first, but if the basic concepts of ventilation are kept in mind, their interpretation should be straightforward. In the FRCA exams, you may be asked to draw graphs of:

- flow against time
- airway pressure against time
- volume against time.

Table. 4.1.2: Comparison of VC, PC and PS modes of ventilation.

	Volume Control (VC)	Pressure Control (PC)	Pressure Support (PS)
Tidal volume	Fixed	Variable	Variable
Trigger	Ventilator (set RR)	Ventilator (set RR)	Patient (variable RR)
Minute volume	Fixed	Variable	Highly variable
Flow	Constant high flow	Decreasing	Decreasing
Airway pressure	Variable	Fixed	Fixed
Inspiration to expiration cycling	When the set tidal volume or maximum inspiratory time* is reached	When the set pressure or maximum inspiratory time* is reached	When the set pressure is reached
Advantages	• Most control over minute ventilation • Tidal volume unaffected by changes in lung and airway compliance	• Reduced barotrauma risk • Compensates for leaks (to an extent) • Decelerating flow is more physiological • Decelerating flow means that a given tidal volume can be achieved using a lower mean airway pressure compared to VC	• Synchronizes with patient effort so better tolerated during respiratory wean • Reduced barotrauma risk, cf. VC/VS • Shares other advantages of PC ventilation
Disadvantages	• Risk of high airway pressures and barotrauma of the lung • Constant high flow during inspiration is difficult for an unsedated patient to tolerate	• Generated tidal volumes unpredictable and dependent on lung compliance/airway resistances • Uncomfortable for patient and may require sedation	• Tidal volume generated is unpredictable and dependent on lung and airway compliance

*The time that the ventilator allocates for inspiration is a function of the respiratory rate and inspiratory: expiratory (I:E) ratio. The I:E ratio is usually set as 1:2. Therefore, if a RR of 10 is set, there will be 6 seconds allocated to one ventilator cycle. If the I:E ratio is 1:2, then the maximum inspiratory time that the ventilator will allow for inspiration is 2 seconds. If the set tidal volume or pressure is not reached before inspiratory to expiratory cycling occurs, the ventilator will alarm.

Pressure

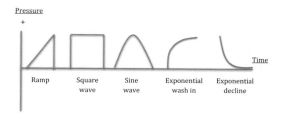

Waveform descriptions
Before describing ventilator waveforms, it is necessary to be familiar with some basic waveforms and the terminology used to describe them (see *Fig. 4.1.1*).

Fig. 4.1.1: Basic ventilator waveform descriptions.

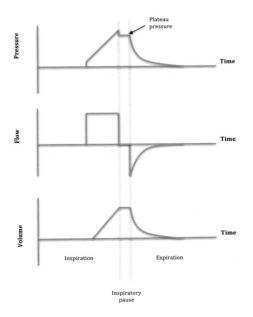

Fig. 4.1.2: VC mode: pressure, flow and volume changes over time.

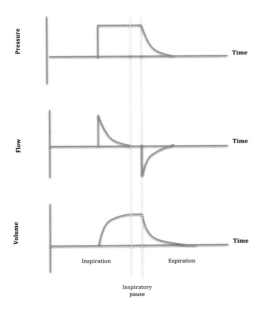

Fig. 4.1.3: PC mode: pressure, flow and volume changes over time.

Volume control

VC produces a fixed tidal volume. To achieve this it applies a constant high flow of gas to the lungs. The volume (and therefore the pressure) in the lungs will ramp up rapidly during inspiration.

Pressure control

PC ventilation delivers a fixed pressure to the lungs during inspiration. The flow will therefore be determined by the pressure difference between the ventilator and the lungs. As the lungs fill, the pressure within them will increase and the pressure gradient will decrease. Therefore flow of air into the lungs will decrease throughout the inspiratory cycle.

Advanced ventilator modes

Microprocessors allow the combination and modification of the basic ventilator modes. It would be confusing and cumbersome to list all advanced modes available on the market, but a brief description of some of the more common and interesting modes is included here.

Pressure regulated volume control

Similar or variant modes: PRVC (Maquet), AutoFlow (Draeger), Adaptive Support Ventilation (Hamilton), Volume Ventilation Plus (Puritan Bennett).

PRVC attempts to combine the best aspects of PC and VC ventilation modes. It attempts to guarantee a set tidal volume without exceeding a set pressure. Like PC, a constant pressure is applied to the lungs and the flow is decelerating. The problem with conventional PC ventilation is that if the patient's lung compliances and resistances suddenly increase, a very low tidal volume may be delivered. PRVC attempts to overcome this by monitoring the achieved tidal volume against the set tidal volume on a breath-by-breath basis. If the tidal volume is less than expected, the ventilator automatically increases the level of pressure for the next breath. The opposite occurs if the tidal volume achieved is greater than the set volume. This is a popular mode of controlled ventilation in intensive care units.

Synchronized intermittent mandatory ventilation

Similar or variant modes: SIMV (Draeger, Hamilton), VCV-SIMV (Puritan-Bennett), Volume SIMV (Viasys); Pressure-SIMV (Viasys), P-SIMV (Hamilton), PRVC-SIMV (Viasys), SIMV-PRVC (Puritan Bennett).

In SIMV mode, a minimum mandatory ventilator rate is set and the patient may breathe between these mandatory breaths without triggering a ventilator-assisted breath. However, SIMV attempts to synchronize mandatory breaths with spontaneous breaths. If the patient makes inspiratory effort during a set time window before a mandatory breath is due to be delivered, a synchronized mandatory breath takes the place of the mandatory breath that was about to be delivered.

SIMV is particularly useful when starting to wean ITU patients from a fully mandatory mode of ventilation. In theory, this mode of ventilation also reduces respiratory muscle atrophy by allowing patients to maintain their use and activity.

In the most basic versions of SIMV, spontaneous breaths are unsupported. Therefore the next logical step in the evolution of SIMV was to combine it with either PS (e.g. SIMV/PS, Draeger) or less commonly, VS. In these versions of SIMV, spontaneous breaths are supported and the settings for supported breaths can be adjusted independently to those for the mandatory breaths. This may facilitate weaning. If a spontaneously breathing patient becomes apnoeic or their minute volume falls, mandatory breaths are delivered at the set backup rate. Of course these mandatory breaths can also be volume controlled, pressure controlled, or a combination of both (e.g. PRVC-SIMV, Viasys).

Bi-phasic positive airway pressure

Similar or variant modes: BIPAP (Draeger), Bi-Vent (Maquet), APRV/ Bi-phasic (Viasys).

BIPAP is a mode of ventilation and should not be confused with BiPAP, which stands for Bi-*level* Positive Airway Pressure and is the proprietary name of a portable non-invasive ventilator produced by Respironics. See *Table 4.1.3* for disambiguation.

Table 4.1.3: WhatPAP?

Abbreviation	Full name	Description
BIPAP	Bi-PHASIC positive airway pressure	An **invasive** ventilation mode (Draega Evita). The ventilator cycles between two different levels of sustained pressure and the patient can breathe spontaneously and unrestricted throughout.
BPAP	Bi-LEVEL positive airway pressure ventilation	A generic **non-invasive** ventilator mode through a tight fitting mask. An inspiratory positive airway pressure (IPAP) and expiratory positive airway pressure (EPAP, i.e. PEEP) can be set. The ventilator is triggered by the patient's inspiratory efforts.
BiPAP	Bi-LEVEL positive airway pressure ventilation	A proprietary name for *Respironics'* **non-invasive** ventilation machines that provide bi-level positive airway pressure ventilation (BiPAP)

BIPAP is a form of pressure controlled ventilation in which there is a time-cycled change between a lower and higher level of sustained airway pressure. The cycling from the lower to the higher pressure generates an inspiratory flow similar to PC ventilation. The magnitude of the step change in pressure can be adjusted depending on the needs of the patient, however, the patient is free to take spontaneous breaths during either phase. BIPAP allows a single mode for controlled ventilation and spontaneous breathing. Proponents of BIPAP argue that it produces a smoother transition from controlled to supported ventilation modes and that the patient can breathe freely and comfortably even when significant controlled ventilation is being delivered.

Note that with most modern ventilators, it is possible to support the spontaneous breaths that are made, independent of the cycling that occurs between the two different levels of sustained pressure.

Automode
Automode is a single ventilator mode that automatically switches between mandatory modes of ventilation (such as PC or VC) and support modes of ventilation (such as PS or VS). When the patient begins to make respiratory effort, the system switches mode entirely, to a support mode. However, if the minute volume falls below a set value, it switches back to a mandatory mode.

Closed loop systems
The holy grail of ventilator research and development is to produce a ventilator system that combines real-time information about respiratory effort, flows, tidal volumes, airway pressures, oxygenation and carbon dioxide removal. It would then use this information to automatically select the best ventilator mode for a given patient at a given time. This would in theory allow a single ventilator mode to be used for the duration of a patient's ventilation.

Automatic tube compensation
ATC (Draeger) or tube resistance compensation (TRC, Hamilton) are spontaneous breathing modes for use with an ETT or tracheostomy. The ventilator uses the length and internal diameter of the tube to calculate and generate just enough support to compensate for the increased resistance caused by the tube.

CPAP versus PEEP

CPAP (continuous positive airway pressure) and PEEP (positive end expiratory pressure) are terms that commonly cause confusion. In some contexts they appear to be interchangeable but in others they do not. It may be helpful to consider the effect they have during spontaneous and positive pressure ventilation modes separately.

CPAP/PEEP in unassisted spontaneous ventilation

When the patient is breathing spontaneously (whether intubated or not) with no assistance from the ventilator, PEEP is the term used for pressure applied to the airway during expiration only. Examples of PEEP include a partially closed APL valve on the breathing system in theatre (when the FGF is insufficient to keep the bag fully inflated between breaths), or more simply, when a person breathes out through pursed lips or a straw. Note that no positive pressure is applied to inspiration in either of these examples.

CPAP is when the pressure is both constant (i.e. of unchanging magnitude) and continuous (i.e. present throughout inspiration and expiration). The classic example of this is when a passenger puts his head out of a car window and faces the direction of travel. There is a positive pressure applied to the airway during inspiration and the same pressure is applied against expiration.

Mechanical ventilation and CPAP/PEEP

The difference between PEEP and CPAP is less clear during positive pressure ventilation, and many argue that there is no difference in this context.

For a tidal volume to be delivered, the airway pressure must be cycled between a higher pressure and a lower pressure. The lower pressure is known as PEEP and the higher pressure is the sum of the PEEP and the set inspiratory pressure (e.g. a set PEEP of 5 cmH$_2$O and a set inspiratory pressure of 10 cmH$_2$O should give a peak inspiratory airway pressure of 15 cmH$_2$O). The same is true when assisted ventilation modes are used and the patient is making respiratory effort. The higher pressure is the sum of the PEEP and the set inspiratory pressure.

PEEP can therefore be thought of as being present throughout the respiratory cycle during mechanical ventilation – during both inspiration and expiration. During mechanical ventilation, therefore, PEEP becomes a misnomer because it is not just present at the end of expiration. The terms PEEP and CPAP are therefore used interchangeably in this context.

CPAP/PEEP can be generated within an ITU ventilator in one of two ways.

- Some ventilators have adjustable expiratory valves that generate a positive back pressure in the breathing system.
- Other ventilators generate a constant and adjustable flow of gas through the breathing system, which is analogous to when a passenger puts his head out of a car window. This method allows better dynamic adaptation of positive airways pressure to the patient's lung mechanics, but increases gas consumption.

Physiological effects of CPAP/PEEP

CPAP and PEEP aim to splint open alveoli and collapsible airways, hence reducing atelectasis and shunt. The added advantages of reducing alveolar oedema and splinting open the pharynx during sleep allow it to be used in the management of pulmonary odema and obstructive sleep apnoea. In left ventricular failure, it is possible that CPAP/PEEP may be beneficial due to a sustained increase in intrathoracic pressure, which reduces venous return and preload. However, excessive CPAP/PEEP may cause hypotension due to an excessive reduction in venous return. Positive intrathoracic pressure also reduces the intramural pressure required to eject blood from the ventricle (see Laplace's law).

Advanced ventilator graphics

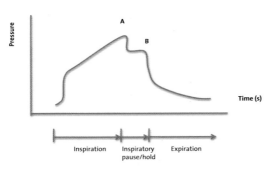

Fig. 4.1.4: A pressure–time curve during VC ventilation. Point 'A' represents the peak inspiratory pressure and point 'B', the plateau pressure.

In *Fig. 4.1.4*, point 'A' represents the peak inspiratory pressure (PIP). It is measured by the ventilator and represents the maximum pressure achieved in the airways during inspiration. As airway resistance increases, so does PIP. Point 'B' represents the plateau pressure (Pplat), which is the pressure within the alveoli and small airways. To measure it, a breath-hold of up to 1 second is required at the end of inspiration. This pause allows time for equilibration of pressures within different conducting airways and distensible alveoli as they vary in size, compliance and resistance. These transient gas flows at the end of inspiration are known as pendelluft (literally, 'oscillating air'). The redistribution of the fixed volume of gas into a larger lung volume during this pause accounts for the drop in airway pressure as measured by the ventilator.

In health, the difference between PIP and Pplat is small and, as tidal volumes increase, they should increase proportionally. Measurement of PIP and Pplat can be useful in the diagnosis of lung disease. In conditions with increased airway resistance (e.g. bronchospasm), an increase in PIP is seen without an increase in Pplat. Conversely, in conditions that give decreased pulmonary compliance (e.g. pulmonary oedema, pleural effusions and ascites) both PIP and Pplat increase proportionally. Pplat should not be allowed to rise above 30 cmH$_2$O so that the risk of alveolar rupture and pneumothorax is minimized.

Gas may be trapped in the alveoli and small airways when larger proximal airways collapse during expiration, blocking its escape. Monitoring of the pressure waveform may provide information

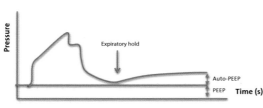

Fig. 4.1.5: A pressure–time curve showing the effects of an expiratory hold.

regarding the degree of gas-trapping. Trapped gas exerts a pressure in the airways known as auto-PEEP. The calculation of this value relies on the ventilator being capable of providing an expiratory hold. During the hold period, the airway pressure measurement will initially show the set value of PEEP. However, if there is gas trapping, the measured airway pressure will slowly rise and settle at a new level. The difference in pressure between the set PEEP and the new value is the auto-PEEP.

The mechanics and classification of ventilators

Whilst there are many different ways of classifying the mechanics of ventilators, the following 4-point method of classification is suggested:

4.3 Oxylog ventilators

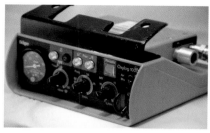

Fig. 4.3.1: The Oxylog 1000 ventilator.

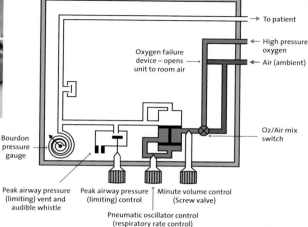

Fig. 4.3.2: Schematic of an Oxylog 1000. Note that if the oxygen supply fails, the ventilator opens to atmospheric air. A more detailed schematic of a pneumatic oscillator can be found in *Section 4.5* on the Penlon Nuffield 200 ventilator.

Overview

The Oxylog series of ventilators was introduced by Draeger in the late 1970s as a robust, intuitive and portable ventilator for use in the emergency department. It has grown in popularity and is used both as a means of ventilation in emergencies and during the transfer of patients. The Oxylog and Oxylog 1000 ventilators are entirely pneumatically driven and controlled, whereas the Oxylog 2000 and 3000 are pneumatically driven and electronically controlled. All except the original remain on the market.

Uses

The Oxylog is primarily used for ventilation outside the theatre and critical care environments.

How it works

The original Oxylog

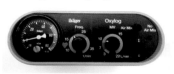

Fig. 4.3.3: The original Oxylog.

The first Oxylog device is an entirely pneumatically driven and controlled, time-cycled constant flow generator. A constant flow of pressurized oxygen from a pipeline or cylinder is divided into aliquots of tidal volume by a pneumatically controlled oscillator. A flow restriction valve limits the pressure at which gas is delivered to the patient to safe levels.

Oxylog 2000

In 1993 the Oxylog 2000 was introduced. It is a pneumatically driven, electronically controlled, time-cycled, flow generator. It incorporates an added spontaneous ventilation mode and enhanced monitoring including an electronic display.

Oxylog 1000

Draeger introduced the Oxylog 1000 in 1997 as a modified version of the original Oxylog ventilator. Even though it was introduced after the Oxylog 2000, it was named the Oxylog 1000 because it was a modification of the original. Like the original, it is an entirely pneumatically driven and controlled, time-cycled flow generator. It retains the simplicity, robustness and portability of the original, but also allows monitoring of airway and gas supply pressures. It includes gas-powered audible and visual alarms indicating high airway pressures. The pressure can be limited but the ventilator is only suitable for individuals who require a minute volume of greater than $3\,l.min^{-1}$.

Oxylog 3000

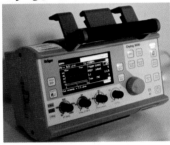

Fig. 4.3.4: The Oxylog 3000.

The Oxylog 3000 ventilator was introduced in 2003. It is a pneumatically driven, electronically controlled, time-cycled, flow or pressure generator, depending on the mode selected. Like the Oxylog 2000, it requires a battery or mains electrical supply to power its display and CPU, but the power for ventilation is primarily derived from pressurized gas. It comprises a graphical interface and multiple ventilator modes such as IPPV, SIMV/ASB, CPAP/ASB and BIPAP/ASB. Dials for adjusting tidal volumes, respiratory rate, FiO_2 (40–100% using solenoid valves) and PEEP are retained on the front of the device. Unlike earlier Oxylog models, the Oxylog 3000 can be used in children because it can deliver tidal volumes as low as 50 ml.

⊕ Advantages

- Intuitive and easy to use.
- Portable.
- The Oxylog and Oxylog 1000 are purely pneumatically driven and controlled, therefore they can be used in environments without a reliable electrical supply.
- Pressurized oxygen may be blended with room air to vary the FiO_2.
- The Oxylog 3000 includes spontaneous and assisted modes.
- The Oxylog 3000 monitors ambient pressure as well as the FGF pressure, allowing it to accurately compensate for low pressure environments, such as in an aeroplane.
- The Oxylog 3000 can be used in paediatric practice.

⊖ Disadvantages

- A limited number of ventilation modes are available.
- The Oxylog 2000 and 3000 models require an electrical supply via mains or an internal battery.

4.4 Manley ventilator

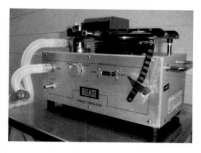

Fig. 4.4.1: The Manley ventilator.
Photo courtesy of Kenneth True;
www.historyofsurgery.co.uk.

Overview

Designed by Roger Manley in 1961 and built by Blease Medical, the Manley ventilator revolutionized anaesthetic practice by providing a reliable and elegant means of ventilating patients. Prior to its introduction, anaesthetists generally preferred to ventilate patients in theatre by hand rather than use the cumbersome and unreliable ventilators that were available at the time. The Manley is a pneumatically powered and controlled, time-cycled, minute volume divider.

Uses

Historically, the Manley ventilator was a popular choice in operating theatres and intensive care units, but it has largely been replaced by more sophisticated ventilators in modern practice.

How it works

This ventilator is a minute volume divider, indicating that the entire FGF is divided into aliquots of tidal volume that are then delivered to the patient, with none of it being wasted. Because additional pressurized gas flow is not required to power a breath, it is highly economical in its use of pressurized gas.

It comprises two bellows and three unidirectional valves controlled by an arrangement of levers, pulleys and mechanical switches. Gas entering the ventilator first passes into a cycling bellow that acts as a mechanical time-cycling device. When the cycling bellow is filled to a set point, a switch triggers the lever system, leading to:

(1) opening of the valve between the cycling bellow and main bellow

(2) closure of the valve between the main bellow and patient

The position of the latch on the lever arm adjusts the tidal volume (i.e. how much the main bellow fills). When the bellow is filled, it triggers a mechanical lever and pulley system that controls three valves.

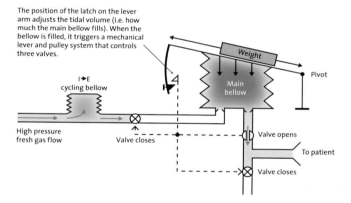

Fig. 4.4.2: Schematic of the Manley ventilator during inspiration.

When the cycling bellow is full, it triggers a series of mechanical pulleys and levers that act on three valves and cycles the ventilator from inspiration to expiration.

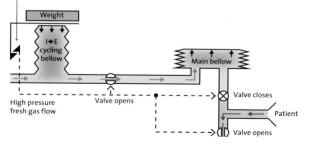

Fig. 4.4.3: Schematic of the Manley ventilator in expiration.

(3) opening of the expiratory valve between the patient and the atmosphere.

The cycling bellow therefore empties, and the main bellow fills with fresh gas, both from the cycling bellow and directly from the piped gas supply. Simultaneously, the patient is isolated from the main bellow and is able to passively expire through the expiratory valve. By adjusting the volume that must collect in the cycling bellow before this lever system is tripped, the inspiratory time (and thus the respiratory rate) can be adjusted.

As the gas enters the main bellows, it also lifts a weight resting on top of it. When the ventilator cycles into inspiration, it is this weight that drives inspiratory flow into the patient's lungs. The position of the mass can be adjusted relative to a pivot; the further the mass is positioned from the pivot, the greater the moment of force applied to the bellows below. Therefore by adjusting the position of this weight, it is possible to alter the inspiratory pressure generated.

The tidal volume delivered by the Manley ventilator is adjusted by a sliding catch on the lever arm of the main bellows. The position of the catch determines how much the main bellows can fill before a second (reciprocal) series of levers and pulleys are triggered. When the set tidal volume is reached, a switch is triggered that ultimately leads to:

(1) closure of the valve between the cycling bellow and main bellow
(2) opening of the valve between the main bellow and patient
(3) closure of the expiratory valve between the patient and the atmosphere.

The main bellows therefore empty into the patient's lungs under the pressure exerted by the weight on top of it. The smaller cycling bellow then begins to fill again and the process is repeated.

The exact changes in the configuration of the valves, latches and bellows is easier to understand by studying *Figs 4.4.2* and *4.4.3*, which show the mechanics of the ventilator during inspiration and expiration.

An APL valve (*Section 3.3*) and reservoir bag (*Section 3.4*) within the breathing system allow manual ventilation without the need to disconnect the ventilator. During spontaneous ventilation through the ventilator breathing system, the configuration is similar to that of a Mapleson D system (*Section 3.5*).

⊕ Advantages

- No electrical power required.
- Simple to use and reliable.
- Does not waste pressurized gas, because all of the FGF is divided and supplied to the patient; no additional gas flow is required to drive the ventilator.
- The ventilator may be used in conjunction with a circle system.

⊖ Disadvantages

- Only a single mode of mechanical ventilation is possible.
- Generates back pressure within the breathing circuit, which can affect the accuracy of vaporizers within the circuit.

4.5 Penlon Nuffield 200 ventilator

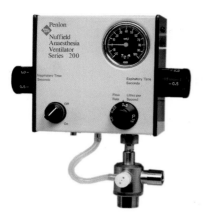

Fig. 4.5.1: The Penlon Nuffield 200 ventilator.

Overview

The Penlon Nuffield 200 is an entirely pneumatically driven and controlled, time-cycled, constant flow generator. It is most commonly used in adults via a Bain breathing system. For use with children under 20 kg, a Newton valve is added which connects with the expiratory limb of a T-piece.

Uses

It is used for short periods of ventilation most commonly in the anaesthetic room, but also sometimes in remote locations such as the radiology department. An MRI compatible unit is available (see *Section 11.3*).

How it works

The Nuffield 200 may be termed an intermittent blower because, in contrast to other ventilators, the driving gas enters the breathing system, but never reaches the patient. Furthermore, fresh gas from the anaesthetic machine (which is used to ventilate the patient) does not pass through the body of the ventilator. This seemingly confusing mechanism is in fact relatively simple when the mechanics of a T-piece breathing system are considered.

When a Nuffield 200 is used with a Bain system, the reservoir bag (*Section 3.4*) is removed and the APL valve (*Section 3.3*) is fully closed. The effective removal of these two components creates a simple T-piece system. In operation, the Nuffield 200 delivers a tidal volume of driving gas into the expiratory limb of the T-piece system. This gas drives fresh gas which is already in the expiratory limb into the patient's lungs. Because the volume of the expiratory tubing exceeds the tidal volume, the driving gas does not reach the patient and is vented during expiration, during which time the expiratory limb fills with more fresh gas from the anaesthetic machine.

There are three control dials on a Nuffield 200. These are used to set the inspiratory flow (in l.sec^{-1}) and the inspiratory and expiratory times (in seconds). It is therefore possible to set respiratory rate, tidal volume and the I:E ratio. For instance, setting inspiratory flow to 0.25 l.sec^{-1}, inspiratory time to 2 seconds and expiratory time to 4 seconds, will deliver a 0.5 litre (0.25 × 2) tidal volume every 6 seconds (i.e. 10 breaths per minute) at an I:E ratio of 1:2. A Bourdon gauge displays the inspiratory pressure on the front of the device.

The ventilator has a removable metal block on its underside called the 'adult patient valve'. This has four ports. One connects to the breathing system in place of the reservoir bag. A second is a pressure relief valve set to vent gas at pressures in excess of 60 cmH$_2$O. A third allows monitoring of the pressure within the valve and is connected with tubing to the Bourdon gauge. The fourth port is found on the underside and vents expired gas. It has a 30 mm connector for connection to the scavenging system. A spring valve within the valve ensures that the driving gas enters the patient breathing system rather than venting through the expiratory port.

Internal mechanism

The mechanism of action of the Penlon is shown in *Figs 4.5.2* and *4.5.3* in simplified form. Pipeline oxygen (at 400 kPa) enters the ventilator through a filter and pressure-reducing valve. During the inspiratory cycle, driving gas flows simultaneously into the breathing system and into an

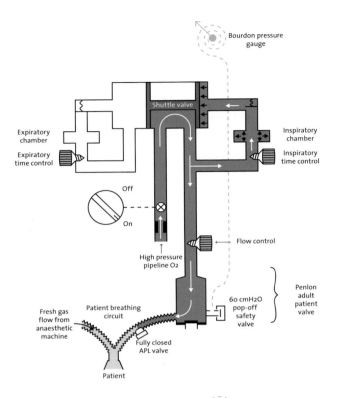

Fig. 4.5.2: Schematic of the Penlon ventilator during inspiration.

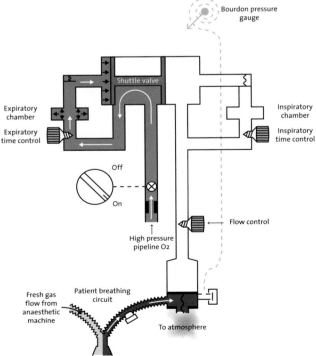

Fig. 4.5.3: Schematic of the Penlon ventilator in expiration.

inspiratory timing chamber. The flow of gas into this chamber is adjusted by the inspiratory time control knob attached to a screw valve. If a short inspiratory time is set, the screw valve opens and allows the inspiratory timing chamber to fill more rapidly. As the chamber fills, the pressure within it increases until it is sufficient to open up an exhaust valve. This exhaust valve connects directly with a second chamber housing a shuttle valve. The pressure of gas entering this chamber pushes the valve across to the opposite end of its housing. In the shuttle valve's new position, the driving gas cannot enter the breathing system or the inspiratory timing chamber. The ventilator therefore cycles from inspiration to expiration.

During the expiratory phase, the patient passively exhales air through the patient valve attached to the underside of the ventilator. During this time, the driving gas is directed to an expiratory timing chamber. Again flow into this chamber is controlled using a screw valve. When the pressure in this chamber increases, it opens an outlet valve that allows gas to escape and enter the housing of the shuttle valve. At this point, the shuttle valve is pushed back to its original position; driving gas is once again directed into the patient's breathing circuit and the ventilator cycles into inspiration again.

With an adult patient valve attached, the lowest tidal volume that can be achieved is 50 ml. A Newton valve should be attached to generate smaller tidal volumes.

Advantages

- Cheap, simple and compact.
- Allows ventilation of most adults and, with the Newton valve attached, children.
- Gases can be scavenged.
- Pneumatically powered and controlled. No electrical connection is required.

Disadvantages

- Requires a pressurized gas source.
- Only volume controlled ventilation is possible – no supported or spontaneous ventilation modes are available.
- The Penlon has no alarms.

4.6 The Newton valve and mechanical thumbs

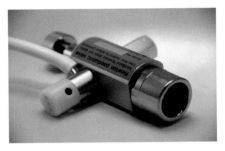

Fig. 4.6.1: The Newton valve.

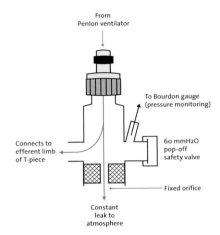

From Penlon ventilator

To Bourdon gauge (pressure monitoring)

60 mmH2O pop-off safety valve

Connects to efferent limb of T-piece

Fixed orifice

Constant leak to atmosphere

Fig. 4.6.2: Schematic of the Newton valve.

Overview

Occlusion of the expiratory orifice of a T-piece with a thumb is a simple method of ventilation which uses the pressure generated by the FGF alone, to inflate a patient's lungs. The expiratory orifice of a T-piece may be fully or partially occluded, depending on the situation. A mechanical thumb ventilator, of which the Newton valve is an example, mimics these actions. Mechanical thumbs are particularly useful where low tidal volumes and low resistance to expiratory flow are necessary, for instance in paediatrics, because they can be used with a valveless breathing system and can vent excess gas by generating a constant leak. More sophisticated mechanical thumbs include some makes of neonatal ventilators.

The Newton valve converts a Penlon Nuffield 200 (*Section 4.5*) ventilator from a pneumatically powered, time-cycled, constant flow generator (or intermittent blower), into a pneumatically powered, time-cycled, pressure generator (or mechanical thumb) ventilator. It is attached in place of the adult patient valve to the underside of the Penlon ventilator.

Uses

The Newton valve is used in paediatric ventilation in conjunction with a Penlon Nuffield 200 ventilator (tidal volumes of 10–300 ml).

How it works

The Newton valve has three main ports and a fourth that connects to a Bourdon pressure gauge (*Section 6.2*). The uppermost port connects to the ventilator and the lower port has a fixed orifice that vents a constant portion of the driving gas into the atmosphere. The third port connects with the expiratory limb of a T-piece (Mapleson E) breathing system.

The Nuffield 200 cycles as normal, but in contrast to when an adult patient valve is used, not all of the driving gas enters the expiratory limb of the attached T-piece – a constant proportion leaks through the fixed orifice on the underside of the Newton valve. As the flow of the driving gas from the ventilator is increased, the pressure generated within the Newton valve increases and generates back pressure along the expiratory limb of the T-piece. This back pressure acts as a 'dam', such that an increasing proportion of the FGF from the anaesthetic machine is diverted into the patient's lungs, rather than into the T-piece.

Partial occlusion of the orifice

When the Penlon ventilator is set to deliver low driving gas flows, the pressure generated within the Newton valve is relatively small and only partially stems the FGF passing along the expiratory limb of the T-piece; the pressure within the expiratory limb increases but some of the fresh gas still flows into the expiratory limb of the T-piece and out through the fixed orifice on the underside of the Newton valve. Under these circumstances, the ventilator and Newton valve behave as a partial thumb occluder, because it is as if a thumb has been partially placed over the orifice of the expiratory limb of the T-piece. The exact tidal volume delivered to the patient is a function of the pressure generated within the Newton valve (by the driving gas from the Penlon ventilator) and the FGF into the inspiratory limb of the T-piece (from the anaesthetic machine).

Full occlusion of the orifice

As the driving gas flow from the Penlon is increased, the pressure within the chamber of the Newton valve will also increase, despite an associated increase in the leak through the open orifice on its underside. As the driving gas flow is increased further, the pressure generated by the gas entering the Newton valve is sufficient to dam the flow of fresh gas from the anaesthetic machine into the expiratory limb of the T-piece. At this point, all of the FGF from the anaesthetic machine is diverted into the patient's lungs, and the lung inflates. The Newton valve in this context behaves as a complete thumb occluder – it is as if the expiratory limb of the T-piece has been completely occluded. Under these circumstances, larger tidal volumes are delivered that are dependent only on the pressure generated by the FGF from the anaesthetic machine.

At even greater driving flow rates, despite a constant leak through the Newton valve's fixed orifice, a proportion of the driving gas from the Penlon will begin to enter the expiratory limb of the T-piece, and force some of the fresh gas within it back into the patient's lungs. Under these circumstances, the Newton valve stops behaving like a thumb occluder (pressure generator) and reverts to operating like an intermittent blower (flow generator). It is therefore important not to set high initial gas flows on the Penlon ventilator when using it with a Newton valve in paediatrics. A low driving gas flow should be chosen initially and this should be increased cautiously until adequate chest movement is seen.

Advantages

- Converts a Penlon Nuffield 200 ventilator from a flow generator into a pressure generator.
- Can deliver very small tidal volumes at safe pressures, which is particularly useful in paediatrics (10–300 ml).
- Simple robust device that can be attached to a Penlon Nuffield 200 ventilator in seconds.
- A PEEP valve can be connected to the expiratory (fixed orifice) port at the bottom of the Newton valve.

Disadvantages

- At high flows, the dynamics of the valve change and it stops behaving as a thumb occluder (pressure generator) and starts acting as an intermittent blower (flow generator).
- Generic disadvantages of the Nuffield 200 (see *Section 4.5*).

Safety

- When first connecting the Penlon ventilator (with a Newton valve attached) to the T-piece, the driving gas flow rate should be set to a minimum and then slowly increased until adequate chest excursion is seen.

4.7 Intensive care ventilators

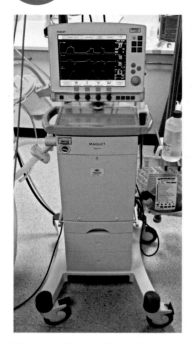

Fig. 4.7.1: A Maquet ITU ventilator.

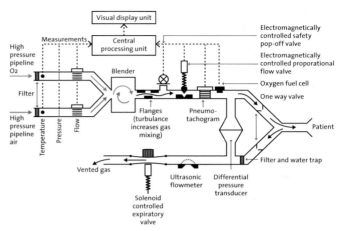

Fig. 4.7.2: Schematic of an ITU ventilator.

Overview

The term 'intensive care ventilator' is likely to eventually become obsolete as ITU ventilator technology is incorporated into anaesthetic machines and portable ventilators. Nevertheless, the term broadly refers to a range of ventilators that can deliver advanced modes of ventilation and are versatile enough to ventilate both children and adults with a range of challenging respiratory pathologies.

Uses

These devices are used to ventilate critically ill patients in the intensive care unit. They can provide both invasive and non-invasive ventilator support. ITU ventilators are not used with volatile anaesthetics and therefore use a simple breathing system with inspiratory and expiratory limbs and venting of all expired gas.

How it works

Modern ITU ventilators cannot easily be classified because they are versatile devices capable of delivering a diverse range of ventilatory parameters. They are usually powered by pressurized gas, whose flow is controlled by electronic solenoid proportional flow valves. These valves are controlled electromagnetically and are able to make many small adjustments every second to the size of an orifice (and therefore the flow through it). ITU ventilators may occasionally be electrically powered using motors and levers to drive bellows filled with gas. Pressure, flow, temperature and oxygen sensors provide constant feedback to the ventilator's CPU, which allow it to adapt to the patient's respiratory mechanics. As a result, a single ventilator can provide a range of ventilator modes, tailored to a multitude of patients with a range of lung pathologies. Two ventilators can even be synchronized to provide different ventilatory parameters to each lung separately, for example, when there is severe unilateral lung disease.

CPAP/PEEP can be generated in one of two ways. Some ventilators have adjustable expiratory valves that generate a positive back-pressure within the breathing system. An alternative method is to generate a constant and adjustable flow of gas through the breathing system, analogous to placing your head out of the window of a moving car, facing in the direction of travel. This method allows better dynamic adaptation of positive airways pressure to the patient's lung mechanics, but also increases gas consumption.

The ventilator has a constant 'bias' flow of gas through it, independent of other ventilatory parameters. This constant flow allows the ventilator to detect a patient's respiratory effort in one of two ways.

- A differential pressure transducer monitors the difference in pressure within the inspiratory and expiratory limbs of the circuit. When the patient makes inspiratory effort, the bias flow will enter the patient lungs so the flow within the expiratory circuit will fall. This is detected by the differential pressure transducer as a drop in the pressure within the expiratory circuit, triggering, for example, a supported breath.
- A more sensitive method is to detect changes in flow within the inspiratory limb of the breathing system using a rapid response pneumotachograph (*Section 6.15*).

⊕ Advantages
- Versatile: can be adapted to support a range of different patients and lung pathologies.
- Advanced ventilator modes are intended to reduce rates of secondary lung injury and assist with respiratory wean.
- Ventilator modes may be upgraded through software updates.

⊖ Disadvantages
- There is no agreed standard nomenclature for ventilator modes between manufacturers.
- Complex, so considerable training is required before use.

4.8 Manual jet ventilators

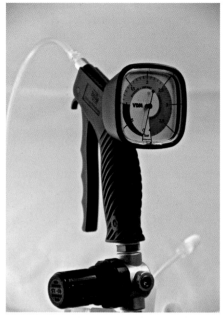

Fig. 4.8.1: A Manujet jet ventilator.

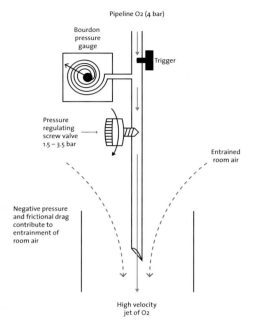

Fig. 4.8.2: Schematic of a manual jet ventilator.

Overview

Jet ventilation was developed in the 1960s and provides a means of ventilating patients when the airway is shared between the anaesthetist and the surgeon. It is also used for emergency ventilation through narrow bore airway devices. Jet ventilators use high pressure oxygen delivered through a small orifice such as a jet needle or cannula.

Manual jet ventilators such as the Sanders injector or Manujet are also known as low frequency jet ventilators. They are pneumatically powered, manually-cycled, flow generators. The Manujet permits alteration of the pressure it delivers, whereas the Sanders injector does not.

High frequency jet ventilators such as the Mistral ventilator are covered separately in *Section 4.9*.

Uses

- Short duration airway surgery, particularly bronchoscopy.
- Prior to the initiation of high frequency jet ventilation.
- Rescue ventilation in a 'can't intubate, can't ventilate' scenario.

How it works

Depending on the model, the jet ventilator is connected to a Schrader valve (wall or cylinder) or a mini-Schrader valve (on an anaesthetic machine), providing a driving pressure of 400 kPa. In a Sanders injector, a manual purge trigger is used to deliver oxygen at 400 kPa, through tubing to a connector, often a Luer lock. This attaches the ventilator to the cricothryoid needle, surgical laryngoscope, bronchoscope or other airway device. The Manujet uses a similar mechanism, but has a pressure regulating valve that permits the pressure delivered to be reduced to between 50 and 350 kPa.

It is important to realize that the pressure delivered by the jet ventilator does not reach the patient, the majority being used to overcome the resistance of the narrow bore cannula; using a typical diameter cannula, peak airway pressure reaches approximately 25 cmH$_2$O.

Entrainment of surrounding air occurs as the oxygen jet exits the jet needle. This entrainment is widely attributed to the Venturi effect (see *Section 1.12*), but there is an increasing body of opinion in favour of the theory that it is the result of the frictional drag on air molecules by the passing oxygen. The tidal volume delivered to the patient is the sum of the injected gas and the entrained air. The FiO$_2$ is also affected by the ratio of injected oxygen to entrained air and is difficult to predict, but is usually between 0.75 and 0.9. Airway pressure and inspiratory and expiratory volumes are not monitored during manual jet ventilation. It is therefore essential that chest movement is carefully observed to ensure adequate ventilation and avoid hyperinflation.

As in standard positive pressure ventilation, exhalation is passive. Importantly therefore, the patient must be seen to fully exhale before the next breath is delivered in order to prevent breath-stacking (further tidal volumes being delivered to an already partially inflated lung). Failure to ensure full expiration may result in volutrauma.

A rate of 10–12 breaths per minute is usually adequate to allow effective removal of CO$_2$. Because this method of ventilation constitutes a semi-open system, end-tidal CO$_2$ is difficult to measure accurately and effective delivery of anaesthetic vapour is not possible. Therefore total intravenous anaesthesia should be used for maintenance. Humidification and warming of inspired gases is also not possible. The technique should therefore only be used for short periods and in emergencies.

Advantages

- Simple and quick to set up and use.
- Effective for rescue ventilation.

Disadvantages

- Cause significant movement of the vocal cords compared to high frequency jet ventilation.
- Can only be used for short periods of time.
- Cannot humidify or warm inspired gases.
- Tidal volumes and FiO$_2$ are variable and impossible to measure.
- Carry a risk of baro- and volutrauma.
- Volatile anaesthetics cannot be delivered.
- Unable to monitor end-tidal CO$_2$ accurately.

4.9 High frequency jet ventilators

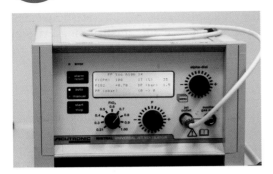

Fig. 4.9.1: The Mistral high frequency jet ventilator (Acutronic Medical).

Overview

Low frequency manual jet ventilation using a Sanders injector or Manujet causes significant movement of the vocal cords, making airway surgery difficult. In the 1970s, automated high frequency jet ventilators (HFJVs) were therefore developed to overcome this problem. These generate low tidal volumes at a high frequency, allowing ventilation with minimal vocal cord movement. As with low frequency manual jet ventilation, high frequency jet ventilation can be delivered via a variety of airway devices (see *Section 2.14*), for example, the Mistral jet ventilator (Acutronic Medical) is in common clinical usage. Other jet ventilators function similarly.

Note that high frequency jet ventilation is not the same as high frequency oscillatory ventilation. High frequency oscillatory ventilation and how it differs from high frequency jet ventilation is discussed in more detail in the next section.

Uses

High frequency jet ventilation is most commonly used in ENT cases and in other surgery where a motionless surgical field is desirable, such as in radiofrequency ablation of hepatic lesions or lithotripsy. It is also possible to use high frequency jet ventilation during one-lung ventilation to improve oxygenation when basic manoeuvres have failed.

How it works

HFJVs are pneumatically powered and electronically controlled, time-cycled, flow generators. They also incorporate a pressure limiting facility. Flow is controlled via a series of solenoid (electromagnetic) valves that open and close at a high frequency. These devices utilize high-pressure pipeline gas at 400 kPa and break up the gas flow into small pulses. Connection to the airway device is through strong, flexible tubing and a Luer lock adapter. The volume of gas delivered to the patient depends on the set frequency, inspiratory time and driving pressure, each of which can be adjusted by the anaesthetist. As with manual jet ventilation, air is entrained as the jet exits the needle or cannula, through a combination of the venturi effect and frictional drag of air.

There are several settings that can be adjusted on the Mistral HFJV:

(1) *Driving pressure:* the (inspiratory) driving pressure is adjustable between 40 and 350 kPa (0.4–3.5 bar). A typical starting driving pressure for an adult is 150 kPa (1.5 bar). This seemingly very high pressure is delivered through a constriction and is therefore dissipated to a safe level before it reaches the airway.
(2) *Frequency:* the frequency of the breaths is also adjustable between 12 and 600 cycles per minute. Unlike conventional ventilation, as the frequency increases, the $PaCO_2$ will paradoxically also increase. A typical starting frequency is 100 cycles per minute.
(3) *FiO_2:* this is adjusted between 0.21 and 1.0 using an oxygen/air blender. The final concentration delivered to the alveoli is harder to predict, because it will be further mixed with entrained air.

(4) *Pause pressure* is the airway pressure at the end of a cycle and approximates to the mean airway pressure. It should ideally be adjusted to less than 20 cmH$_2$O to prevent barotrauma. The ventilator can be set to alarm and automatically cut off until the pressure falls below this set limit.

The tidal volumes generated during high frequency jet ventilation are small and often less than the respiratory dead space. Therefore it is not immediately intuitive how adequate gas exchange is achieved. There are several theories, which may all play a role, to a lesser or greater degree.

- *Convective streaming*: the high velocity inspiratory jet travels down the centre of the airway, whilst gas is simultaneously exhaled around the edge of the stream.
- *Simple diffusion*.
- *Pendelluft*: the high frequency jet stream inflates highly compliant alveoli first. These lung units then empty into alveoli which are less compliant (i.e. have a greater time constant). This process augments ventilation even after the end of the inspiratory phase.
- *Resonance*: when the frequency of the delivered breaths is close to the natural frequency of the lung, the amplitude with which the air moves in and out of distal segments of the lung increases significantly.
- *Cardiogenic oscillations*: as the heart beats, it exerts a vibrational force on the lungs, which may augment gas exchange.

Advantages

- Creates an almost motionless surgical field whilst ventilating the lungs.
- Allows ventilation with reduced alveolar distension and lower mean pressures compared to conventional ventilation and leads to less cardiovascular instability.
- The airway vibration caused by the high frequency ventilation may facilitate clearance of airway secretions.
- Automated, freeing up the anaesthetist.

Disadvantages

- Risk of gas trapping.
- The Mistral is unable to humidify inspired gases, although the newer Monsoon HFJV is capable of humidifying the jet.
- Unable to deliver volatile anaesthetics and so total intravenous anaesthesia is therefore necessary.
- Difficult to accurately measure end-tidal CO$_2$.

4.10 High frequency oscillatory ventilators

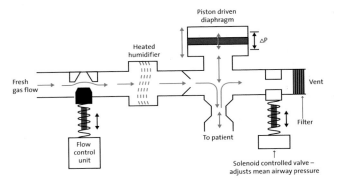

Fig. 4.10.2: Schematic of a high frequency oscillatory ventilator.

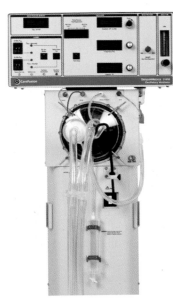

Fig. 4.10.1: A SensorMedics 3100B high frequency oscillatory ventilator.

Overview

Physiologists in 1915 demonstrated that it is possible to obtain adequate alveolar ventilation by delivering tidal volumes that are significantly smaller than the anatomical dead space volume, as long as high respiratory rates are used. This principle is used in both high frequency jet ventilation and high frequency oscillatory ventilation and the theoretical mechanisms of gas movement within the respiratory system are covered in *Section 4.9*. There are, however, significant differences between the two modalities. In high frequency oscillatory ventilation:

- inspiration *and* expiration are active
- ventilation takes place using a sealed breathing system via a standard ETT or tracheostomy; it does not involve jet airway devices
- there is therefore no entrainment of ambient air.

When compared with conventional ventilation, high frequency oscillatory ventilation causes less alveolar distension and smaller shearing forces on the airways.

High frequency oscillatory ventilation is used extensively in neonatal and paediatric intensive care. It has also found use on adult intensive care units. The SensorMedics 3100B model is an example of an oscillator designed for adults (the 3100A model is for use in patients weighing <35 kg). It is an electrically powered and controlled, time-cycled, high frequency oscillator and is described below.

Uses

Whilst there are no strong evidence-based criteria concerning the use of high frequency oscillatory ventilation in ITU, it has been considered most beneficial if it is used early in the management of patients with evidence of acute lung injury or ARDS, although the most recent evidence casts some doubt on this theory.

High frequency oscillatory ventilation can also minimize air leak through a bronchopleural fistulae and promote healing because intrathoracic cyclical pressure and volume changes are minimized.

How it works

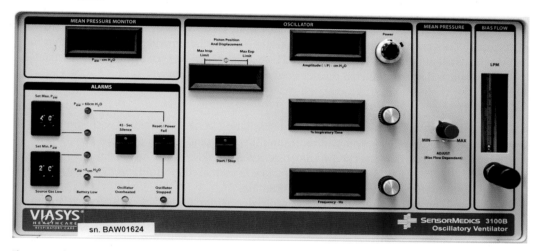

Fig. 4.10.3: The display unit of a SensorMedics 3100B oscillatory ventilator.

The SensorMedics 3100B is a piston-diaphragm oscillator. The diaphragm oscillates at frequencies of 3–15 Hz. The movement of the piston towards and away from the patient means that both inspiration and expiration are active processes. This is in contrast to conventional ventilation and jet ventilation, where only expiration is passive. This reduces the risk of gas trapping.

The dials on the SensorMedics 3100B are divided on its user interface into several areas. These can be seen in *Fig. 4.10.3* and will be covered in turn.

- *Mean airway pressure*: this is set using a dial that varies the resistance of a control valve in the expiratory limb of the breathing system. A common initial setting is 3–5 cmH$_2$O above the mean airway pressure (mPaw) that was observed during conventional ventilation. The mPaw during high frequency oscillatory ventilation can be thought of as having the same function as PEEP during conventional ventilation, but has a higher value (e.g. 25 cmH$_2$O). It is important to note that mPaw will vary depending on the settings for bias flow, power, frequency or % inspiratory time (see below). Adjustment of the control valve will therefore be required following other ventilator settings changes.
- *Bias flow*: this is the flow of fresh gas through the ventilator. It is required to remove carbon dioxide and deliver oxygen. The bias flow is adjusted using a flowmeter to 25–40 l.min^{-1}. Increasing bias flow increases mean airway pressures. Conversely, reducing it may make it difficult to generate the desired mean airway pressure and carbon dioxide removal may also be impaired.
- *Power*: the power dial controls the amplitude of the oscillation (ΔP). The noise of the ventilator and reduced gas movement mean that is difficult to auscultate the lungs during high frequency oscillatory ventilation in a similar manner to conventional ventilation. Instead, one should look for clear and symmetrical vibration of the chest wall and shoulders down to the lower abdomen, known as the 'chest wiggle'. If the pattern suddenly changes, for

example, it becomes unilateral or absent, one should be suspicious of tube migration into an endobronchial position, pneumothorax or accidental extubation. The power is adjusted until adequate 'chest wiggle' is seen and the desired $PaCO_2$ is achieved.

- *Inspiratory time*: this is typically set to 33% of the respiratory cycle.
- *Frequency*: in adults, a typical starting frequency is 3–7 Hz (i.e. 180–420 breaths a minute). Increasing the frequency may worsen carbon dioxide clearance by reducing inspiratory time.
- *Airway pressure alarm*: this will be triggered if the mPaw deviates by more than a set amount (typically +/– 5 cmH$_2$O). When the alarm is triggered, ventilation will cease until settings have been adjusted and the machine is restarted by the user. However, a constant mPaw is usually maintained and so alveolar collapse does not occur immediately.

Advantages

- Traditionally thought to facilitate improved ventilation in ARDS compared with standard ventilatory strategies. However, two recent multi-centre randomized controlled trials contradict this assertion; the OSCAR trial in adults with ARDS found no mortality benefit whilst the OSCILLATE trial was stopped early due to increased mortality in ARDS patients treated with high frequency oscillatory ventilation.
- Both inspiration and expiration are active processes in high frequency oscillatory ventilation.

Disadvantages

- Noisy.
- Not portable.
- Staff training required.
- Vibrations may displace ETT.
- Most patients will require deep sedation with or without muscle paralysis to tolerate high frequency oscillatory ventilation.
- Recent randomized trials suggest that at best there is no difference in mortality and at worst, the mortality is worse in adults treated with high frequency oscillatory ventilation for ARDS.

Other notes

There are various strategies for weaning from high frequency oscillatory ventilation. The manufacturer suggests titrating the FiO$_2$ to patient oxygen saturations of >90%. Once the FiO$_2$ is below 60%, it is then suggested that the mean airway pressure is brought down in 1 cmH$_2$O increments. The power (or ΔP) can also be brought down in 5 cmH$_2$O increments titrated against the $PaCO_2$.

Chapter 5
Delivery of anaesthetic agents

5.1 Introduction to delivery of anaesthetic agents

Delivery of volatile anaesthetic agents

Volatile anaesthetics delivered via the inhalational route are titrated by means of a vaporizer. The vaporizer is incorporated into an anaesthesia delivery system which may be of a continuous flow or draw-over design. Modern anaesthetic machines are continuous flow machines and require a pressurized gas source to drive fresh gas through high resistance vaporizers. This arrangement delivers more accurate anaesthetic concentrations.

In the field, where pressurized gas is unavailable, continuous flow anaesthesia is not possible. A draw-over anaesthesia system such as the Triservice apparatus may therefore be used instead.

Vaporizers

Modern vaporizers are designed to deliver precise and accurate partial pressures of an anaesthetic agent to a patient, irrespective of temperature, atmospheric pressure, the mechanics of the breathing system (e.g. back pressure from a ventilator) and fresh gas composition or flow.

There are a number of ways of classifying vaporizers. We suggest a four-point approach:

- *Mechanism for adding anaesthetic vapour to the fresh gas flow*
  - Variable bypass
  - Measured flow
- *The internal resistance of the vaporizer*
  - High: plenum vaporizers
  - Low: draw-over
- *Temperature compensation*
  - High thermal conductivity and specific heat capacity of the jacket (a 'heat sink')
  - Automatic adjustment of the splitting ratio:
    - Bimetallic strip
    - Bellows
    - Electronically controlled
- *Additional information*

Whilst this method of classification is not exhaustive, it does provide a useful framework to answer questions about a vaporizer during a physics and equipment viva.

Mechanism for adding anaesthetic vapour to the fresh gas flow

Volatile anaesthetics are too potent to be used at their saturated vapour pressure and must therefore be diluted to a safe concentration before being delivered to the patient. This is commonly achieved in one of two ways.

- *Variable bypass vaporizers* (e.g. most modern vaporizers, apart from the Tec 6) split the fresh gas flow into two streams. One stream enters a vaporization chamber and leaves fully saturated with anaesthetic vapour, whilst the remainder of the fresh gas bypasses this chamber. The two gas flows are reunited downstream to produce the desired final concentration. Altering the FGF does not alter the ratio between the flows in the two streams (splitting ratio) and therefore does not alter the final concentration.

- *Measured flow vaporizers* (e.g. the Tec 6 desflurane vaporizer) use a separate heated and pressurized vapour stream that is precisely injected into the FGF. Increasing the FGF dilutes the output and therefore an automated mechanism compensates for this.

The internal resistance of the vaporizer

Draw-over vaporizers have low internal resistances to gas flow. The patient's inspiratory effort is sufficient to draw fresh gas through the vaporizer and draw-over vaporizers are therefore useful in the field where pressurized gas may not be available. Mechanisms to improve the accuracy of anaesthetic delivery, such a baffles and temperature compensation increase resistance and are not usually present in draw-over vaporizers, leading to unpredictable performance. Examples of draw-over vaporizers include the Goldman, the Oxford Miniature Vaporizer (OMV) and Epstein and Macintosh of Oxford (EMO) vaporizers. These vaporizers are used within the breathing system (sometimes called 'vaporizer-in-circle/circuit' or 'VIC', although in practice they are not used with circle systems).

Plenum vaporizers in contrast rely on pressurized gas flow rather than the patient's inspiratory effort (plenum originates from the Latin for 'full' or 'pressurized'). They have a high internal resistance and are used with continuous flow anaesthetic machines. A plenum vaporizer should saturate all gas that passes through the vaporization chamber in order to achieve a consistent output, even at high FGFs. Examples of plenum vaporizers include Boyle's bottle, the Copper kettle, the Tec 5 series and the Aladin cassette. These vaporizers are used outside the breathing system (sometimes called 'vaporizer-out-of-circle/circuit' or 'VOC').

The Tec 6 desflurane vaporizer is a special case. Being a measured flow vaporizer, it functions on entirely different principles but, as with other high resistance vaporizers, it is used outside the breathing system, mounted on the back bar of an anaesthetic machine.

Temperature compensation

As anaesthetic liquid changes state and becomes a vapour, it absorbs heat from its surroundings, which provides the energy to break bonds between the liquid molecules. This energy is known as the latent heat of vaporization. Left unchecked, the temperature of the remaining liquid anaesthetic will fall significantly, along with its saturated vapour pressure and therefore lead to a reduction in the output of the vaporizer. The first method used to compensate for the latent heat of vaporization is to use a heat sink, such as a water bath (Boyle's bottle, see *Section 5.3*) or a large mass of copper (covered in detail in *Section 5.4*). Modern vaporizers are still made of large masses of metal for this purpose.

Invariably though, there will be some drop in temperature within the vaporizer as it is used. To maintain a constant output, this drop in temperature and saturated vapour pressure of the anaesthetic must be compensated for. This is achieved by the use of devices such as bimetallic strips, bellows or electronic control and is discussed further under individual vaporizers later on in this chapter.

Delivery of intravenous anaesthetic agents

Total intravenous anaesthesia (TIVA) may be delivered using standard infusion pumps or even by hand. More accurate dosing may, however, be achieved using specifically designed target controlled infusion (TCI) pumps which use computerized pharmacokinetic models to adjust the infusion rate and therefore achieve specific plasma or effect site concentrations.

The anaesthetic machine

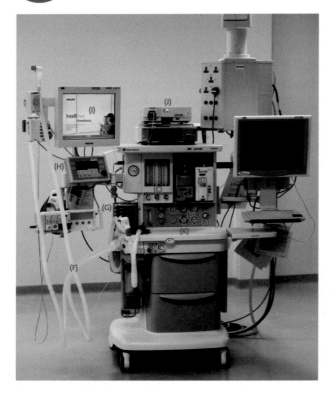

Fig. 5.2.1: A GE Datex Ohmeda Aespire machine. Components include (A) on/off switch, (B) pipeline and cylinder pressure gauges, (C) flowmeters, (D) vaporizers mounted on the back bar, (E) common gas outlet (not in use), (F) circle system, (G) bag in bottle ventilator, (H) ventilator controls, (I) monitor, (J) gas module (for monitoring anaesthetic gases), and (K) suction control.

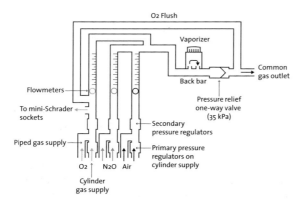

Fig. 5.2.2: Schematic of an anaesthetic machine.

Overview

Fundamental to all anaesthetic machines is the ability to deliver a reliable mixture of gases and anaesthetic vapours to the patient via a breathing system. Most machines also incorporate a ventilator (*Chapter 4*), patient and machine monitoring (*Chapter 6*), suction and scavenging (*Chapter 1*).

Anaesthetic machines must be designed around the vaporizer with which they are to be used. Modern anaesthetic machines are of a continuous flow design, based on the machine introduced by Henry Boyle in 1917. Boyle's machine had a pressurized gas supply, pressure reducing valves, flowmeters, a vaporizer (Boyle's bottle) and a breathing system – features which have endured and remain in modern anaesthetic machines. They are designed for use with high resistance vaporizers, which are more accurate, but require a continuous flow of pressurized gas to overcome their resistance (see *Section 5.5*).

How it works

In order to understand how the anaesthetic machine works, it is helpful to follow the path taken by gas as it flows from its supply, through the machine, to the patient.

The gas supply

Anaesthetic machines are supplied with oxygen, air and often nitrous oxide. There are many design features, covered both here and under Piped medical gas supply (see *Section 1.6*), to prevent cross-connection of these gases, because administration of 100% nitrous oxide leads rapidly to profound hypoxia.

Gases may be supplied from a wall outlet (at 400 kPa), or from cylinders. The wall outlet is a Schrader socket and a non-interchangeable ring collar prevents cross-connection of the hose. The machine end of the hose terminates in a non-interchangeable screw thread (NIST) connecter for attachment to the machine. This colour-coded, anti-kink hose is normally left connected to the machine with disconnection taking place at the Schrader socket if the machine is moved.

Size E cylinders provide an auxiliary (or in some cases, primary) gas supply. They are mounted on the back of the anaesthetic machine via a cylinder yoke. The pin index system prevents cross-connection and a Bodok washer provides a gas-tight seal. There is a pressure gauge and a primary pressure regulator for each cylinder. A full oxygen cylinder has a pressure of 13 700 kPa, which falls as the contents are used, or if the cylinder cools. The pressure regulator reduces this high and variable pressure to a constant 400 kPa, which is the machine's working pressure.

The high pressure system

There is a separate high pressure system for each gas. In order to maintain a continuous flow, the machine relies on a constant pressure of 400 kPa to drive the gas through high resistance flowmeters and vaporizers. Gas from the pipeline or cylinder is therefore passed through a secondary pressure regulator that smoothes fluctuations in pressure.

The high pressure system is also used to supply the emergency oxygen flush, which bypasses the flowmeters and back bar. There may also be connections to mini-Schrader valves used to drive jet ventilators.

An oxygen failure alarm sounds if the oxygen supply pressure falls. In this situation, all gases from the anaesthetic machine are prevented from reaching the patient and instead, room air is allowed into the breathing system.

The low pressure system

The high pressure system for each gas terminates in a needle valve attached to the base of a flowmeter. The needle valve is controlled by rotating a knob on the front of the machine, which alters gas flow. There is an interlink between the oxygen and nitrous oxide valves to prevent the delivery of a hypoxic gas mixture.

Downstream of the flowmeters, the three separate gases are finally allowed to mix, with oxygen being added last to reduce the chance of delivering a hypoxic mixture if there is a proximal leak. The gas mixture passes along the back bar, on which the vaporizers are mounted. When a vaporizer is turned on, the gas mixture is diverted through it and anaesthetic vapour is added. Distal to the vaporizers is a pressure relief one-way valve designed to protect machine components from pressures over 35 kPa.

The final gas and vapour mixture (the FGF) is delivered to the common gas outlet and then to the patient via a breathing system. In most modern machines, the FGF may also be diverted to a built-in circle breathing system by means of a switch. A separate switch controls an built-in bag-in-bottle ventilator.

The FGF is continuously analysed by a paramagnetic and infra-red analyser (see *Chapter 6*). In many machines this electronically switches off the nitrous oxide supply if oxygen concentrations fall below 25%.

Non-interchangeable screw thread connectors

NIST connectors consisting of a probe and a nut are used to connect gas pipelines to the anaesthetic machine.

The probe diameter is gas-specific in order to prevent cross-connection of different gases. Despite the ambiguous name, the nut and its thread are identical for all gases and simply hold the correct probe in place.

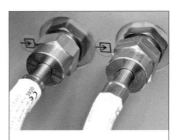

Fig. 5.2.3: NIST connection for pipeline gas on the back of an anaesthetic machine.

Bodok seal

A Bodok seal is a neoprene washer surrounded by a steel reinforcing ring. It provides a gas-tight connection between a gas cylinder and its yoke on the anaesthetic machine.

Frequent changing of cylinders, in combination with the large changes in temperature caused by adiabatic expansion of gas cause alternative seals (such as those made solely of rubber) to leak. Grease and oil are never used because they pose a fire risk in the presence of heat and pure oxygen.

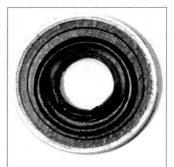

Fig. 5.2.4: A Bodok seal.

Pin index system

The pin index system prevents connection of an incorrect gas cylinder to the yoke on the anaesthetic machine. Pins protruding from the cylinder yoke mate with holes on the correct cylinder valve block.

There are six possible pin positions, divided into two groups of three. One position from the first group and one from the second are used for common anaesthetic gases.

Oxygen	2–5
Nitrous oxide	3–5
Air	1–5
Carbon dioxide	1–6

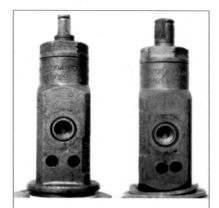

Fig. 5.2.5: Oxygen (left) and nitrous oxide cylinder blocks showing pin index holes.

Oxygen flush

The oxygen flush delivers oxygen at 35–75 l.min^{-1} from the high pressure system upstream of the flowmeters, to the low pressure system downstream of the back bar. It is used when rapid delivery of a high concentration of oxygen is required.

As it is delivered from the high pressure system, it is pressurized at 400 kPa (pipeline pressure) and care must therefore be taken to avoid causing lung baro- or volu-trauma. It does not pass through the vaporizers and will therefore dilute any anaesthetic agent in the breathing system.

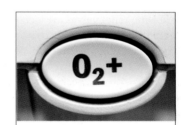

Fig. 5.2.6: A recessed oxygen flush button on the front of an anaesthetic machine.

Pressure regulators

Anaesthetic machines contain several primary and secondary pressure regulators.

Gas in the high pressure chamber of the regulator passes through the valve to the low pressure outlet. As it does so, it exerts a force on a diaphragm that acts to close the valve. The force from a spring acts in the opposite direction on the diaphragm to keep the valve open and the regulator is manufactured so that equilibrium between these two forces is reached at the desired outlet pressure.

Primary regulators reduce high cylinder pressures to a constant pressure of around 400 kPa. In many designs, cylinder primary regulators set the pressure at just below pipeline pressure, so that the pipeline gas is preferentially used. Despite this, regulators may leak cylinder contents, and so the cylinder should be turned off when not in use.

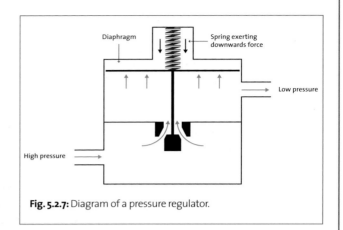

Fig. 5.2.7: Diagram of a pressure regulator.

Secondary regulators are located prior to the flowmeters to smooth out fluctuations in the pipeline supply pressure.

Pressure relief valve

Pressure relief valves are located downstream of each pressure regulator as a backup in case of regulator failure. The relief pressure is set at 700 kPa. They utilize a similar mechanism to the adjustable pressure limiting valve (*Section 3.3*), but are not user-adjustable.

In the low pressure system there is a non-return pressure relief valve situated after the back bar and set at 35 kPa (35 kPa is 357 cmH$_2$O, so this valve offers no protection to the patient). This valve is designed to protect the flowmeters and vaporizers from high downstream pressures and may be activated by occlusion of the common gas outlet. The non-return design also helps prevent back pressure effects when using minute volume divider ventilators.

Needle valve

Needle valves are located at the base of flowmeters. They perform two functions, acting as a control for gas flow and also reducing pressure from the high pressure system (around 400 kPa) to the low pressure system (just over atmospheric pressure).

The pressure drop across the valve occurs because of the high resistance to flow through the narrow lumen.

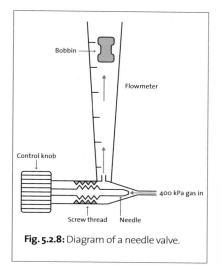

Fig. 5.2.8: Diagram of a needle valve.

Flowmeters

Flowmeters are covered separately in *Section 6.3*.

Back bar

The back bar is part of the low pressure system situated downstream of the flowmeter block. It provides mounts for the vaporizers which are sealed with a rubber O-ring. A missing ring, or poorly seated vaporizer, will result in a leak.

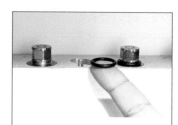

Fig. 5.2.9: Vaporizer mounts on a back bar.

Common gas outlet

The fresh gas leaves the machine via the common gas outlet. This is a tapered 22 mm male, 15 mm female outlet, to which a breathing system may be attached. All machines have a common gas outlet, however, they may also have a built-in circle system, activated by a switch to divert gas flow.

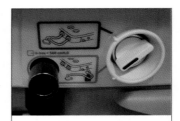

Fig. 5.2.10: A common gas outlet. The switch indicates the gas will exit the outlet rather than being diverted through the built-in circle system.

Mini-Schrader sockets

Auxiliary mini-Schrader sockets are located on most machines and are connected directly to the high pressure system, thus they supply pure oxygen or air at 400 kPa. They are used to drive equipment such as jet ventilators.

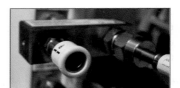

Fig. 5.2.11: A mini-Schrader valve attached to the oxygen supply on an anaesthetic machine. On some machines, the valve is built in.

The anaesthetic machine check

This has been adapted from the Anaesthetic Association of Great Britain and Ireland (AAGBI) guideline '*Checking Anaesthetic Equipment 2012*'. The guidance is available in full on the AAGBI website (www.aagbi.org). The check should take place before every operating session.

Check a self-inflating bag is available
- This is a potentially life-saving alternative means of ventilation in event of gas supply or machine failure.

Perform manufacturer's machine check
- Modern anaesthetic machines may 'self-check' during start up. This is in addition to the checks below.

Check the electrical supply
- The machine should be connected directly to mains supply and switched on. No extension lead should be used.

Check the gas supplies and suction
- Perform a gentle 'tug test' on each gas and vacuum pipeline to check it is securely connected to the Schrader valve.
- Check pipeline pressure gauges read between 400 and 500 kPa.
- Check the cylinders on the back of the machine are filled and turned off.
- Check the flowmeters and hypoxic guard linking the nitrous oxide and oxygen flowmeters.
- Check the oxygen flush.
- Check the suction is clean and generates at least −53 kPa (−400 mmHg).

Check the back bar, breathing system and vaporizers
- Visually inspect the breathing system and 'push and twist' connections.
- Perform a pressure leak test by occluding the patient end and compressing the reservoir bag.
- Check the whole system is patent and leak-free using the 'two-bag' test.
  - Attach a bag to the patient end of the breathing system (a 'test lung').
  - Set the FGF to 5 l.min^{-1} and ventilate manually.
  - Check unidirectional valves (if present) are working.
  - Check the APL valve by squeezing both bags simultaneously.
- Check for small leaks.
  - Turn on the ventilator to ventilate the test lung.
  - Turn off, or minimize the FGF.
  - Open and close each vaporizer – there should be no loss of volume in the system.
- Check the vaporizers are fitted correctly and filled.
- Check the soda lime colour.
- Check the gas outlet is correctly set (*Fig. 5.2.10*).

Ventilator
- Check it is working and configured correctly.

Monitor
- Check it is working and configured correctly.
- Check the alarm limits and volumes set.

Airway equipment
- Ensure the full range required is immediately available.

Record the check

5.3 Boyle's bottle

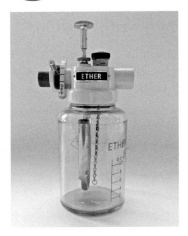

Fig. 5.3.1: A Boyle's bottle.

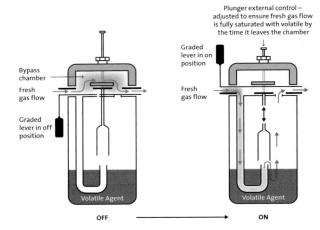

Fig. 5.3.2: Schematic of a Boyle's bottle.

Overview

Boyle's bottle was designed by Henry Boyle in the 1920s and was manufactured by BOC. It is a predecessor of modern plenum vaporizers. It has a relatively high internal resistance and so the FGF through it must be pressurized because the negative pressure generated by the patient's inspiratory effort is insufficient to draw gas through it (cf. draw-over vaporizers).

Uses

Used with early continuous flow anaesthetic machines (which were also invented and eponymously named after Henry Boyle) to deliver ether, trichloroethylene or chloroform.

How it works

Boyle's bottle had a glass reservoir that held a volatile anaesthetic agent. Two levers controlled the FGF. The first lever altered the proportion of FGF that bypassed the vaporization chamber (i.e. it set the splitting ratio). The second lever was a plunger which controlled the saturation of fresh gas with anaesthetic vapour as it passed through the chamber. It worked by adjusting the proximity of the incoming gas to the surface of the volatile liquid. A fully depressed plunger could force the incoming gas to bubble through the liquid and therefore become fully saturated. The plunger had many similarities to baffles in the vaporizing chamber of modern vaporizers, except that it was manually adjustable. Boyle's bottle did not have temperature compensation to counteract the loss of latent heat during vaporization. To some extent, cooling (and the associated reduction in volatile output) could be compensated for by placing the Boyle's bottle in a purpose-made water bath containing water at room temperature, which temporarily stabilized the output (i.e. vapour pressure) of the bottle.

⊕ Advantages

- Could be used with several different anaesthetic agents.
- Full saturation of the vapour chamber gas flow was possible.

⊖ Disadvantages

- No temperature compensation so volatile output fell as the reservoir cooled.
- The concentration of anaesthetic delivered to the patient was imprecise.
- Tipping Boyle's bottle could lead to dangerous rises in anaesthetic concentrations.

5.4 Copper kettle

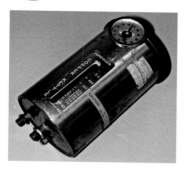

Fig. 5.4.1: A copper kettle vaporizer. Image courtesy of the Anaesthesia Museum, Sheffield Teaching Hospitals NHS Foundation Trust.

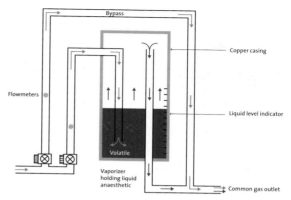

Fig. 5.4.2: Schematic of the copper kettle vaporizer

Overview

The copper kettle is a vaporizer of historical interest and is not in current use. It is classified as a flowmeter controlled, variable bypass vaporizer because the operator controls the flow through the vaporizing chamber and bypass chamber independently using two separate flowmeters.

Uses

The copper kettle was the first vaporizer that allowed precise control of the concentration of volatile anaesthetic administered to a patient. It was used with chloroform, ether and halothane.

How it works

Modern variable bypass vaporizers automatically adjust the splitting of the FGF through the vaporization chamber and bypass chamber, depending on the desired concentration at the common gas outlet. In contrast, the anaesthetist operating the copper kettle had to manually adjust the flow entering and bypassing the vaporization chamber using two parallel flowmeters. One flowmeter controlled gas flow that bubbled through the anaesthetic agent reservoir to become fully saturated with vapour. The second flowmeter controlled the flow that bypassed the vaporization chamber. The bypass flow was then reunited with the fully saturated gas downstream. Determining the exact flows required to deliver a particular partial pressure of vapour to the patient was difficult, but tables were available to assist with these calculations.

Copper was used for the housing of the vaporizer because it has both a high heat capacity and high thermal conductivity. Heat capacity (in joules per kelvin) is the total amount of energy stored in an object, as opposed to the specific heat capacity which is the amount stored per unit mass (in joules per gram per kelvin). Although copper has a much lower specific heat capacity ($0.38\,J.g^{-1}.K^{-1}$) than water ($4.18\,J.g^{-1}.K^{-1}$), which was used as a heat sink by Boyle's bottle, it is much more dense and can therefore hold a large amount of heat energy. Having a high thermal conductivity (which water does not) means that it is able to conduct heat from its surroundings into the vaporizing chamber relatively quickly. Therefore, to a limited extent, the copper housing allows the vaporizer to compensate for fluctuations in temperature within the vaporizing chamber.

Advantages

- Temperature stabilized by the copper heat sink.
- Could be used with any volatile anaesthetic agent.

Disadvantages

- No true temperature compensation.
- Potential to deliver lethal concentrations of anaesthetic agent to the patient by, for example, forgetting to turn on the bypass flowmeter.

5.5 Modern variable bypass vaporizers

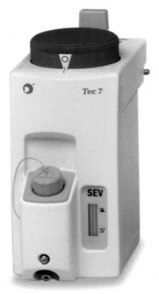

Fig. 5.5.1: A Sevoflurane Tec 7 vaporizer. Image reproduced with permission from GE Healthcare.

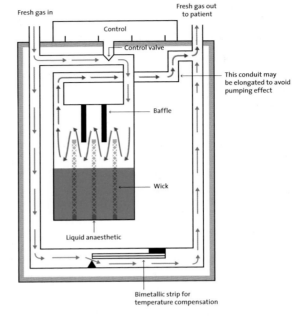

Fresh gas in

Fresh gas out to patient

Control

Control valve

This conduit may be elongated to avoid pumping effect

Baffle

Wick

Liquid anaesthetic

Bimetallic strip for temperature compensation

Fig. 5.5.2: A temperature compensated plenum vaporizer.

Overview

Modern variable bypass vaporizers, such as the Tec 5, are the most commonly used devices for delivering volatile anaesthetic agents in modern practice. They are plenum vaporizers with a high resistance to gas flow and are available for use with sevoflurane, isoflurane, enflurane and halothane. Each vaporizer is calibrated for a specific agent and cannot be interchanged because of the differing physical properties of the volatile agents.

Uses

For the administration of safe, accurate and precise concentrations of a volatile agent via a continuous flow anaesthetic machine (see *Section 5.2*).

How it works

Fresh gas from the flowmeters (*Section 6.3*) enters the vaporizer inlet and is split into two streams. The majority enters a bypass chamber so that it does not come into contact with the liquid anaesthetic, but the other stream (typically less than 20% of the total) is diverted into the vaporizing chamber where the liquid anaesthetic is stored. As the gas flows through this chamber and over the surface of the liquid, evaporation (vaporization) occurs. By the time the gas leaves the vaporizing chamber, it is fully saturated with anaesthetic vapour, which therefore exerts its saturated vapour pressure (SVP). This saturated vapour is then diluted by the gas that bypassed the vaporizing chamber as the two streams are reunited. The vapour pressure of the anaesthetic is therefore reduced to one that produces appropriate anaesthesia and is safe for the patient.

For example, sevoflurane has an SVP of 22.7 kPa at 20°C. Therefore, gas leaving the vaporizing chamber will contain sevoflurane at a vapour pressure of 22.7 kPa. It must then be diluted 10–20 times by the bypass gas to give a useful concentration.

The concentration of anaesthetic produced by the vaporizer therefore depends on the fraction of fresh gas that is diverted into the vaporizing chamber. This fraction is governed by the calibrated control dial. The proportion bypassing divided by the proportion entering the vaporizing chamber is known as the splitting ratio.

In order to ensure that the end concentration is controlled only by the splitting ratio and not by variations in the amount of anaesthetic leaving the vaporizing chamber, the diverted gas must always become fully saturated with vapour before it re-joins the bypass gas. This is achieved using wicks that increase the surface area for evaporation of the anaesthetic liquid and baffles that direct the incoming gas down closer to the surface of the liquid. These features significantly increase the internal resistance of the vaporizer.

Temperature compensation

As liquid evaporates, it loses energy as the latent heat of vaporization, causing cooling. As the temperature falls, so does the SVP of the anaesthetic and therefore the output of the vaporizer. Most modern vaporizers are made of a material such as copper that is a good conductor of heat and which, because of its high mass, acts as a heat sink and helps to keep the temperature inside stable.

Nevertheless, the temperature will eventually fall and modern vaporizers are therefore temperature compensated. Most use a bimetallic strip (see *Section 6.14*: temperature measurement) to automatically make fine adjustments to the splitting ratio. At lower temperatures therefore, the splitting ratio increases slightly and more gas is allowed into the vaporizing chamber to ensure that the end concentration of anaesthetic stays constant.

⊕ Advantages

- Easy to use and reliable.
- Properly calibrated modern variable bypass vaporizers are accurate to +/– 15% of the dial setting for all flows between 200 ml.min^{-1} and 15 l.min^{-1} at 21°C.
- This type of vaporizer does not require a power source.

⊖ Disadvantages

- High internal resistance so must be used 'out of circle'.
- The heat sink makes the vaporizer heavy – another reason why this type of vaporizer is not suitable for use in the field.
- There are no alarms to indicate that the level of liquid anaesthetic inside the vaporizer is low.
- Temperature compensation only works within a reasonable range of ambient temperatures. If the vaporizer is used in an extremely hot or cold environment it will deliver anaesthetic unreliably.

⊘ Safety

- Colour coding indicates which anaesthetic is in which vaporizer.
- There is a key system for filling, so that the vaporizer cannot be filled with the wrong anaesthetic agent.

- Interlocking back bar systems ensure that although more than one vaporizer can be mounted on the anaesthetic machine at the same time, only one can be switched on at a time.
- Internal valves ensure that if the vaporizer is turned upside down, liquid cannot spill into the bypass chamber and dangerously increase the delivered concentration.
- The pumping effect is the increase in delivered anaesthetic vapour concentration caused by intermittent compression and decompression of the gas flowing through the vaporizer. This may occur when mechanical ventilation is used or when the emergency oxygen flush is activated. Gas in the vaporizing chamber is forced backwards and can subsequently flow into the bypass chamber, despite already being saturated with anaesthetic. The effect can be minimized in several ways:
  - lengthening the gas conduits leaving the vaporizer causes damping of the pressure increase caused by the ventilator due to increased volume
  - by ensuring a high resistance is encountered
  - by incorporating non-return valves.

Other notes

It is convenient to refer to *concentrations* of vapour at sea level because atmospheric pressure is approximately 100 kPa. Therefore a vapour pressure of 1 kPa is equivalent to a concentration of 1% (1 kPa / 100 kPa). However, it should be remembered that it is the *vapour pressure* that exerts its anaesthetic effect on the brain and this is particularly relevant when atmospheric pressure changes. Note also that the *saturated vapour pressure* (SVP) of a substance varies with its temperature but not with ambient pressure.

If the atmospheric pressure is altered (for example, at high altitude), the SVP of the anaesthetic does not change, and therefore the *vapour pressure* of the anaesthetic in the gas leaving the vaporizing chamber also does not change. However, the output *concentration* will change because this is the vapour pressure divided by the atmospheric pressure.

For example, at sea level, dialling up 2% on a vaporizer would deliver approximately 2 kPa of anaesthetic (2% of 100 kPa). If the barometric pressure is halved, setting the dial at '2%' will still deliver 2 kPa because SVP does not vary with ambient pressure. Therefore, a vaporizer can be used as normal at altitude because it is the vapour pressure that is clinically important. However, the delivered *concentration* will not be 2% (as read on the dial). If the delivery is 2 kPa at 50 kPa atmospheric pressure, the concentration delivered is actually 4% (2 kPa / 50 kPa = 4%).

Desflurane Tec 6 vaporizer

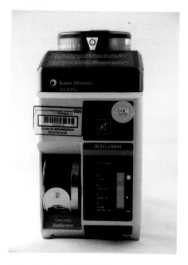

Fig. 5.6.1: The Tec 6 desflurane vaporizer.

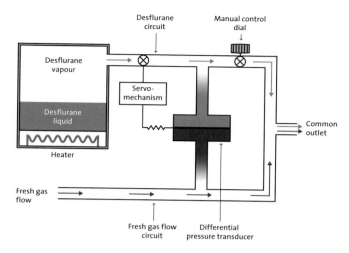

Fig. 5.6.2: Schematic of the desflurane vaporizer. Modified image courtesy of the Anaesthesia Museum, Sheffield Teaching Hospitals NHS Foundation Trust.

Overview

Desflurane is an anaesthetic agent with several desirable properties, such as its low blood:gas partition coefficient. Unfortunately, other physical properties of desflurane mean that it cannot be accurately and safely vaporized using a normal variable bypass vaporizer.

The boiling point of desflurane is 23°C. Because this is close to room temperature, there can be a large and unpredictable change in vapour pressure for a given change in ambient temperature. Therefore, vaporizing desflurane using a standard plenum vaporizer could lead to dangerous and erratic variations in the delivered concentration of anaesthetic. Ohmeda therefore developed the desflurane-specific Tec 6 vaporizer in 1989 as a method for delivering desflurane.

Uses

The Tec 6 vaporizer is specifically designed for the safe administration of desflurane in clinical practice.

How it works

The Tec 6 is an electrically heated, pressurized vaporizer that injects precise quantities of desflurane vapour into the FGF. Unlike variable bypass vaporizers, the fresh gas does not enter a vaporizing chamber.

The desflurane vaporizer has a reservoir chamber that heats desflurane above its boiling point to 42°C and pressurizes it to approximately 2 atmospheres. Temperature compensation is therefore not required in the Tec 6 vaporizer.

There are two mechanisms that govern the release of desflurane vapour into the FGF. The first is the dial that is located on top of the vaporizer that is set to a desired concentration by the anaesthetist. The second is a valve that maintains the set concentration, in response to changes in the FGF (if the FGF increases then the rate of desflurane release must also increase to maintain a constant concentration). This is achieved by a differential pressure transducer which compares the pressure in the desflurane circuit with that in the FGF circuit. When the FGF is increased, its pressure also increases and this is detected by the transducer. A microprocessor then opens the valve enough to increase the amount of desflurane that is injected. The opposite occurs when the FGF is reduced.

Advantages

- Comparable accuracy to variable bypass Tec 5 vaporizers; +/− 15% of dialled setting.
- Unaffected by ambient temperature because the desflurane is heated.
- Automatically compensates for variation in FGF.
- Has visual and audible alarms to alert the anaesthetist that the vaporizer is almost empty or that there is no output.

Disadvantages

- Requires an electrical power supply.
- Requires time to warm up before it is operational.

Safety

- As with other Tec vaporizers, it is very difficult to fill the Tec 6 vaporizer with an anaesthetic other than desflurane due to the key system for filling. There is also a colour coding system that helps prevent filling of vaporizers with the wrong anaesthetic.
- The Tec 6 design prevents desflurane liquid spilling into the FGF if the vaporizer is tilted or inverted.

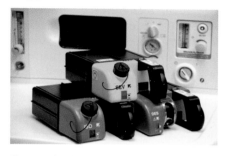

Fig. 5.7.1: The Aladin cassette 2 vaporizers from GE Healthcare. Note that there is integrated housing for the cassettes within the body of the GE Healthcare anaesthetic machine that incorporates the bypass channel.

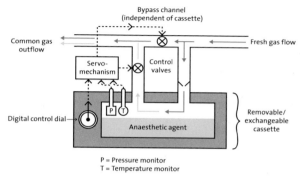

P = Pressure monitor
T = Temperature monitor

Fig. 5.7.2: Schematic of the Aladin cassette vaporizer.

Overview

Aladin cassettes are exchangeable reservoirs of anaesthetic agent that are plugged into an electronically controlled vaporizer housing, through a port on the front of GE Healthcare Aisys anaesthetic machines. Together the cassette and vaporizer housing work in the same manner as a standard variable bypass plenum vaporizer, except that there is second-by-second electronic monitoring and control of the splitting ratio.

Uses

Used with Aisys Carestation anaesthetic machines to deliver halothane, enflurane, isoflurane, sevoflurane and desflurane.

How it works

The cassette is effectively a removable vaporizing chamber that does not incorporate the bypass channels – these are found in the permanent vaporizer housing of the anaesthetic machine. Gas entering the cassette becomes fully saturated with anaesthetic vapour, in the same way as it does in a standard variable bypass vaporizer. On leaving the cassette, it is reunited with and diluted by the gas from the bypass channel to generate the final desired anaesthetic vapour concentration.

As the bypass channel is not located within the cassette, the cassettes can be carried and stored in any orientation, without the risk of anaesthetic agent spilling into the bypass channel and generating unpredictable and dangerous downstream concentrations. Each cassette is specific for a single anaesthetic agent and is magnetically coded so that the vaporizer housing recognizes which cassette has been inserted and automatically makes the necessary adjustments to its bypass flow settings, depending on the potency of the anaesthetic agent within the cassette. The delivered anaesthetic concentration is adjusted electronically and precisely by altering the proportion of FGF that enters the cassette.

The Aladin cassette vaporizer therefore has automated, electronically monitored and controlled FGF, along with temperature and pressure compensation. It is also able to provide on-screen data regarding reservoir levels and precise details of anaesthetic usage. The cassettes are refillable.

The desflurane Aladin cassette works in a different way to standard Tec 6 Desflurane vaporizers; as discussed in *Section 5.6*, desflurane's boiling point is close to room temperature and therefore its output through a conventional variable bypass vaporizer is unpredictable. The desflurane Aladin cassette is not, however, heated or pressurized to the same extent as a Tec 6 vaporizer and instead works in a broadly similar manner to the other (sevoflurane, isoflurane, enflurane and halothane) cassettes. It is able to achieve accurate desflurane output using a variable bypass set up thanks to computerized, second-by-second control of the splitting ratio. Temperature, pressure and agent concentration sensors within and downstream of the vaporizer relay information to a CPU which is capable of rapidly adjusting electromagnetically controlled solenoid valves to alter the flow of fresh gas into the vaporizing chamber many times per second. Accurate and precise output concentrations of desflurane can therefore be maintained, irrespective of ambient conditions.

⊕ Advantages

- Automated recognition of the agent inserted.
- On-screen data showing agent levels and anaesthetic usage.
- Automated, electronically monitored and controlled FGF, temperature and pressure compensation.
- No risk of spillage of anaesthetic agent into the bypass channel.
- Cassette can be carried safely in any orientation.

⊖ Disadvantages

- Specific to a particular branded anaesthetic machine.
- Anaesthetic delivery requires electrical power.

5.8 Goldman vaporizer

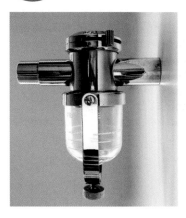

Fig. 5.8.1: The Goldman vaporizer

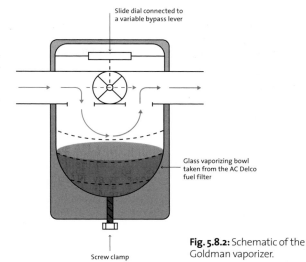

Slide dial connected to a variable bypass lever

Glass vaporizing bowl taken from the AC Delco fuel filter

Screw clamp

Fig. 5.8.2: Schematic of the Goldman vaporizer.

Overview

The Goldman vaporizer is a variable bypass, draw-over vaporizer which is not temperature compensated. It was first manufactured in 1959 by BOC. It was most commonly used with halothane, but it could also be used with trichloroethylene (Trilene). It is no longer used in clinical practice in the developed world.

Uses

Originally designed for use in a non-rebreathing system for dental anaesthesia. Its size, low cost and simplicity made it popular for field anaesthesia and for use in developing countries.

How it works

The Goldman vaporizer has a dome-shaped glass reservoir taken from the AC Delco vehicle fuel filter. It was capable of holding up to 30 ml of halothane or trichloroethylene. The proportion of fresh gas that entered the vaporizing chamber could be adjusted with a ratchet control valve on top of the unit. The vaporizer was designed for use with potent anaesthetic agents like halothane and it was designed to be deliberately inefficient – it was therefore difficult to deliver (dangerous) halothane concentrations greater than 3%. There are therefore no wicks or baffles to improve efficiency of vaporization and the output from the vaporization chamber is not fully saturated with anaesthetic.

⊕ Advantages

- Small and cheap.
- Simple to use and service.
- Lightweight and portable.
- Restricted output prevents halothane overdosing.

⊖ Disadvantages

- Variable output that is difficult to measure.
- No temperature compensation.
- Unsuitable for use with less potent anaesthetic agents, because it is inherently inefficient.
- There is a risk of anaesthetic agent spillage into the breathing system.

5.9 Oxford miniature vaporizer

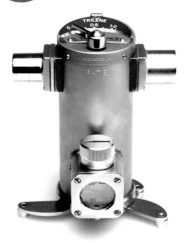

Fig. 5.9.1: The Oxford Miniature Vaporizer. Image courtesy of the Anaesthesia Museum, Sheffield Teaching Hospitals NHS Foundation Trust.

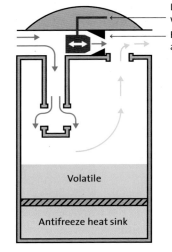

Lever connected to plunger within bypass channel

Bypass channel with adjustable orifice

Volatile

Antifreeze heat sink

Fig. 5.9.2: Schematic of the Oxford Miniature Vaporizer.

Overview

The Oxford Miniature Vaporizer (OMV) is a variable bypass, draw-over vaporizer that is not actively temperature compensated, but it does incorporate an ethylene glycol heat sink. It represented a significant advance in simple, low resistance draw-over vaporizers and can be filled with any agent by exchanging the removable scale on the dial.

Uses

The OMV remains in current use as part of the British military's Triservice apparatus for delivering anaesthesia in the field, typically with isoflurane, but also sevoflurane. It is also still used regularly in parts of the developing world.

How it works

The OMV has a 50 ml vaporization chamber with metal mesh wicks that increase the surface area for vaporization. Like most modern vaporizers, a dial on top of the device controls the proportion of FGF that bypasses or enters the vaporization chamber. However, unlike most vaporizers that can only be used with one agent, the dial on the OMV is removable and may be changed for dials calibrated for other anaesthetic agents. A valve found in the OMV and modern vaporizers prevents the contents of the vaporizing chamber from spilling into the breathing system, even if it is turned upside down.

Whilst the OMV is not temperature compensated, the reservoir is positioned on an ethylene glycol (antifreeze) heat sink that helps reduce the drop in temperature associated with vaporization. The OMV therefore has a more consistent output during operation compared to simpler draw-over vaporizers like the Goldman.

⊕ Advantages

- Portable.
- Robust and easily serviceable.

- Most volatile agents can be used by simply switching the interchangeable dials.
- When the control dial is switched off, volatile agent cannot easily spill into the breathing circuit if the vaporizer is tilted or inverted.
- An ethylene glycol heat sink buffers temperature changes, to an extent.
- Metal mesh wicks help increase the output of the vaporizer.
- Acceptable accuracy over a range of flow rates and tidal volumes.

Disadvantages

- Not temperature compensated.
- Small 50 ml reservoir empties quickly.

5.10 EMO vaporizer

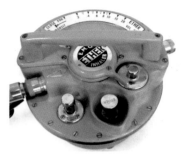

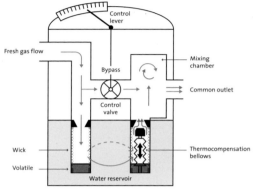

Fig. 5.10.2: Schematic of the EMO vaporizer. Modified image courtesy of the Anaesthesia Museum, Sheffield Teaching Hospitals NHS Foundation Trust.

Fig. 5.10.1: The EMO vaporizer.

Overview

The EMO (Epstein and Macintosh of Oxford) vaporizer was introduced in 1952 and quickly became a popular method for administering ether. It is a variable bypass draw-over vaporizer with temperature compensation using a bellows device. It remains in use in the developing world.

Uses

The accurate and precise delivery of ether irrespective of temperature.

How it works

The EMO vaporizer comprises an anaesthetic reservoir surrounded by a water jacket that acts as a heat sink. A dial on top of the unit is calibrated for ether and varies the splitting ratio. The efficiency with which ether is vaporized is improved by the presence of wicks that increase the surface area.

The feature that was revolutionary at the time was the bellows temperature-compensating valve. The valve is located inside the vaporization chamber next to the outlet. It comprises a plunger attached to air-filled bellows, which expand as the temperature within the chamber increases and contract as it cools. As the bellows expand, the plunger progressively occludes the outlet, reducing the amount of anaesthetic that can leave the chamber. The opposite is true when the vaporizer cools; more anaesthetic is allowed to leave the vaporizing chamber to compensate for a temperature-related drop in the SVP of ether.

The vaporizer is calibrated for an output of 2–20% and is reasonably accurate at room temperature and flow rates of between 4 and 10 l.min^{-1}.

⊕ Advantages

- Temperature compensation.
- Reliable and generally safe.

⊖ Disadvantages

- Bulky and heavy (it weighs 10 kg).
- Requires high gas flow to deliver anaesthetic agents accurately.
- The pumping effect of positive pressure ventilation may lead to dangerous surges in volatile output.
- Designed specifically for use with ether, which is now obsolete in the developed world.

5.11 Triservice apparatus

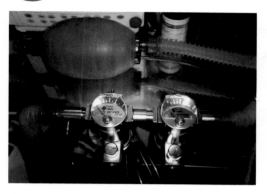

Fig. 5.11.1: The Triservice apparatus is based around two Oxford Miniature Vaporizers and a self-inflating bag. Image courtesy of Dr Mark Reaveley.

Overview

The Triservice apparatus is a draw-over anaesthesia system which may be used without a pressurized gas supply.

The simplest draw-over system would comprise a one way valve and a vaporizer. The vaporizer used must be of very low resistance because it is in the breathing system.

Uses

It is used for anaesthesia in remote areas, often by the military, in situations where the supply of compressed gases is unreliable. It can be used in adults and, with various modifications, can also be used for anaesthetizing children of all ages.

How it works

The Triservice apparatus works by drawing atmospheric air over two Oxford Miniature Vaporizers (*Section 5.9*). Historically, both vaporizers were used simultaneously, one for halothane (for its anaesthetic properties), the other for trichloroethylene (for its analgesic properties). In modern use, isoflurane is the agent of choice. The second vaporizer permits easier refilling whilst maintaining anaesthetic delivery.

Oxygen, if available, may be added upstream of the vaporizers. The anaesthetic gas then passes through tubing and a self-inflating bag (see *Section 3.2*: bag valve mask) to the patient. Exhaled gas is vented through a non-rebreathe valve. The oxygen tubing attached to the self-inflating bag in *Figure 5.11.1* (downstream of the vaporizers) is used only for pre-oxygenation and is not used intra-operatively so that the anaesthetic vapour is not diluted.

If the patient is spontaneously breathing, their inspiratory effort draws gas through the entire system. Positive pressure ventilation may be achieved by squeezing the bag, or a ventilator may be connected upstream of the vaporizers and the system used in a 'push-over' arrangement. However, care is required because there is a risk of very high anaesthetic concentrations in the breathing system using this method.

⊕ Advantages

- Robust, portable and easily modified.
- No pressurized gas supply is required.
- Suitable for paediatric use.

⊖ Disadvantages

- Vaporizer limitations (e.g. no temperature compensation, not suitable for prolonged use).
- Inefficient in anaesthetic gas usage.

5.12 Target controlled infusions

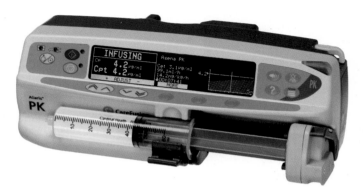

Fig. 5.12.1: The Alaris PK (pharmacokinetic) pump (Carefusion). A target plasma propofol concentration (Cpt) of 4.2 µg. ml⁻¹ has been set. The Cp is also 4.2 µg.ml⁻¹, indicating that the pump has calculated that the plasma concentration has reached this target. This is graphically illustrated on the right of the screen which shows the set concentration (horizontal line) and calculated concentration (shaded area) over the last 5 minutes. The Ce (effect site concentration) is also displayed. At this point the Ce is only 3.1 µg.ml⁻¹, indicating that a steady state at the effect site has yet to be reached. The decrement time is indicated at 7 minutes 41 seconds; this is the predicted time for the target concentration to fall to a set value, usually 1 µg.ml⁻¹. It gives an indication of the time to wake up if the pump is switched off. Image courtesy of Carefusion.

Overview

Total intravenous anaesthesia (TIVA) is the delivery of an anaesthetic entirely by the intravenous route, usually by means of an infusion pump. The simplest method of delivering TIVA is to use a pump programmed in millilitres per hour, adjusted manually. However, the pharmacokinetics of TIVA are complicated and without computer control it is impossible to achieve a known steady plasma concentration (Cp) as the drug redistributes into different body compartments. Specialized infusion pumps have therefore been developed which deliver a target controlled infusion (TCI). In a TCI, the anaesthetist sets a target drug concentration and the pump attempts to achieve it, using an inbuilt mathematical algorithm that is based on the pharmacokinetic behaviour of the drug.

It is worth noting that although a TCI may be used for TIVA, it may also be used as an adjunct to a volatile anaesthetic. The general principles of infusion pumps are covered separately in *Section 9.15*, this section will focus on the specifics of TCI.

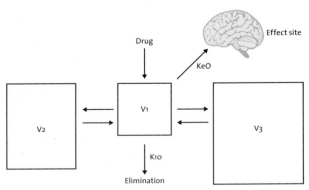

Fig. 5.12.2: The three compartment model, comprising a central compartment (V1) and two peripheral compartments (V2 and V3). The effect site is modelled as a 4th compartment of zero volume.

Uses

A TCI is used to achieve a set target concentration of an anaesthetic drug in the plasma or at the effect site. The most commonly used drugs are propofol and remifentanil, though models for alfentanil and sufentanil are also available.

How it works

In order to achieve a particular target concentration of a drug, TCI pumps are factory programmed with an algorithm based on a pharmacokinetic model for a particular drug. The anaesthetist enters simple data about the patient, such as the age, sex, weight and/or height, and sets the desired concentration. The pump then uses the model to adjust the rate of infusion.

Pharmacokinetics

The pharmacokinetics of most anaesthetic drugs, including propofol and remifentanil may be described using a three compartment model. The compartments are mathematical constructs that allow a model to be created which matches observed effects (such as plasma concentrations and time to onset of anaesthesia); they do not represent actual body compartments. In order to develop a model, a group of volunteers are given known doses of the drug, and plasma concentrations are measured over time. Values for compartment volumes and clearances (both inter-compartment clearance, and elimination from the central compartment) are calculated.

The TCI pump uses these population values adjusted according to the patient demographic data to calculate the predicted concentration of drug in each compartment every few seconds of infusion. Each time it performs the calculation, the TCI pump calculates the amount of drug lost by elimination and transfer. By infusing the same amount, the desired concentration is maintained.

On induction, or if the set concentration is increased, the pump will deliver a bolus dose. Since *volume of distribution = dose/concentration*, it can be seen that the dose required is the initial volume of distribution (Vd) multiplied by the desired concentration.

The rate of infusion at steady state depends on the *clearances* to and from the central compartment. The initial infusion rate will gradually decrease as the peripheral compartment concentrations equilibrate and steady state is achieved.

> Loading dose = Vd × concentration
>
> Infusion rate = concentration × clearance

Effect-site targeting

The effect site for anaesthetic agents is in the central nervous system (CNS), however, for the purposes of the model the effect site is not a physical site or volume but a mathematically useful concept. It is added to the three compartment model as a fourth compartment of zero volume that is in communication with the central compartment. Since it takes time for the plasma concentration (Cp) to equilibrate with the effect site concentration (Ce), there is a delay in achieving the Ce if it is Cp that is targeted. Instead, targeting of effect site concentration aims to reduce this delay. The model achieves this by overshooting the Cp during induction, thus the plasma concentrations may temporarily be very high, with associated side effects.

Ce is also displayed when using plasma targeting modes (see *Fig. 5.12.1*). This

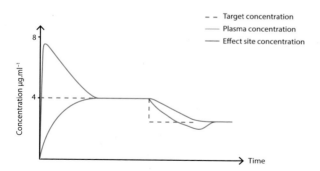

Fig. 5.12.3: Graph illustrating effect-site targeting. At induction, the pump maintains high initial plasma concentrations in order to rapidly achieve the desired effect-site concentration; however, this comes at the cost of increased side effects. When the target concentration is reduced, the infusion stops based on Ce, which reduces at a slower rate than Cp. Cp therefore falls below the target. When Ce reaches the target, the pump administers a small bolus to bring Cp back up.

may be used as a gauge of anaesthetic depth – for instance, during induction Cp will initially rise much faster than Ce. The patient will not be anaesthetized until Ce reaches a certain level (say 2–4 µg.ml^{-1}, depending on co-administration of other agents), irrespective of Cp.

Propofol TCI

The Marsh model was the first propofol TCI model developed, and is still commonly used. It takes into account only the patient's weight, though an age of over sixteen must be entered in order for some models of pump to function. The Marsh model is generally used in plasma targeting mode because, when targeting the effect site, the Marsh model gives a very high initial dose and this may cause cardiovascular instability in elderly or unwell patients.

A later development is the Schneider model, which takes into account weight, height, age and sex, and uses this information to calculate a lean body mass. The Schneider model is generally used in effect-site targeting mode and tends to give lower doses of propofol than the Marsh model, both at induction and during maintenance. This is partly because it uses a much lower value for its central compartment (4 litres rather than 16 litres for a 70 kg patient).

Children have increased central compartment size and rapid clearance; adult models may therefore under-dose them. Child-specific models exist (such as the Kataria and Paedfusor model), however, concerns regarding the development of acidosis and lipaemia associated with prolonged infusions of propofol in children have limited their use. Current evidence suggests that these problems are not significant during short-term infusions in theatre and TCI in children is gradually becoming more popular.

Remifentanil TCI

Remifentanil TCI uses the Minto model, which uses the patient's age, sex, weight and height. It allows for plasma or effect-site targeting.

Propofol and remifentanil are synergistic, partly due to the reduced volume of distribution of propofol when co-administered with remifentanil. A reduced dose of propofol may therefore be used in this situation. No current model takes this into account, though a combination TCI pump is in development.

⊕ Advantages

- Anaesthesia is continuous from the anaesthetic room through to theatre: there is no period of disconnection, as with a volatile agent. For the same reason, TIVA/TCI is useful in procedures involving the airway.
- There may be a reduction in post-operative nausea and vomiting.
- As with all TIVA, theatre and atmospheric pollution is reduced.

⊖ Disadvantages

- Real-time measurement of target concentrations, analogous to the end tidal volatile agent concentration, is not currently possible.
- There are significant differences in rates of drug delivery by different models and modes, the benefits and drawbacks of which must be understood by the anaesthetist.
- TCI models were developed in healthy volunteers and may be inaccurate in obese, unwell, or elderly patients.
- Modelling in children is not as well characterized or established as for adults.

ⓘ Safety

- The pump has no way of knowing if it is delivering anaesthesia to the patient, or onto the floor! A dedicated, visible infusion line should therefore be used for TIVA/TCI wherever possible to reduce the risk of awareness.
- In order to prevent the anaesthetic infusion tracking back up another giving set, anti-reflux valves should be used on *all* infusions attached to the same intravenous access point. Special multi-way connectors and TIVA lines incorporating anti-reflux valves are available.
- Similarly, anti-siphoning valves should also be used to prevent the inadvertent rapid delivery of anaesthetic.

Other notes

Future developments may include 'closed loop' TCI, in which the pump is automatically adjusted according to a measurement of anaesthetic depth, such as the Bispectral index (see *Section 6.17*).

Chapter 6
Monitoring equipment

6.1 Introduction to monitoring equipment

This chapter divides equipment into two categories:

- that used for monitoring the performance of the anaesthetic machine
- that used for monitoring the patient.

However, several pieces of equipment are present in each category that measure the same variable (e.g. pressure or flow). Some exam questions are likely to test knowledge of all equipment that is capable of measuring a single variable, and it is therefore important to have a robust classification in order to provide a good answer.

Measurement of pressure

Pressure is force (in newtons) per unit area (in square meters), and its SI unit is the pascal: $1\,Pa = 1\,N.m^{-2}$. Because 1 pascal is a very low pressure, the kilopascal (kPa) is more commonly used. The units used in this book are those most commonly associated with the context, for example, blood pressure is measured in mmHg and airway pressures in cmH$_2$O (see *Table 6.1.1*).

Table 6.1.1: Methods for measuring pressure and unit conversions.

Methods of measuring pressure	
Direct	**Indirect**
Liquid-containing gauges • Manometer • Barometer	Non-invasive blood pressure measurement, using a cuff
Aneroid gauges • Bourdon gauge • Bellows	Penaz technique
Electronic transduction • Strain gauge	Doppler ultrasound
1 kPa is equal to:	
0.0098 atmospheres (atm) 0.01 bar 7.501 millimetres of mercury (mmHg) 7.501 Torr 0.145 pounds per square inch (PSI) 10.197 centimetres of water (cmH$_2$O)	

Measurement of flow

Flow is the amount of substance moving past a fixed point per unit time and may be laminar or turbulent. In anaesthesia, its units are usually expressed in litres per minute (l.min^{-1}). Laminar and turbulent flow are each governed by different laws, as shown in *Figure 6.3.3*.

An orifice creates a resistance to fluid flowing through it, resulting in a drop in pressure. This can be used to produce a classification of devices that measure flow, depending on whether or not the orifice is of a fixed size and whether or not the pressure difference across the orifice is of a fixed magnitude (see *Table 6.1.2*).

Table 6.1.2: Methods for measuring flow.

Methods of measuring flow		
	Variable orifice	**Constant orifice**
Variable pressure	Watersight flowmeter	Pneumotachograph Water depression flowmeter
Constant pressure	'Bobbin' flowmeter Wright peak flowmeter	Bubble flowmeter
Other methods		
Hot wire flowmeters Pitot tubes Ultrasonic flowmeters Using a device that measures volume (e.g. Wright respirometer) and integrating the result with time		

Measurement of temperature

Temperature is the property that dictates whether heat energy is transferred into or out of a system. Heat will flow from a body with a higher temperature to one with a lower temperature. The base SI unit of temperature is the kelvin (K), but Celsius (°C) is an acceptable derived unit within the system. Several methods can be employed to measure temperature and some of the more commonly used ones are discussed in this chapter. A suggested classification of temperature measurement is shown in *Table 6.1.3*.

Table 6.1.3: Methods of measuring temperature and unit conversions.

Methods of measuring temperature	
Electrical	**Non-electrical**
Resistance thermometer	Fluid expansion thermometers
Thermistor	• Liquid expansion • Gas expansion
Thermocouple	Bimetallic strip
Infra-red thermometers	Liquid crystal thermometers
1 unit of K is equal to:	
1 Celsius (°C) 1.8 Fahrenheit (°F)	
To convert K into...	
Celsius = K − 273.15 Fahrenheit = $\frac{9K}{5} - 459.67$	

Measurement of oxygen

Oxygen is the most important gas that anaesthetists work with. As such, methods used to measure it are commonly asked about in exams. A suggested classification of devices that measure oxygen is provided in *Table 6.1.4*.

Table 6.1.4: Methods for measuring oxygen.

Methods of measuring oxygen		
In vivo	**In a gas**	**In a blood sample**
Arterial • Pulse oximeter (measures saturations, not PO_2) • Transcutaneous PO_2 measurement Venous • Fibreoptics (e.g. jugular venous bulb oxygen monitoring)	Fuel cell Paramagnetic analyser Mass spectrometer	Clark electrode

The blood gas machine

The blood gas machine incorporates several of the components described in this chapter, such as the Clark electrode, Severinghaus electrode and pH electrode. Many calculations can be performed by the machine to derive other variables; a commonly asked question concerns which of the variables provided by the blood gas machine are directly measured and which are calculated based on the measurements and this information is shown in *Table 6.1.5*.

Table 6.1.5: Table showing measured and calculated variables provided by a blood gas machine.

Measured	Calculated
pH	HCO_3^-
PO_2	Base deficit
PCO_2	
Haemoglobin (including Hb, HbO, HbCO, MetHb)	
SaO_2*	
$Na^+ K^+ Cl^-$	
Glucose, lactate	

*The oxygen saturations can be measured directly if the machine has a co-oximeter (and is therefore able to measure concentrations of different haemoglobins). However, machines without this capability may still be able to calculate an approximate value for oxygen saturation by using the oxygen dissociation curve and the measured PO_2.

6.2 Pressure gauges

Pressure is force per unit area, and the SI unit is the pascal (Pa). One pascal is equal to a force of one newton applied over one square metre ($1\,N.m^{-2}$). It is measured using a variety of methods that vary with context.

Atmospheric pressure is directly measured using a barometer that contains a liquid. Similarly, a manometer also contains a liquid and is commonly used to measure blood pressure indirectly and non-invasively.

Aneroid (from Greek *a-* 'without' and *nēros* 'wet' or 'damp') gauges do not contain liquid. They provide a more convenient method of measuring high pressures than liquid-containing gauges.

The difference between gauge and absolute pressures should be noted. A gauge pressure is the measured pressure independent of the atmospheric pressure, whereas absolute pressure includes the atmospheric pressure. In other words, gauge pressure is equal to absolute pressure minus atmospheric pressure. For example, the pressure in a filled oxygen cylinder is usually quoted as 137 bar, and that in an 'empty' oxygen cylinder as 0 bar. Both of these are gauge pressures. An 'empty' oxygen cylinder contains gas at atmospheric pressure – it does not contain a vacuum! Therefore, the absolute pressures of a full and empty oxygen cylinder are 138 and 1 bar respectively.

High pressure aneroid gauges

A common type of aneroid gauge is the Bourdon gauge. This design was patented by Eugene Bourdon, a French engineer in 1849. It consists of a flexible tube that is flattened and coiled inside a metal case. A calibrated dial is found on the front of the case and the tube is connected to a pointer at the centre of the coil via a set of gears. The other end of the tube is exposed to the gas supply pressure.

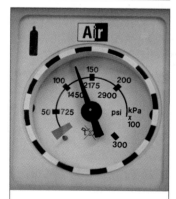

Fig. 6.2.1: A party whistle, like a Bourdon gauge, uncoils as the gas pressure within it increases.

The pressure causes the tube to uncoil (much like a party whistle, *Fig. 6.2.1*) and this rotates the pointer across the dial, indicating the gas pressure (*Fig. 6.2.3*).

 ### Uses
Bourdon gauges are used to measure the high pressure in gas cylinders or pipelines. Those for oxygen, nitrous oxide and air are built into the front of the anaesthetic machine (*Fig. 6.2.2*).

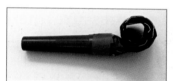 ### Advantages
- Modern Bourdon gauges can be accurate to 0.1–2%.
- Sensitive to small changes in pressure. This sensitivity can be further improved by adding extra gears to amplify small pressure changes.
- The relationship between the extent of uncoiling and the pressure is linear.

Fig. 6.2.2: A Bourdon gauge found on the front of the anaesthetic machine showing air cylinder pressure.

- No electrical power supply required, although Bourdon gauges can be modified to give a digital electronic output.

Disadvantages
- Sensitive to shocks and vibration.
- Demonstrates hysteresis.
- Sensitive to temperature changes.

(a)   (b)

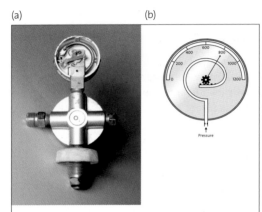

Fig. 6.2.3: (a) A Bourdon gauge with workings visible. Image reproduced with permission from the Anaesthesia Museum, Sheffield Teaching Hospitals NHS Foundation Trust. (b) Schematic of Bourdon gauge mechanism.

Low pressure aneroid gauges

Aneroid gauges used to measure low pressures have some similarities to the Bourdon gauge, for example the bellows gauge. This consists of an elastic chamber (the bellows) through which the pressure to be measured is applied. The bellows expand as the pressure within them increases, causing the movement of a pointer across a calibrated dial via a mechanical link. The range of pressures measured by a particular gauge is dictated by the compliance of the bellows and the configuration of gears in the link.

Uses

These gauges can be used to measure lower pressures such as the patient's airway pressure. Measurements are commonly displayed on the monitor and ventilator in digital form on modern anaesthetic machines.

Outside anaesthetics and medicine, these pressure gauges are used in some aircraft to measure atmospheric pressure and therefore allow the calculation of altitude.

Advantages
- Fast enough response time to allow breath-by-breath measurement of airway pressure.
- Can be modified to give digital electronic output.

Disadvantages
- Large swings in temperature may render the reading inaccurate due to the third perfect gas law (Gay-Lussac's law).

Barometers

A barometer is a device that measures atmospheric pressure (and so is not really a piece of equipment used in anaesthetics), however, the principles of atmospheric pressure measurement are often asked about in examinations. Many different designs of barometer exist, and some are aneroid, but a simple liquid-containing barometer is described here.

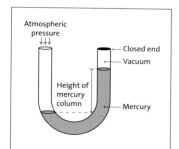

Fig. 6.2.4: A barometer. The height of the mercury column indicates atmospheric (barometric) pressure.

Classically, a barometer is a vertical U-shaped glass tube containing liquid mercury. One end of the tube is closed, and there is a near vacuum in the space between the closed end of the tube and the top of the mercury column. The other end of the tube is open to the atmosphere.

Atmospheric pressure is therefore exerted on the mercury at the open end, forcing the mercury round the U. An increase in pressure causes the mercury column on the closed side of the tube to rise. The height of the column on the closed side above the height on the open side in millimetres is the atmospheric pressure in mmHg. The barometer therefore measures absolute pressure (see *Fig. 6.2.4*).

Technically, the 'vacuum' at the closed end of the tube contains mercury vapour at its SVP. The scale measuring the height of the mercury column should be adjusted to compensate for this – although the effect is small.

Uses
Barometers, by definition, are exclusively used to measure atmospheric pressure.

Advantages
- Very simple to set up and use.

Disadvantages
- The highest atmospheric pressure ever recorded on Earth at the time of writing was 108.57 kPa (814.4 mmHg), and 'normal' atmospheric pressure is considered to be 101.3 kPa (760 mmHg). Therefore, the size of the mercury-containing barometer described above is quite unwieldy.
- Contains toxic mercury, and must have an open end. There is therefore a risk of spillage.

Manometers

Different designs of manometer exist, and many are aneroid; a simple liquid-containing manometer will be described here.

A classic manometer, like a barometer, is a vertical U-shaped glass tube containing a liquid. However, in contrast to the barometer, the liquid is commonly either mercury or water, and both ends of the tube are open.

The pressure to be measured is applied to one end of the tube, and this causes the liquid to move around the U and rise on the opposite side. If the liquid is water then the height difference between the two sides in centimetres is the pressure in cmH_2O, whereas if the liquid is mercury then the height difference in millimetres is the pressure in mmHg. As atmospheric pressure is always being applied to both sides of the tube in a manometer, these devices measure gauge pressure.

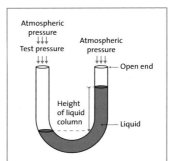

Fig. 6.2.5: A manometer. The pressure to be measured is applied to one side of the tube, forcing the liquid around. The height of the liquid column indicates the pressure being measured. Atmospheric pressure acts on the liquid column from both ends, and is therefore cancelled out.

 ## Uses

The commonest medical use for a liquid manometer is in the indirect, non-invasive measurement of blood pressure.

Advantages

- Simple to use.

Disadvantages

- Although the size of a typical liquid-containing manometer used for blood pressure measurement is not as big as a barometer, they are still bulky. Therefore, aneroid manometers are often used instead.
- Degree of accuracy and precision is lower than some other methods of pressure measurement, and these devices can be operator dependent.

6.3 Flowmeters

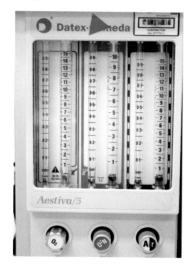

Fig. 6.3.1: A bank of flowmeters mounted on the front of the anaesthetic machine. Small meters read from 0.05 l.min⁻¹ to 1 l.min⁻¹, while the large meters read from 1 l.min⁻¹ to 15 l.min⁻¹.

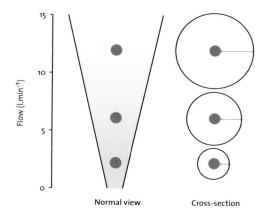

Fig. 6.3.2: Fixed pressure, variable orifice flowmeters showing exaggerated conical shape.

Overview

Constant pressure, variable orifice flowmeters are found on the front of the anaesthetic machine, and also on adaptors that plug into Schrader valves on walls or gas cylinders. Although they appear cylindrical, they are actually conical with their base directed upward. At the apex of the cone there is a needle valve that regulates the flow of gas into the flowmeter. Inside the cone there is a bobbin that moves in the gas flow allowing the flow to be read from a calibrated scale.

The cone of the flowmeter is made of plastic or glass and is coated with a transparent anti-static material; there is also sometimes a conductive strip to prevent the bobbin sticking due to static. The shape of the bobbin varies, but there is often a groove to make them spin in the gas flow and a visual indicator to make it easy to see that they are spinning and have not become stuck. The scale is read parallel with the equator of a spherical bobbin and from the top of a cylindrical one.

Uses

Flowmeters provide a simple visual measurement of each gas as it flows through the anaesthetic machine or out of a gas cylinder or pipeline.

How it works

As the needle valve is opened, gas enters the flowmeter and exerts a force on the bobbin, pushing it upward. The gas flows around the bobbin and on into the back bar, however, the bobbin acts as an obstruction to flow and so there is a pressure drop across it. At equilibrium, the pressure drop is equal to the bobbin's weight (mass multiplied by gravity) divided by its cross-sectional area, and is therefore constant, hence 'constant pressure'. As the bobbin moves upwards inside in the centre of the cone, the gap (or 'orifice') between the bobbin and the side of the flowmeter increases, hence 'variable orifice' (see *Fig. 6.3.2*).

The flowmeter is designed so that at any given flow, the bobbin will reach an equilibrium position where the force of the gas moving in the upward direction is exactly balanced by the force of gravity acting on the bobbin in the downward direction. If the flow is increased, the bobbin rises up the cone due to an increase in pressure between the needle valve and the bobbin. Because the flowmeter is conical, there comes a point where the orifice between the bobbin and the side of the cone has enlarged sufficiently to accommodate the increased flow. This drop in resistance to gas flow reduces the pressure on the bobbin and the force in the upward direction is once again balanced by the force in the downward direction due to gravity. If the flowmeter was cylindrical instead of conical, opening up the needle valve to deliver even a small flow of gas would lead to the bobbin shooting out of the top of the flowmeter, akin to a pea-shooter.

Advantages

- Cheap and simple.
- No electrical power required for use.
- Quick and easy to obtain desired flow and to read the current flow.
- Accurate for flows used clinically (+/− 2.5%). Some machines have a smaller sized flowmeter for lower flows (e.g. 0 to 1 l.min^{-1}) to increase accuracy.

Disadvantages

- Bobbin can get stuck due to static or dirt, leading to inaccurate readings.

Safety

- The oxygen flowmeter is always on the left side of UK anaesthetic machines and the needle valve controller is ribbed so that it can be easily be identified, should you find yourself in the unfortunate situation of delivering anaesthesia in the dark!
- Oxygen always enters the back bar downstream of other gases, which prevents oxygen escaping should a crack develop in one of the other flowmeters.
- The oxygen flow on some anaesthetic machines cannot be reduced below 300 ml.min^{-1} – approximately the theoretical minimum adult oxygen consumption.
- A chain links oxygen and nitrous oxide flowmeters so that N_2O cannot be delivered without also giving a minimum concentration of O_2.

Other notes

The characteristics of the flowmeter at high flows are different to those at low flows. When the bobbin is at the bottom of the meter, the gas flow and velocity are low and the orifice is small. Therefore, flow around the bobbin at the bottom of the meter is laminar and is partially dependent on the viscosity of the gas. When the flow is increased, the gas velocity increases and the orifice becomes larger. The flow around the bobbin at the top of the meter therefore becomes turbulent and the flow is then partially dependent on the density of the gas. Flowmeters are therefore calibrated for a particular gas. The tapering of an air flowmeter will be different to that of a helium flowmeter because although these gases have similar viscosities, their densities are very different.

The density of a gas varies with its temperature and pressure, while its viscosity varies only with its temperature. These variables therefore theoretically introduce a source of error into the flowmeter reading.

Effect of temperature

Because laminar flow of gas is partially dependent on viscosity, and the viscosity varies with temperature, a variation in temperature may result in an inaccurate reading when there is low gas flow. As the temperature of a gas increases, so does its viscosity. From the Hagen–Poiseuille equation (*Fig. 6.3.3*) it can be seen that as viscosity increases, laminar flow decreases. Therefore, a reduced gas

$$Laminar\ Flow = \frac{\pi Pr^4}{8\eta l} = \frac{\pi Pd^4}{128\eta l}$$

$$Turbulent\ flow \propto \frac{\sqrt{P}}{\sqrt{\rho l}}$$

Fig. 6.3.3: The Hagen–Poiseuille equation for laminar flow and determinants of turbulent flow. P = pressure gradient, r = radius of tube, d = diameter of tube, η = viscosity of fluid, l = length of tube, ρ = density of fluid.

flow will occur in the flowmeter if the temperature is high under laminar conditions. However, the scale on the flowmeter cannot change, so although the true flow has decreased, the reading from the scale is higher than the true value – this is known as over-reading. Similarly, at low temperatures the flowmeter will under-read under laminar conditions.

High flow results in turbulence, and the flow then becomes more dependent on the gas density. As the temperature of the gas increases, its density decreases. As the density of a gas decreases, turbulent flow increases. Therefore, an increased gas flow will occur in the flowmeter if the temperature is high under turbulent conditions. Again, the scale cannot change and so although the true rate of flow has increased, the reading is lower than the true value – this is known as under-reading. Similarly, at low temperatures the flowmeter will over-read under turbulent conditions.

Effect of pressure
Gas viscosity is independent of pressure and therefore a change in pressure will have no effect on laminar flow. Flowmeters running at low flows will therefore be accurate, no matter what the ambient pressure.

The density of a gas decreases as its pressure decreases. Turbulent flow increases as the density of the gas decreases. Therefore there will be increased flow in the meter as the pressure falls under turbulent conditions. The meter therefore under-reads as the ambient pressure falls because the true flow is higher than that indicated on the scale. Similarly, should the pressure of the gas increase, the flowmeter will over-read under turbulent conditions.

The Reynolds number
The Reynolds number dictates when flow is likely to be laminar and when it is likely to be turbulent (*Fig. 6.3.4*). The lower this number (especially below 2000) the more likely flow is to be laminar. The equation to calculate the Reynolds number has density as a numerator.

$$Reynolds\ number = \frac{v\rho d}{\eta}$$

Figure 6.3.4: Equation for calculating the Reynolds number. v = fluid velocity, ρ = density of fluid, d = diameter of the tube, η = viscosity of fluid.

During turbulent flow, if the ambient pressure drops sufficiently to cause the Reynolds number to fall below 2000, flow in the meter may become laminar when it would usually be turbulent. Because the flowmeter is calibrated for turbulence at high flows, it would become inaccurate under these conditions. A similar problem would occur if the ambient pressure was very high while using low flows: the flow may become turbulent where they should usually be laminar, making the flowmeter inaccurate.

Figure 6.3.5 shows the changes in flow that occur under different conditions – not a problem during your average surgical list!

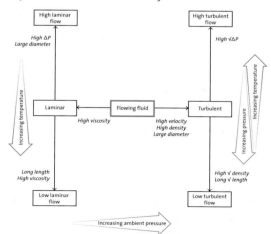

Figure 6.3.5: What affects flow?

6.4 The fuel cell

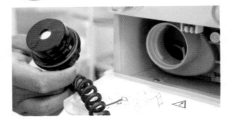

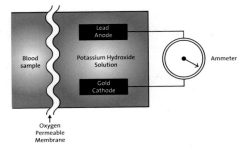

Fig. 6.4.1: The fuel cell removed from covering on anaesthetic machine.

Fig. 6.4.2: Schematic of a fuel cell.

Overview

A fuel cell, also known as a galvanic oxygen analyser, is a device that measures oxygen tension.

Uses

A fuel cell is usually placed at the common gas outlet of an anaesthetic machine to measure the partial pressure of oxygen in the gas entering the breathing system.

How it works

The fuel cell consists of two electrodes, a positive anode made of lead and a negative cathode made of gold, immersed in a solution of potassium hydroxide. The KOH solution is separated from the gas being measured by a membrane that is selectively permeable to oxygen.

The oxygen from the gas diffuses across the membrane and dissolves in the KOH solution until equilibrium is achieved, meaning the partial pressure of oxygen in the solution is equal to that in the gas. At the cathode, oxygen combines with water and electrons to form hydroxyl ions. The reaction at the cathode is therefore:

$$O_2 + 4e^- + 2H_2O \rightarrow 4(OH)^-$$

The hydroxyl ions then react with the lead at the anode to form lead oxide, water and electrons:

$$Pb + 2OH^- \rightarrow PbO + H_2O + 2e^-$$

Electrons are therefore consumed at the cathode and liberated at the anode. This cycle causes an electric current to be generated. The magnitude of the current is measured with an ammeter, and is directly proportional to the rate of these reactions, which in turn are proportional to the partial pressure of oxygen dissolved in the solution. The latter can therefore be calculated.

The above reactions occur spontaneously and no external power is required as the fuel cell behaves as a battery. The response time of a fuel cell is approximately 20 seconds.

⊕ Advantages

- Requires no external power source.
- Small.
- Accurate to within 2–3%.
- Performance of a fuel cell is not affected by water vapour.

⊖ Disadvantages

- Specially adapted fuel cells are required if nitrous oxide is part of the gas mixture, due to the accumulation of nitrogen.
- Fuel cells must be replaced after 6–12 months – they have a limited life span like any battery. The life span is inversely proportional to the oxygen exposure.
- Require regular two-point calibration to maintain accuracy. The fuel cell is calibrated by exposure to air (21% oxygen) and to 100% oxygen.
- Poor response time (approximately 20 seconds).

Other notes

The other device by which the anaesthetic machine measures oxygen tension is the paramagnetic oxygen analyser (see *Section 6.6*).

6.5 Infrared gas analysers

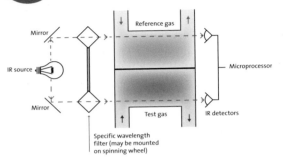

Fig. 6.5.1: A basic infrared gas analyser.

Overview

The infrared gas analyser measures the partial pressure of a gas in a mixture. Molecules that consist of two or more different elements absorb infrared radiation, but those that consist of only one element do not. Therefore, in anaesthetic practice the infrared technique can be used to measure carbon dioxide, nitrous oxide and the volatile agents, but not oxygen, nitrogen or helium.

Uses

The infrared analyser is the method by which the anaesthetic machine measures the partial pressures of volatile agents, nitrous oxide and carbon dioxide. The pressures are usually displayed as a continuous graph of partial pressure against time called the capnograph (see *Section 6.9*).

How it works

The wavelength of visible light ranges from approximately 400 nm to 750 nm. Infrared is invisible to the human eye and has a longer wavelength (but lower frequency, hence *infra*red) than this. Different molecules absorb infrared light to different extents. The analyser uses an appropriate wavelength that is well absorbed by the substance being measured, and that is also sufficiently distant from wavelengths corresponding to the absorption peaks of other substances, since these may cause interference. For example, a convenient carbon dioxide absorption peak is at a wavelength of 4.28 μm, which is a sufficient distance from the nitrous oxide absorption peak at 4.5 μm (see *Fig. 6.5.2*).

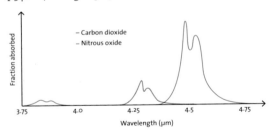

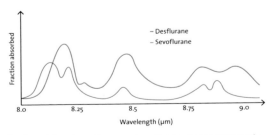

Fig. 6.5.2: The absorption spectra of some gases commonly encountered in anaesthesia.

Light from an infrared source is passed through a filter before entering the analysing chamber, which is made of a substance transparent to infrared such as sapphire (glass is not used because it absorbs some infrared). The filter ensures that infrared light of only one specific wavelength is used, so if the gas in question is carbon dioxide, then the filter will only allow light with a wavelength of 4.28 μm to enter the chamber. As the light passes through the gas, it is absorbed and its intensity decreases. Using a photodetector, the magnitude of the intensity reduction is calculated, and this in turn can be used to calculate the partial pressure of the gas.

One method of reducing potential errors in the system is the use of a reference chamber which is the same design as, and shares the same infrared source as the analysing chamber, but does not contain the gas being measured (it usually contains CO_2-free air). Therefore there is no absorption of infrared at the wavelength of interest, and the intensity of light should not change. If it does, the detected change must be due to something other than light absorption by the gas, such as power fluctuations causing output from the light source to vary. The output from the analysing chamber can be corrected using the output from the reference chamber to reduce errors in the measurement.

⊕ Advantages

- Infrared analysers in clinical use have a good degree of accuracy and precision.
- Simpler than many other methods of gas analysis (e.g. mass spectrometry, see *Section 6.7*).
- Response time is fast enough for breath-by-breath analysis.
- Can analyse the gas mixture for several different gases at once by using different wavelength filters.

⊖ Disadvantages

- Water vapour can interfere with infrared absorption and so gases must be dried before entering the analyser. Gas is therefore conducted to the analyser by Nafion (a modified form of Teflon) tubing, which is selectively and highly permeable to water vapour.
- The analyser must undergo regular two-point calibration.
- Collision broadening (the change in the width of the absorption peak for one gas that occurs when it is mixed with another gas) must be compensated for. This was classically a problem with mixtures of carbon dioxide and nitrous oxide, and caused the older analysers to falsely report a higher partial pressure of carbon dioxide.

Other notes

Modern infrared analysers are able to measure the partial pressure of more than one gas in the mixture as it passes through the analysing chamber. To do this, more than one filter is needed – each allowing a different wavelength of infrared into the chamber and therefore each measuring a different gas.

Not all the different wavelengths can enter the chamber at once, so the filters are mounted on a wheel that spins in front of the light source and allows each wavelength into the chamber one after the other. This gives an intermittent signal for each wavelength – amplification of which is easier than if it were constant. The intermittent system also requires calibration less frequently due to the smaller tendency of the signal to drift.

6.6 Paramagnetic oxygen analysers

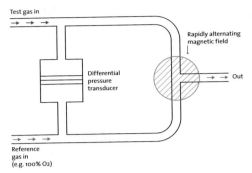

Test gas in

Rapidly alternating
magnetic field

Differential
pressure
transducer

Out

Reference
gas in
(e.g. 100% O2)

Fig. 6.6.1: The paramagnetic oxygen analyser.

Overview

Because gaseous oxygen is a molecule that consists only of oxygen and no other elements, it does not absorb infrared radiation. Therefore infrared gas analysers cannot be used to measure its partial pressure.

Molecular oxygen is, however, paramagnetic. This means that it is attracted by magnetic fields – a property that distinguishes it from many other gases, which are usually weakly diamagnetic and therefore repelled by magnetic fields. Paramagnetism occurs due to the unpaired electrons in the outer shells of the oxygen atoms spinning in the same direction.

The extent to which a gas mixture is attracted by a magnetic field can be used to measure its oxygen content.

Uses

The paramagnetic analyser is used on anaesthetic machines to measure the partial pressure of oxygen in the gas delivered to, and expired by, the patient. The anaesthetic machine may also have other oxygen analysers, e.g. a fuel cell (*Section 6.4*).

The paramagnetic analyser helps prevent a hypoxic mixture being delivered, which is especially likely when low gas flows are employed. The anaesthetic machine monitor alarms when the detected partial pressure of oxygen falls below a set limit.

How it works

In modern paramagnetic oxygen analysers, the gas to be tested flows into one tube and a reference gas with a known oxygen concentration flows into a parallel tube. The gases then pass through flow restrictors and subsequently into a magnetic field that is rapidly switched on and off (at approximately 100 Hz). The higher the oxygen content of the gas, the more it moves towards the magnetic field. Due to the flow restrictor, the faster flowing gas leaves an area of low pressure behind it and a differential pressure transducer can be used to compare the gas pressure between the test tube and the reference tube. The pressure difference between the test gas and the reference gas is used to calculate the oxygen content in the test gas.

Older paramagnetic analysers use a gas-tight chamber with a set of two glass balls containing nitrogen gas connected by a bar in a 'dumb-bell' arrangement. The dumb-bell is exposed to a uniform magnetic field and is suspended by a wire so it can rotate. Rotation occurs when the test gas passes through the chamber and is attracted into the magnetic field. The extent of the rotation is proportional to the partial pressure of oxygen in the mixture.

There are two methods of measuring the angle of rotation of the dumb-bell. One is to have a mirror on the dumb-bell that reflects a beam of light and a photodetector array can then measure the angle of the reflection of this beam. The other method is to use an electric motor to resist the rotational movement. The magnitude of the current required by the motor to stop the dumb-bell rotating is then proportional to the oxygen partial pressure. The latter is a null-deflection method and is more accurate.

Older paramagnetic analysers often have a much slower response time of up to 60 seconds.

➕ Advantages

- Highly sensitive, accurate and precise.
- Modern analysers have a fast response time and can measure the partial pressure of oxygen on a breath-by-breath basis.
- Do not require regular calibration.

➖ Disadvantages

- Analysers are potentially made inaccurate by condensation of water vapour, but have a water trap incorporated to avoid this.
- In theory, the magnetic properties of other gases will cause interference. However, there are very few other substances in anaesthetics that are paramagnetic. Nitric oxide is the only other paramagnetic gas that may occasionally be encountered clinically and it does not interfere for two reasons: one is that nitric oxide is used in tiny quantities (up to 150 ppm) and the other is that the magnitude of its paramagnetic properties is small compared with oxygen. Oxygen has a magnetic susceptibility more than twice that of nitric oxide. Similarly, the diamagnetic properties of gases such as carbon dioxide, nitrous oxide and the volatile anaesthetics are of such a small magnitude that they are not able to significantly affect the paramagnetic analyser. The magnetic susceptibility of oxygen is more than 160 times that of CO_2 and N_2O.

❗ Safety

- Paramagnetic analysers are very reliable, but failure may risk exposure of the patient to a hypoxic gas mixture.

Other notes

A method of indirectly measuring carbon dioxide concentration in a gas mixture by measuring the change in oxygen concentration with a paramagnetic analyser before and after the gas passes through soda lime was suggested in the 1970s. It is not used in clinical practice today.

6.7 Other methods of gas analysis

Raman scatter

When photons of light collide with a substance, scattering (deviation of the photons from their original course) takes place. Most scattering is elastic, resulting in no change in the photons' energy state; this is known as Rayleigh scatter. A tiny proportion (approximately 0.00001%) of photons will be scattered inelastically, causing the release of a photon with a different, usually lower energy (and therefore wavelength). This is known as Raman scatter and, because the change in wavelength is specific to the substance, it can be used to analyse a mixture of gases.

In a Raman analyser, an argon laser is passed through a chamber containing the gas mixture. Being a laser, the incident light is all of the same wavelength. Some of the light undergoes Raman scatter. The change in wavelength will be specific to the gas (e.g. the wavelength of light scattered after colliding with oxygen will be different to that scattered after colliding with carbon dioxide). The analyser then uses narrow-band filters to collect the scattered photons. By using separate filters and photodetectors, the intensity of light at different wavelengths can be individually measured. The intensity of light at a given wavelength will be proportional to the concentration of the gas in the mixture that produced it.

Advantages
- Fast enough response time for breath-by-breath analysis.
- Despite the fact that a small amount of volatile anaesthetic is burned by the laser in the analysis process, the sampled gas can be returned to the breathing system.
- Can analyse a mixture for many different gases at the same time.

Disadvantages
- Currently very expensive to produce. No products are currently available in the UK.

Colorimetric analysis

Colorimetric analysers are simple tools used to detect the presence of carbon dioxide. They can be used to help confirm correct position of an endotracheal tube when formal capnography is not immediately available. They consist of a transparent plastic case with a pH indicator inside. Carbon dioxide dissolves in condensed water vapour and forms carbonic acid. This leads to a fall in the pH, which causes the indicator to change colour (see *Fig. 6.7.1*).

Advantages
- Cheap and simple to use.
- Disposable.

Disadvantages
- Semi-qualitative measurements only.
- Limited accuracy.

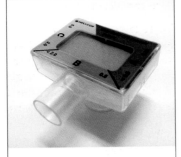

Fig. 6.7.1: A colorimetric carbon dioxide detector. The device can be incorporated into a breathing system using the connectors.

Mass spectrometry

The use of this technique for clinical work has been abandoned due to expense, the size of the machine, and the availability of more practical methods of gas analysis in theatre (e.g. infrared). The mass spectrometer works by first ionizing the gas, and then separating the ions on the basis of their mass-to-charge ratio (*Fig. 6.7.2*).

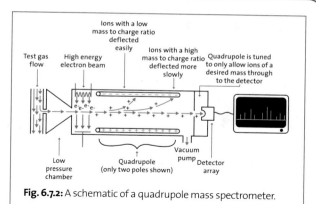

Fig. 6.7.2: A schematic of a quadrupole mass spectrometer.

A tiny sample of test gas is drawn into a low pressure chamber and some of this sample is then allowed to leak into an adjacent ionization chamber, within which there is a near vacuum. A high energy electron beam is passed across the gas as it enters this chamber, causing the molecules to break up (or 'crack') into positively charged fragments of different masses. The cracking pattern is the molecule's fingerprint, and it allows the spectrometer to distinguish between gases of the same molecular weight (e.g. CO_2 and N_2O). Due to their ionization, the fragments can be accelerated by electric and magnetic fields. They are drawn into a region of static and oscillating electromagnetic fields, the quadrupole, that is tuned to allow only ions of a particular mass-to-charge ratio to reach the detector. The tuning is varied so that a spectrum of mass-to-charge ratios is scanned, and from this the composition of the original gas mixture can be reconstructed. Response times of approximately 100 milliseconds are possible.

In principle, mass spectrometry can be used to identify unknown compounds and this is the reason that NASA includes such devices on exploratory spacecraft such as Voyager and the Mars Rovers. However, these machines are likely to only encounter small, simple molecules. The analysis of larger molecules (e.g. anaesthetic vapours and organic compounds) can become very complicated, and so knowledge of which gases are likely to be present in the mixture makes the task much easier.

Where mass spectrometry has been employed in anaesthesia, there was often only one machine per department. Gas samples from each theatre therefore had to be analysed one at a time, meaning continuous analysis of gas from any one patient was not possible. This, along with the fact that gas had to travel a considerable distance from a patient to the machine, also meant that (despite the machine's fast analysis time) there was a delay before information was available for the anaesthetist and therefore results were not contemporary.

Advantages
- The technique is capable of rapidly producing very accurate and precise results.

Disadvantages
- Although the mass spectrometer itself has a fast response time, the way it was used in anaesthesia meant that breath-to-breath analysis was not possible.
- Expensive.
- Relatively large and bulky.
- Gas sample cannot be returned to the breathing system.

Piezoelectric absorption

A crystal of quartz can be made to resonate at its natural frequency by the application of an alternating current. This is the piezoelectric effect, and the oscillation frequency can be measured. A piezoelectric gas analyser is designed to measure the concentration of volatile anaesthetic agents in a gas mixture. In the analyser, a crystal is coated in silicone oil in which volatile agent dissolves. The amount of anaesthetic dissolved is proportional to the concentration in the gas mixture, and as it dissolves the anaesthetic causes a change in the resonant frequency of the crystal. This change in frequency can be measured and compared to the resonant frequency of a second crystal that is not coated in oil which acts as a reference. The concentration of anaesthetic can then be calculated.

Advantages
- Good response time, although not as fast as infrared analysers.
- Cheap.

Disadvantages
- Cannot detect oxygen, nitrous oxide or carbon dioxide.
- Cannot differentiate between the different volatile agents.
- Nitrous oxide will also dissolve in the oil, making the measurement of volatile anaesthetic inaccurate. This must be compensated for.

Gas chromatography

The gas mixture to be analysed is transported by an inert carrier gas (such as helium, argon or nitrogen) through a column containing stationary microscopic solid fragments covered in a thin layer of a liquid such as polyethylene glycol. The constituents of the gas mixture dissolve in the liquid to differing degrees, depending on their solubility. The flow of each different constituent through the column is therefore slowed by a different amount, resulting in the separation of the mixture into its component gases. The individual gases are then detected as they leave the column, and the concentrations in the original mixture can be calculated by reference to standard samples. Many different types of detector are used, depending on the chemistry of the gases being analysed.

Advantages
- Very accurate and can detect tiny concentrations of a substance.

Disadvantages
- Unable to continuously analyse a flowing gas, as would occur in an anaesthetic breathing system.
- Need to have some knowledge of which gases are present in the mixture before analysis to measure their concentrations.
- Impractical for clinical purposes, but is used as a research tool.

Laser refractometry

Although this method of gas analysis is not used routinely in the operating theatre, it is the principal method used by manufacturers of anaesthetic vaporizers to ensure accurate calibration of their products. They are also used to measure environmental concentrations of anaesthetic vapours in operating theatres in order to check they are below safe levels.

The speed of light is reduced as it passes through a transparent substance such as a gas and the magnitude of the reduction depends on the concentration of gas present. The ratio of the speed of light in a vacuum to the speed of light through the gas is the refractive index of the gas.

In a laser refractometer, a coherent monochromatic light beam (i.e. a laser) is split into two. Half travels through a chamber containing the test gas, and half passes through a reference chamber that contains a near-vacuum. The light passing through the test gas is slowed so that it becomes out of phase with the light passing through the reference chamber. When the beams of light are reunited and focused onto a screen, an interference pattern is produced. Bright lines occur where the light from the two chambers is in phase, and dark lines ('fringes') where it is out of phase. The appearance of the fringes will depend on the refractive index of the gas, and this in turn depends on the concentration of the gas. Therefore, the lines can be used to determine the gas concentration in the mixture.

Advantages
- Portable analysers are available.
- Tiny concentrations of anaesthetic can be detected (down to 0.0001%).

Disadvantages
- Unable to perform breath-by-breath analysis.
- Must know the refractive index of the substance being analysed in order to measure its concentration.

Ultraviolet spectrometry

This is very similar to infrared absorption analysis, but uses absorption of ultraviolet rather than infrared light to analyse the gas mixture. Gases that contain only one element (such as O_2, N_2 and He) can be analysed as well as gases containing several elements (such as CO_2, N_2O and the volatile agents). The only analyser based on ultraviolet spectrometry available for clinical use was for the measurement of halothane. They are therefore obsolete and of historical interest only.

Disadvantages
- Ultraviolet light has sufficient energy to cause breakdown of halothane, yielding molecules that are toxic. The sampled gas cannot therefore be returned to the breathing system.

- Activation of the alarm opens the breathing system to the atmosphere, so that at least 21% oxygen is delivered.
- It is not possible to prevent the alarm sounding in the event of an oxygen supply failure.
- It is not possible to reset the alarm or anaesthetic supply until the oxygen pressure is reinstated.

Other notes

Oxygen delivery is so important that there are several different mechanisms on anaesthetic machines that help prevent failure. The alarm described above is one, but others include the following.

- Oxygen is the last gas to be added from the flowmeters. This helps to prevent hypoxic mixtures in the event that a flowmeter is damaged.
- The pin-index system, colour coding, NIST system and collars on Schrader valves help prevent connection of the wrong gas to the oxygen inlet on the anaesthetic machine.
- The chain-link device that links the oxygen and nitrous oxide flowmeters.
- The monitor has an alarm that signals if the paramagnetic analyser and/or fuel cell indicate a low inspired fraction of oxygen.
- The monitor has an alarm that signals if the pulse oximeter indicates a low oxygen saturation in the patient.

6.9 Capnograph waveforms

The capnograph is a plot of the partial pressure of carbon dioxide against time. Measurement of carbon dioxide in expired gas is achieved using an infrared gas analyser. These may be classified as main stream or side stream, depending on the part of the breathing system that the gas is sampled from.

A main stream capnograph is an infrared analyser that is attached to the breathing circuit close to the patient. It analyses the gas mixture *in situ* without the need to remove a sample. Main stream analysers have an almost instant response time but are heavy, add bulk to the breathing system and increase its dead space. They usually measure only carbon dioxide, and not other anaesthetic gases.

A side stream capnograph is located at a distance from the breathing system, usually incorporated in a gas module on the monitor, with the ability to measure other anaesthetic gases. Gas is aspirated from the breathing system via a 1.2 mm internal diameter Nafion tube at rates of approximately 50–150 ml.min^{-1}. Nafion is a type of Teflon, and is used because it is inert and does not react with volatile agents. It is impermeable to carbon dioxide but not to water vapour, allowing the gas to be dried as it travels to the analyser. The gas passes from the breathing system, down the Nafion tubing, through a moisture trap before being analysed. It is then either returned to the breathing system (which is necessary for true low-flow anaesthesia), or vented into the scavenging system. Side stream capnographs have a slower response time because the gas has to travel from the patient to the analyser; however, the delay of usually less than a second is acceptable.

Normal

The normal capnograph trace is split into four phases. Phase one represents the end of inspiration and the beginning of expiration, when the CO_2-free gas that occupied dead space in the airway is exhaled. Phase two represents a rapid rise in PCO_2 as alveolar gas appears. In normal lungs there is then a plateau (phase three) where expiration continues but PCO_2 does not rise any further. The end of this phase is taken as end-tidal CO_2 (EtCO$_2$), just prior to phase four which is a sharp drop in PCO_2 to zero, representing inspiration.

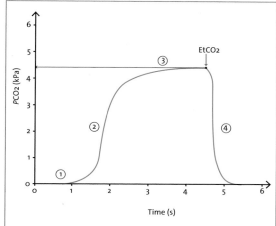

Fig. 6.9.1: A normal capnograph trace divided into four phases.

Hyperventilation

Hyperventilation causes the EtCO₂ to fall. The shape of the capnograph trace is otherwise preserved. A fall in EtCO₂ may be caused by reduced production as well as over-ventilation. See capnograph trace during cardiac arrest (*Fig 6.9.9*).

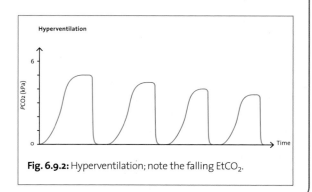

Fig. 6.9.2: Hyperventilation; note the falling EtCO₂.

Hypoventilation

Hypoventilation causes the EtCO₂ to rise. The shape of the capnograph trace is otherwise preserved. A rise in EtCO₂ may be caused by increased production as well as under-ventilation. Increased production is associated with hypermetabolic states and may occasionally be a sign of malignant hyperthermia.

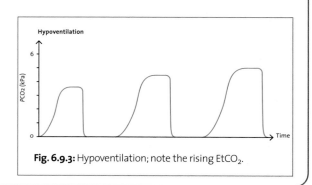

Fig. 6.9.3: Hypoventilation; note the rising EtCO₂.

Rebreathing

Rebreathing occurs when the fraction of inspired CO₂ (FiCO₂) rises above zero. The shape of the capnograph wave form is otherwise preserved, except that EtCO₂ will also rise as a consequence. Causes of rebreathing include exhausted soda lime in a circle breathing system, or insufficient FGF in Mapleson systems. *Figure 6.9.4* shows the FiCO₂ at a constant level above zero. However, in some circumstances, the baseline may rapidly rise.

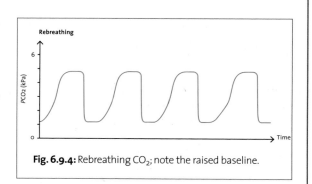

Fig. 6.9.4: Rebreathing CO₂; note the raised baseline.

Lower airway obstruction

The capnograph representing lower airway obstruction is seen in patients with chronic obstructive lung diseases such as emphysema and asthma. It is also seen acutely during bronchospasm. Phase two of the capnograph is seen to have a reduced gradient, and phase three may be missing altogether. This effect is caused by areas of lung with obstructed bronchi emptying more slowly than areas of lung with normal bronchi.

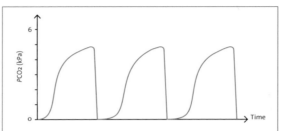

Fig. 6.9.5: Lower airway obstruction; note that the plateau is upward sloping and never levels out.

Loss of neuromuscular blockade

As the effect of neuromuscular blocking drugs wears off, the patient may begin to breathe out of synchrony with the ventilator. If the patient takes a breath during the ventilator expiratory time, this will be seen on the capnograph as a reduction in PCO_2 – which looks like a notch in the plateau phase. These notches are also sometimes known as curare clefts. They may be small, or reach down to a PCO_2 of zero and split the plateau in two.

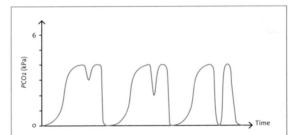

Fig. 6.9.6: Loss of neuromuscular blockade. The 'curare clefts' occur as the patient takes spontaneous breaths.

Cardiac oscillations

These are most easily seen when there is a very slow respiratory rate, or long expiratory time. Instead of phase four being a clean downward stroke, it gradually falls and there are oscillations in the trace. These are due to the pulsations of the heart compressing the airways slightly and moving gas back and forth.

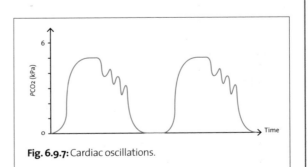

Fig. 6.9.7: Cardiac oscillations.

Oesophageal intubation

Capnography is a highly reliable method of detecting oesophageal intubation. Very little CO_2 is present in the oesophagus. In the event that the endotracheal tube is incorrectly placed in the oesophagus, the capnograph either remains flat during ventilation or small abnormal waveforms will be produced that diminish in height over 2–3 cycles until they are lost altogether. If there is any suspicion that this is what has happened, the tube should be removed immediately.

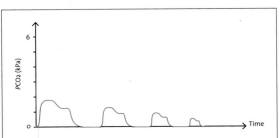

Fig. 6.9.8: Oesophageal intubation; note the irregularly shaped waves and the rapid decline in $EtCO_2$.

Loss of cardiac output

At the point of cardiac arrest, the delivery of CO_2 to the lungs by the circulation stops. Therefore, despite an unchanged minute volume the $EtCO_2$ on the capnograph progressively falls, and will soon become almost undetectable. Capnography is still recommended during resuscitation if the patient is intubated, because chest compressions should restore some blood flow, and therefore CO_2 delivery, to the lungs.

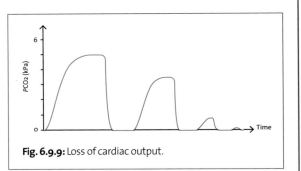

Fig. 6.9.9: Loss of cardiac output.

6.10 Pulse oximeters

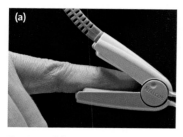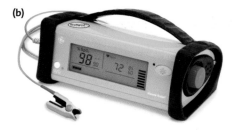

Fig. 6.10.1: (a) A pulse oximeter on a finger. **(b)** The TruSat pulse oximeter. Image reproduced with permission from GE Healthcare.

Overview

Pulse oximeters were introduced in the mid-1980s. They calculate the amount of oxyhaemoglobin (HbO) as a percentage of the total haemoglobin in arterial blood. Pulse oximeters provide a continuous reading of plethysmographic oxygen saturation (SpO$_2$), in other words, the oxygen saturation of pulsatile blood. They also indicate the pulse rate, and many display the tracing of pulsatility against time, known as a plethysmograph.

Uses

AAGBI guidelines state that the continuous monitoring of SpO$_2$ is essential during the administration of any general anaesthetic or sedation. SpO$_2$ monitoring is also essential in critical care areas and in recovery. It is also measured intermittently in patients in non-critical care areas.

How it works

$$I = I_0.e^{-(DC\varepsilon)}$$

$$log \frac{I_0}{I} = DC\varepsilon$$

Fig. 6.10.2: The Beer–Lambert equations. I_0 = incident light, I = emergent light (light after it has passed through the substance), D = distance light travels through the substance, C = concentration of the substance, ε = molar absorption coefficient (a measure of how efficiently a substance absorbs light at a given wavelength). The expression $log(I_0/I)$ in the second equation is known as absorbance.

The pulse oximeter relies on two physical laws, whose combined equation is shown in *Fig. 6.10.2*.

Beer's law
The absorption of radiation as it passes through a substance increases exponentially as the concentration of the substance increases.

Lambert's law
The absorption of radiation as it passes through a substance increases exponentially as the distance it travels through the substance increases.

Detecting the saturation
The pulse oximeter consists of a clip that is usually attached to a finger, toe or earlobe. On one side of the clip are high intensity monochromatic light emitting diodes (LEDs), and on the other is a photo detector. Light from the LEDs passes through tissue before hitting the detector, and the amount of light absorbed by the tissue can be calculated. There are two LEDs, one that emits light at 940 nm (in the infrared spectrum), and one that emits light at 660 nm (in the red spectrum).

Light at 940 nm and 660 nm is absorbed by both HbO and deoxyhaemoglobin (Hb), but with differing efficiency. HbO absorbs more light at 940 nm than Hb, whereas the situation is reversed at 660 nm. *Figure 6.10.3* shows the absorption spectra of Hb and HbO.

The two LEDs are cycled on and off and absorption of each wavelength is measured. Both LEDs are switched off completely after each cycle so that interference from ambient light can be subtracted.

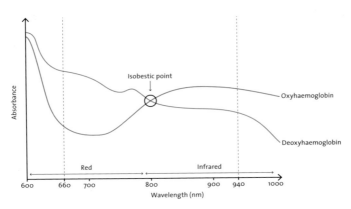

Fig. 6.10.3: The absorption spectra of oxyhaemoglobin and deoxy-haemoglobin. The isobestic point (805 nm) is the wavelength that both types of haemoglobin absorb to the same degree. Another occurs at 590 nm. Older pulse oximeters used the isobestic points as a reference, as absorption of light at these wavelengths is independent of oxygen saturation.

The ratio of absorption at 660 nm to the absorption at 940 nm is calculated, and this ratio can then be used to derive the oxygen saturation using an algorithm. This algorithm corrects the Beer–Lambert equations for the fact that light is not passing through a simple vial of pure haemoglobin, but through living tissue. It is based on data collected from healthy volunteers breathing low-oxygen gas mixtures.

It is important to realize why two wavelengths are used instead of just one. In accordance with the Beer–Lambert laws, if a single wavelength was used alone (e.g. 660 nm) and the system detected a change in light absorption, it would be impossible to decide whether this was due to a change in Hb concentration, HbO concentration, overall haemoglobin concentration, or a change in the thickness of the tissue. The thickness of the tissue may be altered if the cardiac output changes or if vessels in the tissue dilate or constrict for any reason (e.g. due to temperature). The addition of a second wavelength that has different absorption characteristics to the first allows differentiation between these possibilities. Any variation in light absorption caused by a change in tissue thickness or overall haemoglobin concentration would cause the absorption of both wavelengths to change by the same percentage and in the same direction. The ratio of absorbance would therefore be unaltered. In contrast, if the absorbance of light at 660 nm changes differently to that at 940 nm the ratio will shift. The only reason why absorption at one wavelength should change differently to absorption at the other is a change in the relative concentrations of Hb and HbO.

Detecting the pulse

The method described above must be applied to the peak of the pulse wave only, in order that the oximeter measures only the saturation of arterial blood. To do this, the oximeter must measure only the pulsatile component of the absorption signal.

As a pulse of blood enters the tissue during systole, both the concentration of HbO and the distance through the tissue increase. According to the Beer–Lambert law, therefore, the absorption of light rises during systole and then falls back to a baseline during diastole. This diastolic baseline is due to light absorbed by tissues such as venous blood, muscle and skin. The pulsatile signal is obtained by subtracting the diastolic baseline from the total signal.

The whole waveform of the pulse must be captured in order to accurately detect the peak light absorbance, and therefore measurements must be made very frequently throughout the cardiac cycle. The LEDs are therefore switched on and off at a frequency of several hundred hertz. The saturation is calculated using only the absorption ratio at the peak of the pulse.

Technically speaking, the pulse oximeter therefore measures the pulsatile, or 'plethysmographic' oxygen saturation rather than the arterial oxygen saturation. This is the difference between SpO_2 as measured by the pulse oximeter and SaO_2 as measured by the blood gas analyser.

Advantages

- Easy to use, safe, non-invasive.
- Reliable and accurate (+/− 2%) between saturations of 70% and 100% in sinus rhythm.
- Gives a continuous measurement of oxygen saturation and pulse rate.
- Is not affected by the presence of different haemoglobins (e.g. HbF, HbA_2, HbS, etc.) or haemoglobin concentration.

Disadvantages

- The algorithm used to convert the absorption ratio into the saturation is derived from data from healthy volunteers. Because it is considered unethical to reduce a volunteer's oxygen saturation to less than about 75%, the algorithm becomes much less accurate at saturations below this.
- Measurements can become inaccurate in irregular heart rhythms such as atrial fibrillation, or where there is peripheral vasoconstriction and little pulsatile flow in the tissue.
- Interference from movement or nearby electrical devices can cause loss of signal.
- False high measurements may be caused by carboxyhaemoglobin, because it has a similar absorption spectrum to HbO. Readings tend towards 96–97%.
- False low measurements can occur in the presence of methaemoglobinaemia (readings tend towards 85%) and dyes such as methylene blue and indocyanine green. Nail polish (especially if coloured black, green or blue) may also interfere with the reading.

Safety

- Pressure sores and burns may be caused by the oximeter clip, particularly in young children, if the site is not altered at regular intervals.
- It must be remembered that pulse oximetry gives no information about oxygen delivery. A saturation of 100% may be present in a patient who is very anaemic. Similarly, due to the plateau at the top of the sigmoid-shaped oxyhaemoglobin dissociation curve, pulse oximeters are insensitive in detecting hypoxaemia. A patient with normal saturations may have a relatively low PaO_2.

Other notes

Co-oximeters use different wavelengths of light to a standard pulse oximeter to differentiate between different types of haemoglobin (e.g. HbA, HbA_2, HbF, HbS, HbCO, etc.). They tend to be found on blood gas machines and used to analyse blood samples, instead of making measurements *in vivo*.

6.11 Electrocardiographs

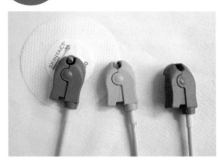

Fig. 6.11.1: ECG electrode and connectors. The red electrode is placed on the right arm, yellow on the left arm, and green on the left leg to form Einthoven's triangle.

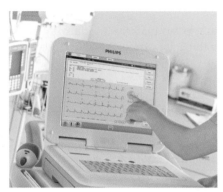

Fig. 6.11.2: The Pagewriter ECG machine. Image supplied by and reproduced with permission from Philips Healthcare.

Overview

The typical resting potential of the interior of a cardiac myocyte may be −80 to −90 mV as compared to the exterior, and this will rise to approximately +30 mV during an action potential. Different groups of cells in the heart are depolarized at different times during the cardiac cycle, and an electrical wave travels through the myocardium. This wave can be detected at the skin surface and displayed as an electrocardiograph (ECG). The ECG is therefore a graph of myocardial electrical potential against time.

Although the change in the membrane potential of an individual myocyte during an action potential is approximately 120 mV, the average signal from the whole heart is attenuated before it reaches the skin surface so that the amplitude of a normal QRS complex is of the order of 1–2 mV.

Uses

The AAGBI considers continuous ECG monitoring as essential during the administration of any general anaesthetic or sedation, and also in critical care areas. The ECG can also be used to obtain a snapshot of electrical activity in the heart.

Continuous ECG monitoring provides some information about the heart rate and rhythm, while a snapshot '12-lead' ECG (see below) is a more sensitive indicator of rhythm, axis, ischaemic changes and subtle electrical abnormalities.

How it works

ECG electrodes

Electrodes are required for the detection of the small electrical changes at the skin surface caused by the heart. There are three electrodes used in the most basic ECG and ten used in a 12-lead ECG (see below).

Electrodes are disposable and consist of thin layers of silver and silver chloride covered in a gel that is rich in chloride ions. Small changes in potential difference at the skin surface cause polarization of the silver/silver chloride electrode and this is transmitted via a cable to the ECG machine where the signal is amplified. *Figure 6.11.1* shows typical ECG electrodes.

Each electrode is referred to by its position, for example, right arm (RA) or left leg (LL). In some cases, the signal from more than one electrode is averaged and treated as a single virtual, or 'indifferent', electrode.

ECG leads

A lead is a measure of the potential difference between two electrodes. For example, lead I measures the difference between LA and RA. The simplest arrangement of three electrodes (RA, LA and LL) produces three bipolar limb leads – I, II and III. These form the approximately equilateral Einthoven's triangle (*Fig. 6.11.3a*).

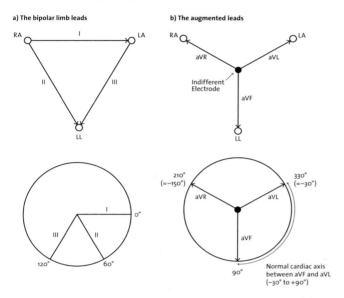

a) The bipolar limb leads

b) The augmented leads

Figure 6.11.3: (a) The bipolar limb leads forming Einthoven's triangle. (b) The augmented leads, formed using an indifferent electrode.

Three more leads can be constructed from Einthoven's triangle. An indifferent electrode can be formed by averaging the signal from all three electrodes and then the signal from each individual electrode measured against this. The signals from these leads have a smaller voltage and require more amplification and are therefore referred to as the augmented leads. For example, aVF is a lead comparing the indifferent electrode and the LL electrode. Because they use an indifferent electrode, they are also sometimes known as the unipolar limb leads (see *Fig. 6.11.3b*).

In a 12-lead ECG, six more leads are added to those already described by adding six more electrodes (C1 to C6) positioned over the anterior chest wall. The signal from each electrode is compared with that from the indifferent electrode to form leads V1 to V6. Because the indifferent electrode is used, these leads are also regarded as unipolar.

The electrode at one end of the lead acts as a positive terminal while the other acts as a negative terminal. Whether a particular electrode is positive or negative depends on the lead. For example, the LA electrode is positive in lead I, but negative in lead III. Indifferent electrodes always act as the negative terminal.

If a depolarization wave travels towards the positive terminal (or a repolarization wave travels away), there will be an upward deflection seen on the ECG in that lead. Similarly, a depolarization wave travelling away from the positive terminal will cause a downward deflection. Because of this directional information, each lead is able to give information about a different anatomical aspect of the heart. Those leads with a positive terminal towards the left of the body (aVL, I, II, V5 and V6) are said to be lateral leads because they give information about the lateral side of the heart. Similarly, II, aVF and III are inferior leads, V1 and V2 are septal leads and V3 and V4 are anterior leads.

This is particularly useful in identifying the coronary vessels responsible for regional ischaemia and anticipating possible complications. For example, acute ST elevation in leads II, III and aVF suggests inferior infarction. The inferior territory is supplied by the right coronary artery and usually this vessel also supplies the atrio-ventricular node. A likely complication of acute inferior myocardial infarction is therefore atrio-ventricular conduction delay or blockade and this can be anticipated thanks to the ECG. Similarly, the anterior territory is supplied by the left anterior descending artery and the lateral territory by the circumflex artery in most people. In a standard 12-lead ECG there is no lead that is orientated to the posterior cardiac territory, although certain inverted changes in the anterior leads may be interpreted as being due to posterior territory pathology in some cases.

While it may appear obvious, it is worth restating that an ECG 'lead' does not refer to any physical wire or cable. It is simply terminology for the comparison of electrical activity detected in two electrodes.

Output
The output from a 3-lead ECG is often displayed on a monitor with no permanent record being kept. Conversely, the 12-lead ECG is usually printed onto a piece of graph paper. Each lead is printed as a separate graph of voltage against time.

The ECG machine is usually calibrated so that each centimetre on the y-axis represents 1 mV, while each 25 mm on the x-axis represents 1 second (i.e. the 'paper speed' is 25 mm.sec^{-1}). This calibration can be deliberately altered to aid resolution of more subtle ECG abnormalities if necessary.

Interference
In order to detect very small amplitude biological signals such as the ECG, the electrical activity of interest (the signal) needs to be distinguished from the interference (the noise). There are several ways of improving the signal to noise ratio.

As stated earlier, a 12-lead ECG uses ten electrodes: RA, LA, LL, C1 to C6 and a ground electrode. The ground electrode is used to reduce interference. The activity in the lead of interest is compared to the activity in the ground electrode and only the differences between these are likely to be due to the ECG signal. Therefore, anything common to both inputs can be discarded as noise. The signal to noise ratio is improved using this method which is known as common mode rejection.

Amplifiers also have a role in reducing interference. The ECG has a frequency of 0.5–100 Hz, and the amplifier in the ECG machine can be set to ignore anything with a frequency outside this range by using high- or low-pass electrical filters.

ECG machines can also be set in 'monitor' or 'diagnostic' mode. In monitor mode, the amplifier only responds to frequencies between 0.5 and 40 Hz and this further reduces interference (due to the narrower bandwidth) at the expense of resolution. In diagnostic mode, the amplifier responds to frequencies between 0.05 and 100 Hz. This allows more accurate interpretation due to higher resolution, but the ECG is more at risk of interference. In practice, diagnostic mode is therefore used almost exclusively for 12-lead ECGs.

ECG cables are shielded with an insulator that helps to reduce induction currents being produced by external sources running on mains electricity.

Interference from surgical diathermy is difficult to eliminate.

⊕ Advantages

- Improved patient safety under anaesthesia.
- Allows rapid detection of changes in heart rate and rhythm, as well as allowing detection of ischaemia and other abnormalities.
- Simple to set up and cheap.

⊖ Disadvantages

- Interference from patient movement and diathermy.
- Misplacement of the electrodes can lead to difficulty in correct interpretation of the ECG, especially when 12 leads are used.

ⓘ Safety

- If the diathermy plate is improperly applied during surgery, so that there is only a small contact point between it and the skin, diathermy current may flow through the ECG electrodes, causing burns to the skin.

Other notes

Alternative electrode placement

Although the electrode configurations described above are the standard ones, others may also be used. Some commonly seen electrode positions include:

- CM5: this is a variation of the 3-lead ECG where the RA electrode is placed on the centre of the manubrium (hence CM) and the LA electrode is placed in the C5 electrode position. CM5 is therefore a variation of the electrode positions used to acquire lead I. It is said to be more sensitive in detecting left ventricular ischaemia than the standard configuration, detecting more than 80% of cases.
- CB5: in this configuration the RA electrode is placed over the right scapula (central back) and the LA electrode is place in the C5 position. This gives better resolution of the P wave and QRS complex and is therefore useful for detection of arrhythmias.

The 'five lead' ECG

The naming of this type of ECG confuses everyone! In a 5-lead ECG, the term 'lead' is used incorrectly because it refers to the cables used to connect the electrodes to the machine.

The 5-lead ECG really should be called a 5-electrode ECG because RA, LA, LL electrodes are used plus a ground electrode, and a single chest electrode instead of C1–C6. This configuration can therefore monitor seven leads: I, II, III, aVR, aVL, aVF and a unipolar chest lead.

This configuration is often used in theatre when high vigilance to the ECG is required. The 5-electrode ECG allows continuous monitoring of more than the standard three leads.

EASI 12-lead

The EASI ECG is a system produced by Philips that uses five electrodes to produce a 12-lead ECG. The electrodes are all placed on the precordium, and a computer uses an algorithm to derive all 12 leads from the data it collects. Philips warn that the EASI system gives an approximation of a conventional 12-lead ECG and that it should not be used for diagnostic purposes.

6.12 Non-invasive blood pressure measurement

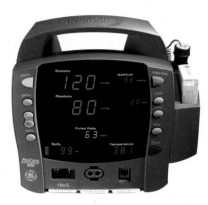

Fig. 6.12.1: A DINAMAP non-invasive blood pressure machine. Image reproduced with permission from GE Healthcare.

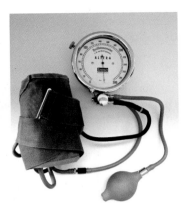

Fig. 6.12.2: An example of Von Reckinghausen's oscillotonometer.

Overview

Arterial blood pressure is usually measured non-invasively using either a cuff and a stethoscope, or an oscillometric device such as the device for indirect non-invasive automated mean arterial pressure (DINAMAP). Both of these methods rely on a cuff that temporarily occludes blood flow through the brachial (or other) artery, but other non-invasive methods also exist.

Uses

The AAGBI considers the monitoring of blood pressure as essential during the administration of any general anaesthetic or sedation. Non-invasive measurement is usually sufficient.

How it works

Auscultation

One of the simplest methods of measuring the blood pressure requires a mercury manometer or aneroid gauge that shows the pressure in a cuff, and a stethoscope. Sounds heard through the stethoscope when it is held over the brachial artery as the cuff pressure is slowly reduced are used to deduce the blood pressure. The sounds were first described by the Russian army surgeon, Nicolai Korotkoff in 1905. There are several theories regarding how the sounds are produced, and the most commonly encountered one is described below.

The cuff must have a width that is 20% greater than the diameter of the arm. It is wrapped around the upper arm and manually inflated while a distal pulse is palpated. The point at which the pulse becomes impalpable is the point at which the systolic pressure is no longer able to overcome the pressure on the artery exerted by the cuff. This is therefore an estimate of the systolic blood pressure.

The cuff is then deflated and the stethoscope is placed over the brachial artery distal to it. The cuff is inflated again to approximately 20 mmHg above the estimated systolic pressure before the pressure is slowly reduced once more while the operator listens through the stethoscope.

When the cuff pressure falls just below systolic, the artery will begin to open and allow blood flow during systole. During diastole, the artery collapses again under the pressure of the cuff and no blood flows. The turbulent blood flow is heard as a rushing noise and the highest pressure where this is audible is taken as the systolic pressure. As the pressure in the cuff continues to fall, more blood is allowed to flow during systole. Eventually, the cuff pressure falls below diastolic pressure and the artery no longer collapses under it. When this occurs, the blood flow becomes laminar again and is therefore not audible. The point at when the sound of turbulent blood flow disappears is taken as the diastolic pressure. The appearance and disappearance of the noise of turbulent blood flow are known as Korotkoff sounds one and five respectively. Korotkoff sounds two, three and four are also described (see *Table 6.12.1*). The mean arterial pressure can be calculated (see *Fig. 6.12.3*).

Table 6.12.1: The sounds heard through the stethoscope during the different Korotkoff phases. In practice, phases 1 and 5 (and occasionally 4) are most important.

Korotkoff phase	Description
1	Onset of clear, crisp, short tapping tones – this is taken to be systolic pressure
2	The crisp tap becomes a softer murmur. There may be an auscultatory gap during this phase where no sound is heard at all. This is why systolic pressure should first be estimated by palpation before the cuff is re-inflated and auscultation is then used. If auscultation is used as the sole method of measuring blood pressure, the auscultatory gap in this phase may be mistaken for the silence above systolic. Systolic pressure would then be underestimated.
3	The sound becomes clearer and more crisp again
4	There is a muffling or muting of the sound
5	The onset of silence. In some patients, particularly some pregnant women this phase does not exist (i.e. sounds continue even with a cuff pressure of zero). In this case, onset of phase 4 should be taken as diastolic pressure.

Oscillometry

The DINAMAP uses a similar system to the one described above, but it is automatic and no auscultation is necessary. The cuff is inflated by a machine and then allowed to fall at a rate of 2–3 mmHg per second. As the turbulent flow begins the artery repeatedly opens and collapses, producing small oscillations in the pressure in the cuff. An electronic pressure gauge connected to a microprocessor detects these oscillations. The point at which they are first detected is taken as systolic pressure, while mean arterial pressure is taken to be the point at which the oscillations are at their greatest amplitude. The diastolic pressure is then calculated. See *Figures 6.12.3 and 6.12.4*.

$$MAP = DP + \frac{SP - DP}{3}$$
$$= \frac{PP}{3}$$
$$= \frac{2DP}{3} + \frac{SP}{3}$$

Fig. 6.12.3: Some different methods of calculating mean arterial pressure (MAP). SP = systolic pressure, DP = diastolic pressure, PP = pulse pressure.

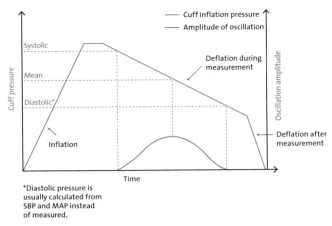

*Diastolic pressure is usually calculated from SBP and MAP instead of measured.

Fig. 6.12.4: The oscillatory method of measuring blood pressure. The blue curve shows the pressure in the cuff and the red curve shows the amplitude of oscillations detected.

Advantages

- Simple to use and gives reliable, accurate measurements.

Disadvantages

- Cuffs that are too small will over-read, while oversized cuffs will under-read.
- Inaccurate measurements obtained if heart rhythm is not regular, especially with automated equipment such as the DINAMAP.
- Difficult to obtain accurate readings (or any readings) if the blood pressure is very high or very low.
- Measurement frequency is limited to a maximum of approximately one reading per minute.

Safety

- Very frequent measurements have been known to cause a petechial rash or neuropraxia of nerves under the cuff, especially if the blood pressure is high.
- Care should be taken in patients with severe peripheral vascular disease.

Other notes

Other methods that are seldom seen in clinical practice are sometimes asked about in exams:

- The Von Recklinghausen oscillotonometer (*Fig. 6.12.2*) was used prior to the invention of the microprocessors used in the DINAMAP. It uses two cuffs, each with an aneroid pressure gauge. The proximal cuff is used to occlude the artery, while the distal cuff is used to measure the oscillations.
- The Penaz technique permits continuous non-invasive measurement of blood pressure, and can be combined with algorithms that allow approximation of cardiac output. One such system is the Finometer (Finapres Medical Systems).

6.13 Invasive blood pressure measurement

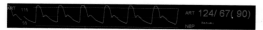 ART 124/ 67(90)

Fig. 6.13.1: A normal arterial blood pressure trace.

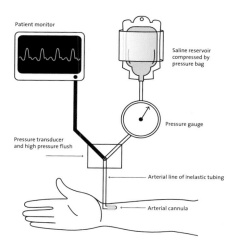

Fig. 6.13.2: A schematic of invasive blood pressure monitoring using a radial artery cannula.

Overview

Invasive blood pressure monitoring refers to techniques that involve direct access to the arterial system in order to obtain the measurement.

Uses

Indications for invasive blood pressure monitoring include the use of vasoactive or inotropic drugs, expectation of large changes in intravascular volume or pressure, and when frequent sampling of arterial blood is required. Invasive monitoring may also be considered in situations when non-invasive readings are likely to be inaccurate, such as when monitoring patients in atrial fibrillation or with morbid obesity.

How it works

A cannula, most commonly 20G, is placed in a peripheral artery and connected to a transducer via a column of pressurized saline. The pressure of this column must be above the systolic blood pressure (300 mmHg is typical). The transducer should be positioned level with the patient's heart. A system for continuously flushing the cannula with saline is incorporated into the transducer set. A flow of approximately $4\,ml.h^{-1}$ is used to prevent occlusion by blood, although it can be manually activated to flush much more rapidly.

The pressure from the artery is transmitted through the fluid column to a thin diaphragm. The movement of the diaphragm caused by the arterial pressure is detected by a strain gauge; as the diaphragm is stretched, wires in the transducer are also stretched and their electrical resistance changes. The resistance signal is converted to a pressure signal by a calibration. In practice, this system is made more accurate by the use of a Wheatstone bridge (see *Section 12.6*). The signal from the transducer is then amplified and displayed as a continuous waveform.

Advantages

- Considered more accurate than non-invasive techniques.
- Gives beat-to-beat measurement of blood pressure and is not affected by heart rate or rhythm.
- Allows easy sampling of arterial blood.
- Some invasive blood pressure systems can be connected to cardiac output monitors (see *Chapter 9*) that analyse the arterial waveform.

Disadvantages

- Complications of arterial cannulation, such as:
  - bleeding and haematoma formation
  - infection – either local or systemic
  - ischaemic complications distal to the cannulation site.

- Potential for accidental intra-arterial injection of drugs.
- Risk of blood loss if cannula is disconnected and this is not noticed.
- Inaccurate readings can be caused by damping in the system or kinking of the cannula.
- It can take considerable practice to learn the skill of arterial cannulation.
- The system must be calibrated at a zero point and may be subject to drift over long periods of time. Regular recalibration by opening the system to atmospheric pressure is required.

! Safety

Allen's test can be performed before cannulation of the radial artery. The test ensures that the hand has an intact collateral arterial supply via the ulnar artery. The patient clenches their fist while pressure is applied over both radial and ulnar arteries. The fist is then unclenched. The hand will be white due to occlusion of its blood supply. The pressure over the ulnar artery is then released, and the whole hand should turn pink within five seconds. If it does not, the collateral supply may not be sufficient.

Other notes

There are two properties of the invasive blood pressure monitor (and almost all other electronic monitoring systems) that dictate how accurately it is able to reproduce the arterial pressure wave. These are the natural frequency and the damping coefficient.

Natural frequency and resonance

The natural frequency of an object is the frequency at which it oscillates or vibrates after something causes it to move. For example, a child's swing will swing back and forth at a particular frequency once it is pushed. This frequency is dictated by some of the swing's physical properties, such as the length of the chain it hangs from and the local strength of gravity.

If an energy wave is applied to an object, and the wave has a frequency equal to the object's natural frequency, it will cause the object to vibrate or oscillate. If the application of energy continues, the amplitude of the oscillation will increase. This is known as resonance. The classic example of this is the opera singer producing a note at the natural frequency of a wine glass and causing it to first vibrate and subsequently shatter.

Like all other objects, the arterial pressure monitoring equipment has a natural frequency. It is therefore important that the monitoring system is constructed in such a way that its natural frequency is significantly different from the frequency of the patient's pulse. If this were not the case, then the pulse wave would cause the system to resonate and it would become impossible to reproduce the pressure waveform accurately. However, the situation is more complex than this.

Although the pulse rate is usually quoted in beats per minute (bpm), for the purpose of this topic it is usually converted to beats per second (hertz). A normal adult pulse rate is therefore between approximately 1 and 2 Hz (60–120 bpm). The maximum pulse rate the monitor could encounter might be between 3 and 4 Hz (180–240 bpm) in a tachycardic neonate or during supraventricular tachycardia. The pulse rate is known as the fundamental frequency of this monitoring system.

Like all complex waveforms, the arterial pressure wave can be broken down into a series of simple component sine waves of different amplitudes and frequencies using Fourier analysis. The frequencies of these sine waves are always whole number multiples or 'harmonics' of the fundamental frequency. If the original arterial pressure waveform includes high frequency components (e.g. a fast upstroke), then the monitoring electronics need to be capable of detecting and responding to this frequency. Therefore, the system must be constructed in such a way that its natural frequency is not only significantly different from the heart rate, but also significantly different from the high frequency component of the pressure waveform. Again, if this were not the case then the system would resonate and distort whenever the pressure wave contained these high frequency components.

As a result of this, in order to ensure that resonance does not occur, the natural frequency of the arterial pressure monitoring system must be at least ten times the maximum pulse rate (i.e. at least the tenth harmonic of the fundamental frequency), or at least 40 Hz. In practice, this can be made more likely by using short pieces of non-compliant tubing with a large internal diameter for the arterial cannula and saline column, avoiding the inclusion of three-way taps in the system, and ensuring that there are no bubbles present.

Damping

While the natural frequency of an object or system is the property that dictates when it will oscillate, the damping coefficient is the property that dictates how much it resists oscillation. In other words, it is a measure of the frictional forces within the system. Different amounts of damping cause different effects (*Fig. 6.13.3*).

Critical damping

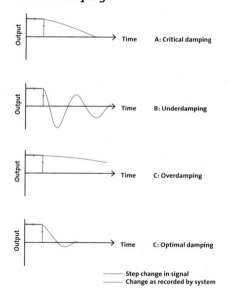

Fig. 6.13.3: Damping.

Following a step change in the signal to zero, a critically damped system is one whose measurement of the signal returns to zero at the fastest possible rate without any overshoot. The damping coefficient in a critically damped system is 1.

Underdamping

If the frictional force in the system is not enough to stop it overshooting the zero point following the step change in signal, the system is said to be underdamped and the damping coefficient is less than 1. An underdamped monitor will exaggerate signals and, in arterial pressure monitoring, the systolic pressure may read much higher than it actually is. Artefactual detail may appear with increased prominence.

Overdamping

An overdamped system will not overshoot the zero point because the frictional force is more than sufficient, but the time taken to reach zero will be prolonged. An overdamped system has a damping coefficient greater than 1. An arterial pressure monitor that is overdamped will miss fine detail in the wave and the amplitude will be artificially reduced resulting in an abnormally high diastolic pressure and low systolic pressure. Overdamping may occur due to bubbles or blood clots in the tubing.

Optimal damping

Although a critically damped system does not overshoot the zero point and takes a shorter period of time to return to zero than an overdamped system, for the purposes of arterial pressure monitoring it is still too slow. A compromise between the amount of overshoot (accuracy) and response speed is known as optimal damping and this occurs when the damping coefficient is 0.64 (64% of critical damping). Following a 'square wave' flush of saline, an optimally damped arterial pressure monitor will overshoot once in each direction, before settling back to the patient's waveform.

6.14 Temperature measurement

The measurement of temperature is performed for several reasons and using several methods. It is necessary for devices to measure the temperature of fluids or gases (e.g. in fluid warmers and hot air patient warmers). It is also necessary to measure the patient's temperature, because changes may help in making diagnoses and can also be responsible for certain complications (e.g. bleeding).

Liquid expansion thermometers

These thermometers rely on the volumetric expansion or contraction of a liquid such as mercury or alcohol in response to a change in temperature. These liquids are chosen because they display linear expansion over the temperatures of interest. As the liquid warms, it expands and rises from a reservoir into a glass column alongside a calibrated scale, from which the temperature can be read.

Advantages
- Easy to read and simple to use.
- Accurate for the purposes of measuring body temperature.

Disadvantages
- Slow response time.
- Glass can break, causing injury and toxicity if mercury is employed.
- Inaccurate at very low temperatures if mercury is used (it freezes at −38.8°C) and at high temperatures if alcohol is used (it boils at 78.5°C).

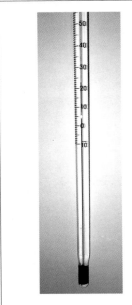

Fig. 6.14.1: An alcohol liquid expansion thermometer.

Gas expansion thermometers

The volume of a gas is related to its temperature by Charles' law: as its temperature increases, so does its volume. The absolute change in the volume of a gas with a known thermal expansion coefficient can be used to determine the temperature. However, if the volume of the system is fixed then the pressure of the gas will increase as the temperature increases, obeying the 3rd perfect gas law. The pressure in the system can then be measured using an aneroid gauge calibrated for temperature.

Advantages
- Sensitive and accurate over a wide range of temperatures.

Disadvantages
- Slow response time.
- Large and bulky.

Bimetallic strips

The bimetallic strip consists of strips two different metals joined together. The metals have different coefficients of thermal expansion, and they are wound into a coil. As the temperature increases, one metal will expand more than the other, causing the coil to loosen. Similarly, the coil will tighten as the temperature decreases. At the centre of the coil is a pointer, which moves across a calibrated dial as the coil tightens or loosens so that the temperature can be read.

When your consultant sends you to buy coffee, you may see your local barista using a bimetallic strip thermometer to measure the temperature of the steamed milk.

Advantages
- Cheap.

Disadvantages
- Limited accuracy and slow response times.

Liquid crystal thermometers

Liquid crystals are substances that behave in some ways like liquids and in other ways like solid crystals. One use for them is the measurement of temperature, because a change in temperature affects their optical properties and can make them change colour.

A liquid crystal thermometer used for measuring body temperature consists of a plastic strip that contains several liquid crystals that change colour at different temperatures, in the range 35–40°C. The strip is held on the forehead and the temperature can be determined by which crystals change colour. Lower range thermometers of this type are available for measuring room temperature.

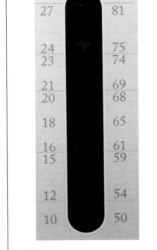
Fig. 6.14.2: A liquid crystal thermometer for measuring room temperature.

Advantages
- Easy to use.

Disadvantages
- Slow response time.
- Usually cannot display the temperature in units smaller than one degree celsius.

Infrared thermometers

The wavelength and intensity of infrared radiation that an object gives out varies with its temperature. The pyroelectric effect is the generation of a temporary polarization in the molecules of some substances when they are exposed to infrared at certain frequencies. The potential difference that is generated is proportional to the change in temperature.

Ceramic crystals with pyroelectic properties are therefore used in infrared tympanic thermometers. The voltage generated across the crystal in response to infrared radiation from the tympanic membrane is used to determine the temperature.

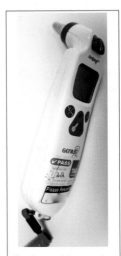
Fig. 6.14.3: A tympanic infrared thermometer.

Advantages
- Very fast response time.

Disadvantages
- Can be rendered inaccurate if not directed at the tympanic membrane properly, or if there is wax in the external auditory canal.

Resistance thermometers

The electrical resistance of a metal increases linearly with its temperature between 0 and 100°C. In a resistance thermometer, a fixed voltage is passed across a metal wire. The current that flows is measured and the resistance is calculated using Ohm's law. The temperature of the wire can therefore be determined. A Wheatstone bridge (see *Section 12.6*) is often added to the system to improve accuracy. Resistance thermometers are seldom used in clinical practice.

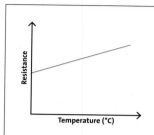

Fig. 6.14.4: The relationship between a metal's electrical resistance and its temperature.

Advantages
- These thermometers can measure changes in temperature as small as 0.0001°C.

Disadvantages
- Slow response time.
- Bulky.

Thermistors

A thermistor works on a similar principle to the resistance thermometer, except that a metal oxide is used rather than a metal. The electrical resistance of a metal oxide falls exponentially as its temperature increases. A Wheatstone bridge is used to improve accuracy.

Thermistors are small and robust, permitting their use in a range of anaesthetic equipment including nasopharyngeal temperature probes and pulmonary artery catheters (see *Section 9.6*).

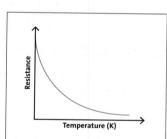

Fig. 6.14.5: The relationship between a metal oxide's electrical resistance and its temperature.

Advantages
- Fast response time.
- Can be made very small if necessary.

Disadvantages
- Require calibration and output is subject to drift.

Thermocouples

When two conductors made from dissimilar materials are joined together, a potential difference is produced at the point of contact, the magnitude of which depends on the temperature. This is known as the Seebeck effect. By measuring the voltage across the junction of the two metals, the temperature can be determined.

Further electrical connections to the thermocouple must be made to complete a circuit and allow measurement of the voltage. The other connections are held at a constant temperature so that any variation in the measured voltage through the circuit must be due to the temperature in the thermocouple.

The thermocouple is used in some body temperature probes (although thermistors are also commonly used for this purpose) and in intravenous fluid warmers.

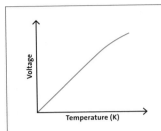

Fig. 6.14.6: The Seebeck effect. The potential difference that occurs at the junction of two dissimilar metals varies with temperature.

Advantages
- Fast response time.
- Cheap, small.

Disadvantages
- Requires slightly more complicated electronics than some other devices. The circuitry must be kept at a constant temperature and the measured signal is small and requires amplification.

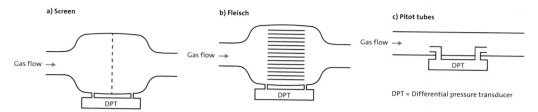

Fig. 6.15.1: The main types of pneumotachograph.

Overview

A pneumotachograph is a device used to measure gas flow. In contrast to the constant pressure, variable orifice flowmeters described in *Section 6.3*, the pneumotachograph is a constant orifice (or 'constant resistance'), variable pressure flowmeter.

There are several types of pneumotachograph available, including 'screen' and 'Fleisch'. 'Hot wire' flowmeters and Pitot tubes are also discussed here.

Uses

Pneumotachographs are found on anaesthetic machines and ventilators and are used to measure respiratory flows.

How it works

Screen and Fleisch pneumotachographs

A screen pneumotachograph consists of a widening of the tube that the gas is flowing through with a perforated gauze screen within it. The wider tube causes a reduction in velocity, and flow is more likely to be laminar. The resistance of the screen causes a pressure drop across it, which is measured by a differential pressure transducer. The resistance offered by the screen does not change and therefore the detected drop in pressure must be proportional to flow.

A Fleish pneumotachograph has a set of parallel fine bore tubes through which the gas flows. These offer a resistance to flow in the same way as the screen above. A pressure differential is then used to calculate flow.

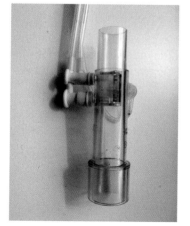

Fig. 6.15.2: Pitot tubes. This connects to a breathing system. The yellow tubing connects to the differential pressure transducer.

Hot wire flowmeter

A hot wire flowmeter consists of two thin metal wires set at 90° to each other that are heated to a constant temperature by an electric current. The electrical resistance is dependent on the temperature of the wires. As the gas flows over the wires, they are cooled. The change in electrical resistance due to cooling is proportional to the flow.

Pitot tubes

Two small tubes fixed in the gas flow are orientated so that one faces directly into the oncoming gas and the other faces directly away. The pressures in the tubes are measured. The pressure in the tube facing the oncoming gas flow is higher than that in the tube facing the opposite direction. This pressure differential is proportional to the flow (see *Fig. 6.15.2*).

Advantages

- Accurate and rapid measurement of flow.
- Also commonly used to calculate volumes by integrating the flow measurement with time.
- Some pneumotachographs are heated in order to prevent water vapour condensing inside them and causing errors in reading the pressure differential.

Disadvantages

- In order to be able to draw conclusions about flow from a pressure differential, the flow must be laminar. Anything that alters the flow characteristics may cause an error in the reading. Changes in ambient temperature, or addition of other gases to the mixture, thereby changing the overall viscosity or density, may cause flow to become turbulent.
- Some larger pneumotachographs may add dead space and resistance to a breathing system.

Other notes

As explained above, pneumotachographs are constant orifice, variable pressure flowmeters. Constant pressure, variable orifice flowmeters are discussed in *Section 6.3*.

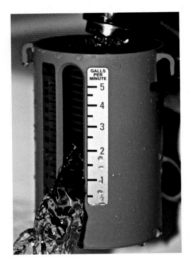

Fig. 6.15.3: A variable pressure, variable orifice flowmeter for measuring liquid flow.

The watersight flowmeter is a variable pressure, variable orifice device. A tube with holes along its length is vertically submerged in water and the gas flows through the tube before bubbling out of the holes. As the flow increases, the gas bubbles out of deeper holes and each is labelled to indicate a particular flow. The sum of the areas of the holes with gas bubbling from them therefore increases as the flow increases – this is the variable orifice. The pressure required to force gas through deeper holes also increases as the flow increases – this is the variable pressure. A very similar device can be used to measure flow of liquid and is shown in *Figure 6.15.3*.

In contrast, a bubble flowmeter is a constant pressure, constant orifice device and is used to measure low flows. A bubble of soap is carried along a tube by a gas. The distance the bubble travels in a set time is used to calculate the flow. The orifice is the diameter of the tube, which does not vary, and therefore the pressure of the gas is also constant.

None of these flowmeters are often used in modern clinical practice.

6.16 Wright respirometer

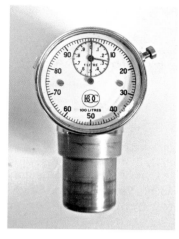

Fig. 6.16.1: A Wright respirometer.

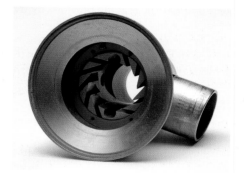

Fig. 6.16.2: A Wright respirometer with front removed so that workings can be seen. Image reproduced with permission from the Anaesthesia Museum, Sheffield Teaching Hospitals NHS Foundation Trust.

Overview

The Wright respirometer is used to measure gas volumes. It is a compact device that consists of a vane encircled by a housing that contains angled slits. There is a gas inlet on one side and an outlet on the other. A calibrated dial with a pointer is found on the front of the device that is connected to the vane via mechanical gears.

Uses

The Wright respirometer is an older method of measuring gas volumes. It was previously the most common way of measuring tidal volumes from anaesthetized patients. A modern version of the device also exists and is found more frequently in contemporary anaesthetic machines (see below).

How it works

Gas enters the respirometer through the inlet and has to move through the slits in the housing. Due to the angle of the slits, the gas exerts a rotational force on the vane in the centre of the device and causes it to spin. Via a set of gears, the spin of the vane moves the pointer over the calibrated dial so that the volume can be read.

⊕ Advantages

- Simple, cheap.
- Mechanical – requires no electrical power source.

⊖ Disadvantages

- Over-reads volumes at high gas flows and under-reads volumes at low flows.
- There is no facility for electronic output or recording of volumes over a period of time.
- The respirometer will only measure the volume of gas flowing through it in one direction. If gas flows backwards through the device, the volume cannot be measured. Therefore separate respirometers, mounted in opposite orientations, are required for inspiratory and expiratory volumes.

- When the gas flow is optimal, the reading provided by the respirometer still has an error of 5–10%.
- There is no mechanism preventing the condensation of water vapour on components such as the moving pointer and this may lead to large errors in the readings.
- Having the device in the breathing system modestly increases the dead space and resistance.

Other notes

Modern versions of the Wright respirometer overcome many of the disadvantages of the original device described above.

Newer respirometers allow gas to travel through in both directions, making the vane spin in opposite directions depending on the flow. It is therefore possible to measure both inspiratory and expiratory volumes with a single device. Furthermore, these modern versions use an infrared light beam to count the rotations of the vane, and this information can then be used to provide an electronic measure of the gas volume.

6.17 Depth of anaesthesia monitors

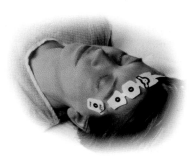

Fig. 6.17.1: The correct placement of BIS electrodes. Image used by permission from Nellcor Puritan Bennett LLC, Boulder, Colorado, doing business as Covidien.

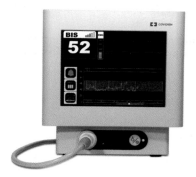

Fig. 6.17.2: The BIS monitor. Image used with permission from Nellcor Puritan Bennett LLC, Boulder, Colorado, doing business as Covidien.

Overview

Awareness during anaesthesia can have serious long-term consequences. Unfortunately there is no universally reliable indicator of anaesthetic depth. Clinical signs of sympathetic nervous system activity provide some information, but have been shown to be unreliable when used alone. Measurement of end-tidal volatile anaesthetic concentration provides useful information, but suffers from significant inter-patient variability and does not take into account intravenous drugs. The isolated forearm technique (which involves a tourniquet inflated above systolic blood pressure to prevent neuromuscular blocking drugs from reaching the forearm, allowing the patient to use their hand to communicate if they are aware) is a research tool and is not yet applicable to clinical practice.

The logical approach to developing a true depth of anaesthesia monitor lies in analysis of the electroencephalograph (EEG), and monitors that analyse the EEG are therefore becoming more common. These monitors are currently the source of much debate. An ideal monitor would predict explicit and implicit awareness as well as movement in response to a surgical stimulus, regardless of the patient or anaesthetic agent used. No monitor is currently able to do this. Nevertheless, some studies have shown a reduction in awareness, and a reduction in the adverse effects of excessive anaesthesia has also been demonstrated.

In 2012, the National Institute for Health and Care Excellence (NICE) in the UK issued guidelines that recommend, as an option, the use of depth of anaesthesia monitors in patients at higher risk of awareness, or of excessively deep anaesthesia (see *Table 6.17.1*). They also concluded that although there was more uncertainty about the clinical benefits of E-Entropy (GE Healthcare) and Narcotrend-Compact-M (MT MonitorTechnik) monitors than about Bispectral index (Covidien), all these monitors were broadly equivalent.

Uses

Monitors based on EEG analysis are used alongside other methods to estimate the depth of general anaesthesia. It is hoped they will reduce the incidence of awareness, and the adverse effects of deep anaesthesia.

Table 6.17.1: Factors suggesting that the patient may be at risk of either awareness under anaesthesia, or of excessively deep anaesthesia.

Risk factors for awareness	Risk factors for excessive anaesthesia
Patient factors	
Younger age group	Patients with hepatic disease
Chronically high opiate or alcohol intake	High BMI
Previous experience of awareness	Older age group
Risk of haemodynamic instability	Poor cardiovascular function
Co-morbidity (e.g. hyperthyroidism)	
Anaesthetic factors	
Use of neuromuscular blockers	Unrecognized equipment failure
Use of TIVA?	
Difficult intubation	
Unrecognized equipment failure	
Surgical factors	
Cardiac surgery	
Obstetric surgery with GA	
Emergency / trauma surgery	

BMI = body mass index; TIVA = total intravenous anaesthesia.

How it works

Raw EEG

The EEG is a graph of electrical activity in the brain against time and is obtained by placing approximately 20 electrodes on the scalp and recording the potential difference between 16 combinations of these. EEG waves vary between 50 and 200 μV in amplitude and can be over 100 Hz in frequency. This generates a massive quantity of raw data, and analysis is extremely complicated. Changes in frequency and amplitude of the waves may be caused by many things other than anaesthetic agents. For these reasons the raw EEG is not appropriate for routine monitoring of anaesthetic depth.

During deep anaesthesia, a pattern called *burst suppression* is discernable. This is when there is a burst of electrical activity followed by a period of almost isoelectric EEG. Electrical activity subsequently resumes.

Compressed spectral array

The compressed spectral array (CSA) is a method of analysing the complex data from the raw EEG and condensing it into a more manageable and easily interpretable form. In this method, short periods of EEG recording are performed, each of 5–10 seconds in length. Each recording is known as an epoch. The epochs are then subjected to Fourier transformation, which breaks down the complex waveforms of the EEG into a set of simpler sine waves of different frequencies. As anaesthesia deepens, low frequencies become more common than high ones. The abundance of each frequency can be displayed using a histogram called the CSA.

The spectral edge is the frequency below which 95% of the CSA occurs and is therefore a marker of the highest occurring frequencies. It has been suggested as a single number that can be monitored to give an indication of the depth of anaesthesia, and it will fall as anaesthesia deepens. However, it does not correlate well with drug concentration, especially during emergence.

The median frequency has an improved (although certainly not perfect) correlation with drug concentration. It is the frequency below and above which 50% of the CSA occurs. Unfortunately it is not consistent between patients and differs depending on which anaesthetic agent is used.

Bispectral index

As well as a tendency for frequencies in the EEG to become lower as anaesthesia deepens, there is also a tendency for the signals from different parts of the brain to fall out of phase with each other. The biocoherence is a measure of how the phase differs between signals, with 0 being completely random in their relationship to one another and 1 indicating an invariable phase relationship.

The Bispectral index (BIS) is a dimensionless number between 0 and 100 that is derived from the CSA, the biocoherence, the level of burst suppression and other parameters. The BIS algorithm is proprietary, but was derived from analysis of the recordings of EEGs of healthy volunteers who underwent general anaesthesia several times. The system has been validated in other healthy volunteers and in patients.

The equipment used to monitor BIS consists of a disposable strip that incorporates three or four electrodes (depending on the model) that is placed on the patient's forehead. This strip is then plugged into a cable that connects to a computer. A BIS score of 0 indicates an isoelectric EEG, whereas 85–100 indicates the normal awake and alert pattern. A BIS score of 60–85 suggests sedation and 40–60 suggests appropriate general anaesthesia. Below 40, burst suppression increasingly occurs and the anaesthetic is likely to be too deep.

In addition to the BIS score, three other variables are commonly displayed.

- *SQI* (signal quality index) indicates the reliability of the signal displayed either as a bar or a dimensionless number from 0 to 100. There is no recommendation regarding what represents an adequate signal.
- *EMG* (electromyograph) reports the power contained in the frequency range 70–110 Hz. This includes the EMG from frontalis muscle activity which may cause a falsely high BIS score, particularly during emergence.
- *SR* (suppression ratio) indicates the percentage of the last 63 seconds in which there has been an isoelectric EEG. Under general anaesthesia, this should ideally be 0.

Although BIS is one of the preferred monitors of this type, it does have some problems. It appears that nitrous oxide does not significantly alter the BIS score with inhaled concentrations of up to 70% having little effect, despite causing clinical sedation. Similarly, ketamine has excitatory effects on the EEG despite causing dissociative anaesthesia. Therefore BIS is generally unreliable in the presence of ketamine or nitrous oxide. The effects of opioids on the BIS score have not yet been fully elucidated. It is also not possible to predict when a particular patient will lose or regain consciousness, as there is considerable variation in BIS scores between patients with these events.

There is conflicting evidence regarding whether the use of BIS reduces the incidence of awareness under general anaesthesia. The B-Aware randomized controlled trial conducted in 2004 showed a reduction in the risk of awareness in patients who were monitored with BIS. However, a follow-up trial (B-Unaware) in 2008 compared the use of BIS with monitoring of the end-tidal volatile anaesthetic concentration and found no difference in the incidence of awareness. Both of these trials were criticized for their design.

E-Entropy

E-Entropy monitors are similar to BIS in that they analyse the raw EEG obtained via three forehead electrodes and produce a score, which is interpreted in a very similar way to that obtained from BIS, with 40–60 suggesting appropriate anaesthesia.

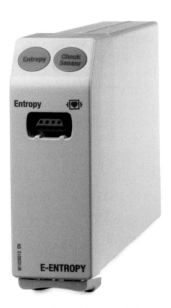

Fig. 6.17.3: The E-Entropy module. Image reproduced with permission from GE Healthcare.

The difference is in how the entropy monitor calculates its score. Instead of using the CSA and biocoherence, the entropy monitor gives a score based on how chaotic the EEG signal is. As the patient's level of anaesthesia becomes deeper the EEG becomes less chaotic or, in other words, has less entropy. A lower score therefore indicates a deeper level of anaesthesia.

The monitor reports two scores. One is the State Entropy (SE, range 0–91) that analyses the lower frequencies from the EEG and the other is the Response Entropy (RE, range 0–100) that analyses the EEG, but also higher frequencies from the frontalis muscle EMG. This is an attempt to separate the monitoring of anaesthesia and analgesia, because the activation of frontalis muscle is associated with nociception. A rise in the difference between RE and SE is said to reflect this. RE is difficult to interpret in the presence of neuromuscular blocking agents. E-Entropy modules may also display burst suppression ratio (BSR); as with SR in BIS, the target value for BSR is 0.

E-Entropy suffers with many of the same problems as BIS, such as inter-patient variability and the lack of effect of some drugs such as nitrous oxide on the score. The E-Entropy module is shown in *Figure 6.17.3*.

Auditory evoked potentials

Evoked potentials are EEG waveforms detected in specific areas of the central nervous system (CNS) in response to different stimuli. These stimuli may be visual, somatosensory or auditory. The latter are the most studied for use in depth of anaesthesia monitors.

Audible clicks of a fixed intensity, frequency and duration are played to the patient through headphones while they are under anaesthesia. Electrodes on the skin surface record the EEG response to the clicks from different parts of the auditory pathway between the acoustic nerve and the primary auditory cortex. As well as the frequency and amplitude of the responses, the delay between the stimulus and the response (the latency) is also measured.

The responses are divided into three phases: brain stem (latency up to 10 msec after the stimulus), early cortical (middle latency of 15–80 msec) and late cortical (long latency of over 80 msec). Under the influence of the volatile general anaesthetic agents, the latencies of all three phases become longer and the amplitude of their response waves diminish. The intravenous anaesthetics tend to have a smaller effect on the brainstem, but alter the cortical latency and amplitude in a similar way to the volatile agents. Nitrous oxide produces a reduction in amplitude of the responses, but has no effect on latency.

The change in response under the influence of general anaesthetics can be used to give an idea of the depth of anaesthesia. However, the use of auditory evoked potentials (AEPs) has some drawbacks: the response may be difficult to interpret if sounds other than the standardized clicks are heard, the age and gender of the patient may affect the response, as may the choice of anaesthetic agent.

Advantages

- These monitors produce a regularly updated number indicating depth of anaesthesia.
- The effect of total intravenous anaesthesia (TIVA) on risk of awareness has been disputed. NICE state that patients receiving TIVA are not considered to be at a higher risk of adverse outcomes than those receiving inhaled anaesthetics. However, they recommend the use of depth of anaesthesia monitors if TIVA is being used because it is cost-effective and it is not possible to measure anaesthetic concentration while using this technique.
- Some studies have shown them to reduce both awareness and the consequences of excessively deep anaesthesia (for instance post-operative cognitive dysfunction).

Disadvantages

- The displayed score does not always have a good clinical correlation.
- Certain anaesthetic agents cannot be used with certain monitors (e.g. ketamine and BIS), or make interpretation difficult.
- Factors such as hypothermia, hypoxia and hypercarbia, may cause changes in the reading that are not due to the anaesthetic agent.
- Interference from the ECG or EMG may affect the reading, as may other electrical sources such as diathermy.
- BIS and E-Entropy not fully validated for use in young children, and there are few data available evaluating their use in people with neurological disorders.

Other notes

Awareness under anaesthesia is not commonly detected, and so studies that have sufficient numbers of patients to be adequately powered can be difficult to conduct. Depth of anaesthesia monitors should be used alongside the other tools that are available to assess the likelihood of awareness, particularly clinical judgement.

Accidental awareness under general anaesthesia was the subject of the fifth National Audit Project (NAP5), conducted between June 2012 and June 2013, by the Royal College of Anaesthetists and the Association of Anaesthetists of Great Britain and Ireland.

Coagulation testing: TEG and Rotem

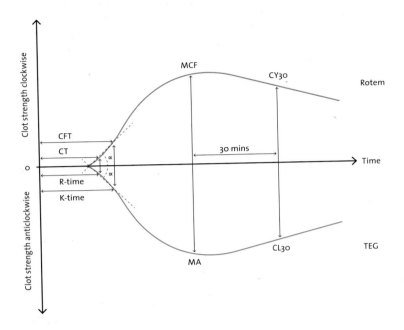

Fig. 6.18.1: A representation of data obtained from TEG and Rotem machines.

Overview

TEG and Rotem machines use a technique that measures both the time taken for blood to clot and the strength of the clot as it forms, in order to assess coagulation. The method was first described in 1948, but was used primarily as a research tool until recent years when rotational thromboelastometry (Rotem, Tem International) and thromboelastography (TEG, Haemonetics) machines became available.

These techniques have several advantages over traditional clotting assays, and give a more complete picture of the function of the coagulation system.

Uses

These machines are used in many clinical situations when rapid assessment of a patient's coagulation function is useful. These include during cardiac surgery, obstetrics, trauma, liver transplantation and any situation involving major haemorrhage.

How it works

While traditional coagulation assays such as the prothrombin time (PT) and activated partial thromboplastin time (APTT) test specific enzymatic pathways within the clotting cascade, the TEG and Rotem machines measure clot formation in whole blood.

A small volume of whole blood is added to a cup containing a clot activator. It is possible to perform the test without a clot activator, but it takes much longer to obtain the results and the reference ranges are different. Alternative cups that contain heparinase (an enzyme that breaks down heparin) with the clot activator, and other reagents are also available.

The cup is placed on the machine, and a sensor pin is inserted into the blood. There is rotational movement between the pin and the cup in one direction, followed by a short pause. Rotation then occurs in the opposite direction. This back and forth rotation continues throughout the analysis, and is intended to represent sluggish venous blood flow. The whole system is kept at 37°C. As the clot begins to form, the blood becomes more viscous and exerts more resistance to rotation. This resistance is detected and plotted on a graph of clot strength against time (see *Fig. 6.18.1*).

The normal thromboelastogram begins with a horizontal line, and then becomes cigar-shaped as the clot begins to form. There are two symmetrical arms to the cigar part of the graph, as rotation occurs in two directions.

None of the measurements made by these techniques can be directly related to measurements made in standard laboratory coagulation assays. Similarly, it should be appreciated that although TEG and Rotem work in similar ways, their reference ranges and terminology are different and cannot be interchanged. An attempt to interpret a reading from a TEG machine using the Rotem reference ranges, for example, may lead to the incorrect treatment being given.

TEG

In the TEG system, 360 μl of fresh whole blood should be added to the cup within 5 minutes of it being taken. If citrated blood is used, it can be taken at a distant site and brought to the analyser within 2 hours; calcium (20 μl of 0.2 M calcium chloride) must also be added to the cup before the assay is started if citrated blood is used. The system uses kaolin as the clot activator. Once the assay is started, the cup takes 10 seconds to rotate by 4°45′, before pausing and then rotating back in the other direction. A torsion wire on the pin detects the frictional force generated as a result of the blood clotting.

(a)

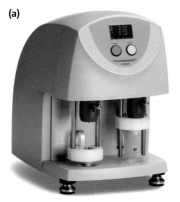

(b)

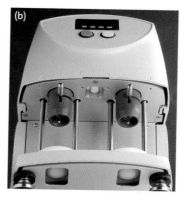

Fig. 6.18.2: (a) A TEG machine and **(b)** underside of machine, showing pins. Images used with permission from Haemonetics Corporation.

The R-time (reaction time) is the time taken between the beginning of the assay and the point where the graph amplitude is 2 mm. It represents the time taken for fibrin formation to begin.

As the clot strengthens, the graph moves further from its baseline and the arms become wider. The time taken from the R-time to where the graph is 20 mm wide is known as the K-time (coagulation time); 20 mm is an arbitrary point, but the time taken to reach it is used as a measure of how quickly the clot is strengthening. The α-angle is the angle to horizontal made by a straight line between the 2 mm point and the 20 mm point. It provides similar information to the K-time and is a measure of how quickly the clot is forming.

The maximum amplitude (MA) is reached when the graph becomes no wider, representing the maximum strength of the clot. Eventually thrombolytic mechanisms will begin, and the graph will begin to narrow again as the clot breaks down. The CL30 (clot lysis) is the percentage reduction in amplitude of the graph 30 minutes after the MA. The CL60 is the same measurement an hour after the MA. These numbers give an idea of the stability of the clot once it has formed, and whether thrombolysis is occurring. The lysis time is similar, and is the time after MA that the graph amplitude has fallen by 2 mm.

Generally speaking, a prolonged R-time represents the presence of anticoagulants, or deficiency of clotting factors. The K-time is dependent on platelets and fibrinogen, as is the α-angle and the MA. A shortened lysis time or high CL30 indicates activation of the fibrinolytic system or poor platelet function. Therefore a prolonged R-time may indicate the need for treatment with clotting factors or fresh frozen plasma, a prolonged K-time, low α-angle or low MA may indicate the need for treatment with platelets or cryoprecipitate, and a high CL30 or low lysis time may indicate the need for treatment with an antifibrinolytic agent.

TEG PlateletMapping
The standard TEG masks the effects that anti-platelet drugs such as aspirin and clopidogrel have on clot formation. This is because kaolin is responsible for the generation of large quantities of thrombin, which activates all platelets regardless of the presence of these drugs. Therefore, TEG must be used in a different way to reveal how well platelets are functioning and the extent to which they have been pharmacologically inhibited.

Platelets can be activated via a number of pathways. Thromboxane is derived from arachidonic acid, and binds to a specific receptor on the surface of the platelet. Similarly, ADP is another substance that causes platelet activation and has its own receptor. These pathways are blocked by aspirin and clopidogrel, respectively. However, platelets inhibited by these drugs can still be activated by thrombin.

The PlateletMapping system measures the MA of clots formed in several circumstances. Blood is taken from a patient who is taking aspirin and divided between three TEG cups.

- In the first cup, the blood is exposed to kaolin – the thrombin produced as a result activates all platelets, regardless of the presence of aspirin, and elicits a maximum response.
- The second cup contains heparin to ensure that thrombin is not active, and an enzyme (reptilase) that cleaves and activates fibrinogen but has no effect on platelets – a fibrin-only clot is therefore formed.
- The third cup also contains heparin and reptilase, but arachidonic acid is added. The arachidonic acid is able to activate the platelets that are not inhibited by aspirin. Therefore, the MA of the clot that forms is a reflection of the proportion of platelets not affected by aspirin. If a patient is taking clopidogrel instead of aspirin, ADP is included in the cup instead of arachidonic acid. This is able to activate any platelets that have not been inhibited by clopidogrel. If a patient is taking both aspirin and clopidogrel, then a combination of the cups described above can be used.

The system can then calculate the platelet function as a percentage of maximum by comparing the MA of the clots formed in each of the three cups.

Rotem
Rotem is a very similar system, although there are some differences. In this system, 300 μl of citrated blood are added to the cup, and it stays stationary while the pin rotates within it. Different clot activators and reagents can be used (see below). An optical system is used to measure the developing frictional force; light from an LED is reflected onto a detector by a mirror that is

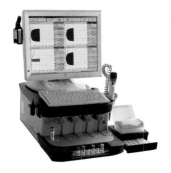

Fig. 6.18.3: The Rotem-delta. Image reproduced with permission from TEM International GmbH.

mounted on the pin. As the pin rotates in the slowly clotting blood, a varying amount of light will fall on the detector. The rotation of the pin, which is stabilized by a ball bearing mechanism, is said to be more stable and less sensitive to vibration and mechanical shock.

The results obtained from Rotem are very similar to those from TEG, but are given different names and have different reference ranges. The R-time becomes Clotting Time (CT), K-time becomes Clot Formation Time (CFT), and MA becomes Maximum Clot Firmness (MCF). The name of the α-angle is the same as in TEG. *Table 6.18.1* shows the different measurements made by each system and their definitions.

Several different calcium-containing reagents and clot activators are available for use with Rotem. The most commonly used are the INTEM and EXTEM reagents that cause clot formation by activation of the intrinsic and extrinsic pathways, respectively. Abnormalities in the individual pathways can then be detected. The FIBTEM reagent contains a platelet inhibitor (cytochalasin D) and so is used to determine how well a clot forms using fibrin alone. It can therefore detect abnormalities of fibrinogen concentration or function. Also, the comparison of results obtained using EXTEM with those using FIBTEM can be used to assess the contribution of platelets to the clot firmness. The HEPTEM reagent contains heparinase and comparison of results from this reagent and those from the INTEM reagent can be used to detect residual heparinization. Finally, the APTEM reagent contains the anti-fibrinolytic agent aprotinin, and comparison of results from it and the EXTEM reagent can be used to more easily detect hyperfibrinolysis than if using EXTEM alone.

Table 6.18.1: Equivalent measurements made by TEG and Rotem machines.

TEG measurement	Rotem measurement	Description
R-time	Clotting time (CT)	Time taken from start of analysis to when amplitude is 2 mm. Represents time taken for clot formation to begin.
K-time	Clot formation time (CFT)	Time taken for amplitude to rise to 20 mm. Represents how rapidly the clot is gaining strength.
α-angle	α-angle	In TEG, this is the gradient of a line between the R-time and the K-time. In Rotem this is the angle of a tangent to the curve at 2 mm amplitude. Another representation of how quickly clot is forming.
Maximum amplitude (MA)	Maximum clot firmness (MCF)	Where the amplitude of the graph is at its maximum. Represents the maximum strength the clot achieves.
CL30, CL60	LY30, LY60	The amplitude of the graph at 30 or 60 minutes (which will be less than MA/MCF due to clot lysis). Therefore gives representation of how rapidly lysis is occurring.

⊕ Advantages

- Machines can be located in theatres or critical care areas facilitating rapid bedside testing of coagulation.
- Most results are available in a shorter time than lab assays.
- Tests clot formation in whole blood.
- Able to detect hypercoagulable states as well as hypocoagulation.
- Provides information about fibrinolysis as well as clot formation.
- Able to determine the contribution of platelets to clot formation – a measurement of platelet function rather than just number.
- The operating temperature of the machine can be altered so that it is the same as a particular patient's body temperature. By doing this, and comparing the result to an assay performed at 37°C, the effect of hypothermia on clotting can be ascertained.

⊖ Disadvantages

- Because blood is analysed *in vitro*, clotting abnormalities caused by the endothelium cannot be detected. These systems therefore cannot detect von Willebrand's disease.
- The use of these machines can take a while to learn, as may interpretation of the results. These problems will become less frequent as the machines become more commonly used.
- Measurements made by TEG and Rotem do not always correlate.

Other notes

Many other systems are available for bedside assessment of coagulation, including the following.

- The Sonoclot (Sienco).
- Devices that measure platelet function:
  - Platelet Function Analyser (Siemens)
  - Multiplate (Dynabyte)
  - VerifyNow (Accumetrics).
  - Plateletworks (Helena Laboratories).
- Devices that specifically measure INR:
  - CoaguChekProDM (Roche).
- Devices that measure activated clotting time:
  - Hemochron Junior Signature (ITC).

6.19 Activated clotting time measurement

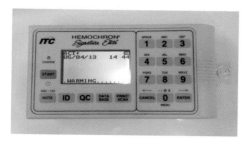

Fig. 6.19.1: The Hemochron Signature Elite ACT machine (ICT).

Overview

The activated clotting time (ACT) is a simple, non-specific bedside test of clotting function. The normal range is 100–140 seconds, although this varies depending on how the test is performed.

Uses

The ACT is used most commonly to monitor the effect of high dose unfractionated heparin before and during cardiopulmonary bypass in cardiothoracic surgery. Doses of 300–400 IU.kg^{-1} heparin are used to keep the ACT above 400 seconds. It may also be used to monitor the effect of heparin in patients being treated with extracorporeal membrane oxygenators (ECMO, see *Section 9.11*), and during some endovascular procedures.

Low dose heparin therapy is usually monitored using the APTT. This is unsuitable for monitoring the effect of high dose heparin because the blood will not clot at all using the reagents, so ACT is used instead.

How it works

Historically, the ACT test was performed manually by adding a clot activator to a test tube of whole blood and incubating it in a water bath at 37°C. The tube would be removed every 5 seconds to see if the blood was still liquid. The time at which the blood was first deemed to be clotted would be taken as the ACT.

The process is now automated and less operator dependent. However, the ACT remains a crude test of clotting function. It can be used to monitor the effect of heparin during surgery, because heparin is assumed to be the only variable affecting clotting. In reality, the ACT may be affected by many other variables such as hypofibrinogenaemia, clotting factor deficiencies, thrombocytopenia and haemodilution, and (for some ACT machines) the presence of aprotinin, an antifibrinolytic drug.

There are several machines available to measure ACT. However, they all differ slightly in their methods and also in the type of clot activator used (a variety are available, including kaolin, Celite, glass beads, silica or other substances). Because of this, they will give slightly different results and a particular patient must be monitored by the same type of machine throughout their treatment, otherwise it is impossible to compare one result with the next.

An early ACT machine was the Hemochron, developed in 1966. A 2 ml sample of whole blood is added to a test tube in a well in the machine that has been warmed to 37°C. The tube contains Celite and a vertical magnetic bar. The timer is then started and the test tube is rotated within the well. While the blood remains liquid, the magnetic bar does not move. As clotting occurs, the bar becomes lodged in the blood clot and begins to rotate with the tube. A magnetic sensor detects the movement of the bar and stops the timer. This time is taken to be the ACT. Under- or over-filling the test tube may affect the result.

A more modern hand held device called the Hemochron Signature Elite is also available. A glass cuvette that contains the clot activator (a mixture of kaolin, silica and phospholipids in this case) is placed in the machine, which warms it to 37°C. A 50 µl whole blood sample is placed in the cuvette and the machine aspirates 15 µl of this for testing, with the rest being drawn into a waste channel. The timer is started when the test sample is mixed with the clot activator. It is then moved to and fro in front of an optical sensor. As the blood clots, the machine can no longer move it along the test channel. The optical sensor detects this and stops the timer.

The clot activator used in the Hemochron Signature Elite causes the blood to clot approximately twice as fast as it would if Celite was used. However, the result is mathematically converted into Celite equivalents before being displayed as a time in seconds. This is the reason that 'timer' on the machine appears to be counting in faster units than seconds while a sample is being analysed.

Other ACT machines are also available that use different methods of measurement.

Advantages

- Fast, easy test to perform and the machine is usually kept available in theatres so immediate results are available.
- Some machines are small, battery or mains powered and portable.
- Results are available quickly.

Disadvantages

- Non-specific. Changes in ACT assumed to be due to heparin, but may not be.
- No standardized clot activator, so the ACT measured by one type of machine may be different to that measured on the same sample by a different type of machine.
- No correlation between ACT and other laboratory coagulation tests such as APTT or PT.
- Aprotinin interferes with ACT results if the clot activator is Celite, and the result is falsely prolonged. This does not occur to a significant extent if kaolin or other activators are used.

6.20 The Clark electrode

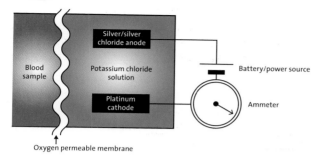

Fig. 6.20.1: The Clark electrode.

Overview

The Clark electrode, also known as the polarographic electrode, is a device that measures oxygen tension in a gas or liquid.

Uses

The Clark electrode is used by blood gas analysers to measure the partial pressure of oxygen.

How it works

The Clark electrode works using a similar principle to the fuel cell (see *Section 6.4*). A positive anode made of silver and silver chloride and a negative cathode made of platinum are immersed in a solution of potassium chloride. The KCl solution is separated from the blood sample by a membrane that is permeable to oxygen. A potential difference of approximately 0.6 V is applied across the electrodes, causing the silver anode to react with chloride ions in solution. This oxidation reaction produces silver chloride and liberates electrons:

$$4Ag + 4Cl^- \rightarrow 4AgCl + 4e^-$$

Oxygen from the blood diffuses across the membrane and into the KCl solution until equilibrium is achieved, meaning that the partial pressure of oxygen in the solution is equal to that in the blood sample.

At the cathode, the oxygen then reacts with water and the electrons that were liberated at the anode to produce hydroxyl ions:

$$O_2 + 2H_2O + 4e^- \rightarrow 4OH^-$$

Electrons are therefore consumed at the cathode and liberated at the anode. This cycle causes an electric current to be generated. The magnitude of the current is directly proportional to the partial pressure of oxygen dissolved in the solution.

⊕ Advantages

- Accurate to less than 0.5 kPa.
- Can be made very small to fit alongside other analysers in the blood gas machine.
- Acceptable response time for bedside testing.

⊖ Disadvantages

- The system must be kept at 37°C, because the reactions are temperature sensitive. Corrections for the patient's temperature can calculated after measurement.
- Some Clark electrodes are made inaccurate in the presence of halothane, and give a falsely high reading for oxygen tension. This is avoided by either not using halothane, or by the use of a membrane separating the electrolyte solution and the blood that is impermeable to halothane.
- The membrane is delicate and damage to it will cause the reading to be inaccurate.

- The system requires regular two-point calibration.
- Cannot be used for continuous *in vivo* measurement.

Other notes

The potential difference of 0.6 V applied across the two electrodes in this system is required to start the chemical reaction. This is in contrast to the fuel cell where the reaction at the anode is spontaneous.

Maintaining a very precise and stable potential difference across a system is difficult and there are usually small fluctuations. The value of approximately 0.6 V is used because this is in the middle of the range where small fluctuations in voltage will have no effect on the current produced. Therefore, any change in the current must be due to a change in oxygen tension in the sample. There is also a linear relationship between current and oxygen tension at this voltage.

6.21 The pH electrode

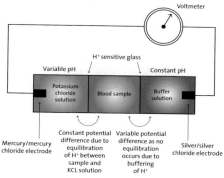

Fig. 6.21.1: The pH electrode.

Labels in figure:
Voltmeter
H⁺ sensitive glass
Variable pH
Constant pH
Potassium chloride solution
Blood sample
Buffer solution
Mercury/mercury chloride electrode
Constant potential difference due to equilibration of H⁺ between sample and KCL solution
Variable potential difference as no equilibration occurs due to buffering of H⁺
Silver/silver chloride electrode

Overview

The pH electrode, sometimes known as the glass pH electrode, is a device that measures the concentration of hydrogen ions (H^+) in a solution and so allows the calculation of its pH.

Uses

The pH electrode is used by blood gas analysers to measure the pH of a blood sample.

How it works

The pH electrode actually consists of two electrodes: a silver/silver chloride measuring electrode and a Calomel (mercury/mercury chloride) reference electrode.

The measuring electrode contains a buffer solution separated from the blood sample by pH-sensitive glass. The glass acts as a semi-permeable membrane that only hydrogen ions can cross: H^+ diffuses from the blood sample across the glass and into the solution. The buffer ensures that the pH of the solution does not change and no equilibrium is reached, so the concentration gradient is maintained, and H^+ continues to diffuse across the glass. This concentration gradient of a charged ion across a semi-permeable membrane, results in the presence of a potential difference across the membrane that is proportional to the H^+ concentration in the blood sample.

In order to judge the magnitude of the potential difference in the measuring electrode, the reference electrode is used to complete the circuit. The reference electrode contains 20% potassium chloride solution, which is in contact with the blood sample via another semi-permeable membrane. The KCl solution has no buffering properties and so the pH falls as H^+ diffuses into it. Eventually, an equilibrium is achieved and the pH of the KCl solution is equal to that in the blood sample.

The potential difference between the measuring electrode buffer solution and the reference electrode KCl solution can then be measured. The voltage is a reflection of the H^+ concentration (and therefore pH) of the blood sample.

⊕ Advantages

- Accurate.
- Can be made small enough to fit alongside other analysers in the blood gas machine.
- Acceptable response time for bedside testing.

⊖ Disadvantages

- Like other analysers, the system must be kept at 37°C in order to obtain accurate results.
- Any damage to the glass membrane will result in other ions diffusing into the buffering solution in the measuring electrode. This will result in inaccurate measurements.
- Two-point calibration is required regularly.
- Cannot be used for continuous *in vivo* measurement.

Other notes

Note that while the fuel cell and Clark electrode produce a *current* that is proportional in magnitude to the oxygen tension they are measuring, the pH electrode (and the Severinghaus electrode) produce a *voltage* that is proportional in magnitude to the H^+ concentration they are measuring.

6.22 The Severinghaus electrode

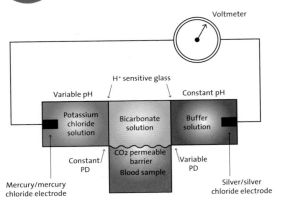

Fig. 6.22.1: The Severinghaus CO_2 electrode.

Labels in figure:
Voltmeter
H⁺ sensitive glass
Variable pH
Constant pH
Potassium chloride solution
Bicarbonate solution
Buffer solution
Constant/ PD
CO2 permeable barrier
Blood sample
Variable PD
Mercury/mercury chloride electrode
Silver/silver chloride electrode

Overview

The Severinghaus electrode is a device that measures the carbon dioxide tension in a sample of liquid. It is a modified pH electrode.

Uses

The Severinghaus electrode is used by blood gas analysers to measure the partial pressure of carbon dioxide in a blood sample.

How it works

The pH electrode is modified so that instead of the blood sample coming into direct contact with the pH-sensitive glass of the measuring electrode, there is a semi-permeable barrier, through which only carbon dioxide (and not hydrogen ions) can pass. The CO_2 diffuses through this barrier into a solution of sodium bicarbonate in water contained within a nylon mesh.

The increase in carbon dioxide in this solution causes a fall in its pH due to the increase in hydrogen ions produced as it reacts with the water:

$$CO_2 + H_2O \leftrightarrows H_2CO_3 \leftrightarrows H^+ + HCO_3^-$$

The bicarbonate solution takes the place of the blood sample in the pH electrode: H⁺ ions diffuse from it into the buffering solution in the measuring electrode and into the KCl solution in the reference electrode. The concentration of H⁺ can then be measured and the pH of the solution calculated.

However, in the Severinghaus electrode, the calculated pH can only be due to the carbon dioxide that has diffused across the semi-permeable membrane from the blood sample. Therefore the PCO_2 in the blood sample can be deduced.

⊕ Advantages

- Can be made small enough to fit alongside other analysers in the blood gas machine.
- Acceptable response time for bedside testing, although slightly slower than the pH electrode due to the extra barrier to diffusion and extra reactions that take place.

⊖ Disadvantages

- Like other analysers, the system must be kept at 37°C in order to obtain accurate results.
- More parts are present that could be damaged and affect the accuracy of the instrument, e.g. the pH-sensitive glass and the carbon dioxide permeable membrane.
- Two-point calibration is required regularly.
- Unsuitable for continuous *in vivo* measurements, although modifications have been made that do allow this, either transcutaneously or via an intra-arterial cannula.

6.23 Jugular venous oximetry

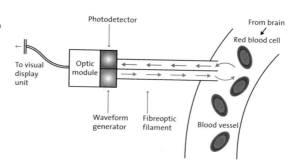

Fig. 6.23.2: Reflectance spectrophotometry. The tip of the fibreoptic catheter should sit in the centre of the jugular venous bulb.

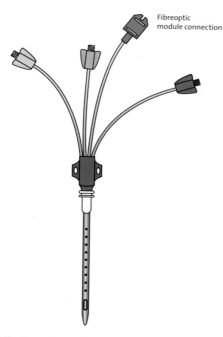

Fig. 6.23.1: A central venous fibreoptic catheter.

Overview

The internal jugular vein originates from the jugular venous bulb at the base of the skull, which is in turn formed from the confluence of the inferior petrosal sinus and sigmoid sinus. The jugular bulb drains blood from both hemispheres of the brain, with approximately 30% derived from the contralateral hemisphere.

Jugular venous oximetry measures the oxygen saturation of blood in the jugular venous bulb. It indirectly allows estimation of the adequacy of oxygen delivery to the brain. The main factors that affect oxygen delivery are cerebral blood flow, arterial oxygen saturations and the level of haemoglobin in the blood. If oxygen delivery falls due to either reduced cerebral blood flow or arterial oxygen content, but the oxygen demand remains constant then the venous oxygen content will fall. Similarly, if the brain's demand for oxygen increases but delivery does not increase proportionally, then more oxygen will be extracted leading to reduced venous oxygen content. Both of these scenarios are reflected by a reduced jugular venous oxygen saturation (S_jvO_2).

In health, the jugular venous saturation is approximately 55–75%.

Uses

Jugular venous desaturation is an early harbinger of cerebral ischaemia, whether intracranial or cardiorespiratory in origin.

It is primarily used in intensive care units to guide the management of head injured patients or those with raised intracranial pressure. It may also have a role in monitoring patients during neurosurgery or those being weaned off cardiopulmonary bypass.

How it works

Fibreoptic technology allows continuous *in vivo* monitoring of S_jvO_2. A fibreoptic catheter is placed through the internal jugular vein and passed retrogradely into the jugular venous bulb. The correct positioning of the catheter can be confirmed using a lateral radiograph of the neck, which should show the catheter tip at the level of the mastoid process.

The catheter utilizes reflectance spectrophotometry using two or three different wavelengths of light, not dissimilar to pulse oximetry (see *Section 6.10*). The catheter contains two fibreoptic cables. The first emits light of specific wavelengths intermittently into the surrounding blood, whilst the second transmits reflected light back to a photosensor. When saturations are low, there is less oxyhaemoglobin to absorb light. Therefore the proportion of reflected light with a wavelength preferentially absorbed by oxyhaemoglobin, increases.

⊕ Advantages

- Provides an early indicator of cerebral ischaemia.
- Continuous measurements are possible.

⊖ Disadvantages

- Malposition may give spurious results.
- Incomplete mixing of venous run-off from the brain may mean that saturations are not representative of oxygen demands of the entire brain.
- The jugular venous bulb also drains some blood from the scalp and skull.
- May not identify regional/ focal cerebral ischaemia.
- Generic complications of internal jugular vein catheterization.

Other notes

If the S_jvO_2 falls below 50–55%, the following strategy may be useful.

(1) Ensure that the catheter is in the correct position.
(2) Check calibration of the device by running a jugular venous blood gas sample.
(3) Diagnose and treat anaemia or arterial hypoxia.
(4) Increase cerebral blood flow by, for example, increasing systemic blood pressure with vasopressors, treating cerebral vasospasm and optimizing the $PaCO_2$.
(5) Treat causes of raised cerebral metabolic oxygen demands ($CMRO_2$) e.g. seizures, pyrexia or inadequate sedation.
(6) Treat increased intracranial pressure, e.g. using mannitol, cerebrospinal fluid drainage, cooling or decompressive craniectomy.

6.24 Hygrometers

Hygrometers are used to measure humidity, which may be absolute or relative:

- **absolute humidity** is the amount of water vapour per unit volume of air (measured in $g.m^{-3}$)
- **relative humidity** is the ratio of absolute humidity to the total amount of water vapour that would be present if the air were fully saturated, expressed as a percentage.

The maximum amount of water vapour that air can hold falls as the temperature decreases. Relative humidity is therefore dependent on the temperature.

The relative humidity in operating theatres is usually kept at 50–60%, because higher values are uncomfortable and lower values increase the risk of sparks.

Hair hygrometer

In a hair hygrometer, a human or animal hair is linked to a spring gauge. The hair lengthens as it absorbs water, moving the pointer across a non-linear scale.

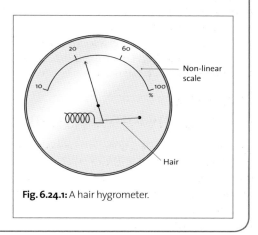

Fig. 6.24.1: A hair hygrometer.

Wet and dry bulb hygrometer

A wet and dry bulb hygrometer consists of two standard mercury thermometers. One has its bulb exposed to the air, and thus reads the true temperature. The other thermometer's bulb is kept wet by a wick submerged in water. As the water evaporates, the bulb cools due to the latent heat of vaporization and the temperature reading therefore falls.

In humid environments, only a small quantity of water evaporates and the thermometers read a similar temperature. If the humidity is low, there is a large difference in readings due to a lot of evaporation. Tables are used to look up the relative humidity from the two temperatures.

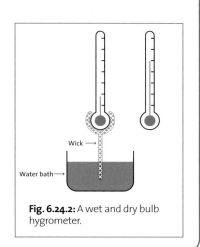

Fig. 6.24.2: A wet and dry bulb hygrometer.

Dew point hygrometer

The dew point is the temperature at which water vapour condenses to form liquid water. As air is cooled, the maximum amount of water vapour it can hold also falls and therefore relative humidity rises. The dew point is reached when relative humidity reaches 100% and therefore water vapour begins to condense. Dew point hygrometers rely on cooling a mirrored surface until dew forms, and using tables to look up the relative humidity at the ambient temperature.

Regnault's hygrometer is a dew point hygrometer in which air is bubbled through a mirrored tube containing ether (ether is used because it is highly volatile). As ether evaporates, the tube is cooled. The temperature at which dew forms on the outside of the tube is noted by the operator.

Electronic dew point hygrometers are extremely accurate, relying on electronic detection of dew on a chilled mirror. Electronic feedback varies the temperature to maintain a dynamic equilibrium between evaporation and condensation on the mirror.

Electronic humidity sensors

A polymer whose capacitance alters with humidity is incorporated into an electric circuit, thus allowing an electronic display of humidity. Capacitative hygrometers are less accurate than electronic dew point hygrometers, but are simpler and more robust.

Resistive sensors are also available.

Mass spectrometry

Mass spectrometry permits very rapid and accurate measurement of absolute humidity, but requires extremely expensive equipment and is unsuitable for routine use (see *Section 6.7: Other methods of gas analysis*).

Chapter 7
Filters and humidifiers

7.1 Passive humidifiers

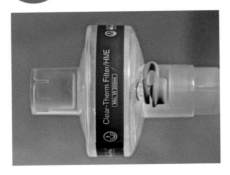

Fig. 7.1.1: A heat and moisture exchange filter (HMEF).

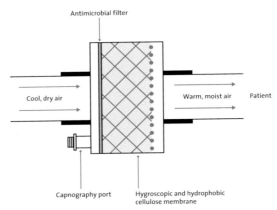

Fig. 7.1.2: Schematic of an HMEF.

Overview

Humidifiers add heat and moisture to cool dry inspired gases. Passive humidifiers do not require external energy to function. The heat and moisture exchanger (HME) is the commonest passive humidification device used in anaesthesia. It is used in patients whose nasal passages (the body's own HME) are bypassed by an airway device such as an endotracheal tube (ETT) or laryngeal mask. Mechanical ventilation with cool, dry gases is known to impair mucociliary clearance of sputum, contribute to airway plugging and atelectasis, as well as exacerbating intra-operative heat loss. HMEs are simple, efficient devices that provide a solution to these problems.

Uses

HMEs are incorporated into breathing systems in most ventilated patients. They are also attached to tracheostomy tubes in patients who no longer require a breathing system. These are known by several different terms, including: Swedish nose, Thermal Humidifying Filter, Artificial nose, Thermovent T and the Edith Trach.

HMEs can also be combined with electrostatic microbial filters (HME filters, HMEF) so that they also protect the ventilated patient and equipment from particulate matter, including some bacteria.

How it works

An HME is a passive device that recovers and retains heat and moisture during expiration and then returns it to cool, dry gas that passes in the opposite direction on inspiration. An HME comprises a core of material within a plastic casing. The ability of an HME to recover and transfer heat and moisture depends largely on the characteristics of the material within its core. HMEs can be classified into three groups, each with their own particular performance characteristics, based on the nature and configuration of their core material:

- hydrophobic (water repelling) HMEs
- hygroscopic (water retaining) HMEs
- combined hygroscopic–hydrophobic HMEs.

The simplest and earliest HMEs were hydrophobic. These models have an aluminium core, which provides a surface that rapidly cools warm, humid expired gases. The cooling causes water vapour to condense and collect between the aluminium inserts. During inspiration cool, dry inspired gas passes through this insert in the opposite direction and absorbs heat and moisture from it. This returns the aluminium to its cooled state and the cycle repeats itself during the next expiration. Hydrophobic devices are the simplest and cheapest, but least efficient, HME devices, producing a modest moisture output of 10–14 mg $H_2O.l^{-1}$ at tidal volumes of 500–1000 ml. In addition, they can suffer from problems caused by the pooling of condensed water.

The efficiency of HMEs was increased by the development of a hygroscopic core. A material with a low thermal conductivity such as paper or foam is impregnated with hygroscopic salts such as calcium or lithium chloride. Instead of moisture being stored as condensed water droplets, the moisture is preserved by a chemical reaction with the salts. These HMEs are more efficient and can produce higher absolute humidities of 22–34 mg $H_2O.l^{-1}$ at tidal volumes of 500–1000 ml.

Newer devices combine hygroscopic, hydrophobic and electrostatic filters in varying configurations to produce even more efficient devices.

Advantages

- Cheap and simple.
- Do not require a power source.
- Produce 60–80% humidification of inspired gases.
- Reduce heat and moisture loss from the conducting airways and therefore improve mucociliary function and sputum clearance.
- When combined with a filter, can be very efficient at removing bacteria and viruses. Some studies show a reduction in rates of ventilator-associated pneumonia in critical care.

Disadvantages

- Increase the dead-space of the breathing system. Smaller HMEs are therefore used for children.
- Increase the resistance of the breathing system.
- A progressive increase in resistance through the HME is seen after several hours of use due to an increase in the material density of the HME.
- Add bulk to the patient end of the breathing system.
- HMEs can become occluded with secretions, blood or water.
- The efficiency falls as tidal volumes and inspiratory flow rates increase.
- It can take 10–20 minutes for HMEs to equilibrate and reach maximal efficacy.

7.2 Active humidification

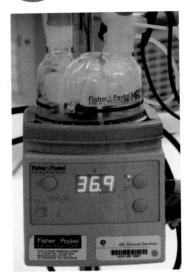

Fig. 7.2.1: A surface water bath humidification device used in ITU.

Overview

Active gas humidifiers humidify (and often warm) cool, dry inspired gases using an energy-dependent process. This is in contrast to passive humidification where no external energy source is required. Active gas humidification is used to prevent the effects of breathing cool, dry gases for long periods. These effects are known to include atelectasis, exacerbation of intra-operative heat losses, and impaired mucociliary function. Active humidification is generally more effective (in terms of the relative humidity achieved) than passive humidifiers like HMEs.

Uses

Used in patients who are mechanically ventilated or require oxygen therapy for significant periods, or have respiratory problems and are at risk of airway plugging (e.g. asthmatics).

How it works

Gases that are fully saturated with water at body temperature (37°C) have an absolute humidity of $44\,g.m^{-3}$. An approximate comparison of the absolute humidity achieved by various devices is shown in *Table 7.2.1*. Note that values quoted by the manufacturer are usually measured under optimal conditions, and the actual humidity achieved may be less in clinical practice. Note that if the absolute humidity achieved in the lungs is greater than $44\,g.m^{-3}$, water may precipitate within the alveoli.

Table 7.2.1: Absolute achievable humidities for active and passive humidifiers.

Humidifier	Achievable absolute humidity $(g.m^{-3})$
Cold water bubble active humidifier	10
Heat and moisture exchanger (NB. a passive humidifier)	25–30
Warm water bubble active humidifier or warm water surface humidifier	40
Gas-driven nebulized active humidifier (with anvil or rotating disc)	50–60
Ultrasonic nebulized active humidifier	80–90

Surface water bath humidifiers

Inspiratory gas is passed over the surface of a heated water bath. As it does so, it picks up water vapour from above the surface of the water and carries it to the patient. The water bath is usually heated to 40–45°C, but may be increased to 60°C to reduce bacterial growth.

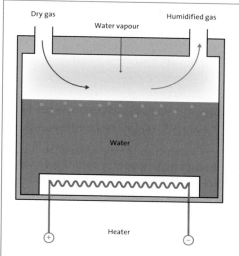

Fig. 7.2.2: Schematic of a surface water bath humidifier.

Advantages
- In contrast to aerosolized water droplets, water vapour does not usually carry microbes. Therefore, in comparison with nebulizers and bubble humidifiers there is, theoretically, a reduced risk of infection.
- The humidifier does not significantly increase resistance to gas flow.
- Usually located some distance from the patient. This reduces the risk of liquid water entering the inspiratory limb of the breathing system.

Disadvantages
- Condensation can build up in the inspiratory limb of breathing system.
- Thermostat failure could lead to airway scalding.
- Bacterial and fungal colonization of the water reservoir can occur.

Bubble humidifiers

Fresh gas is directed through a reservoir of sterile water via a fine capillary network or nozzle with multiple apertures. As the gas bubbles through and out of the reservoir, it becomes saturated with water vapour and transports it to the patient. The absolute humidity achieved by the bubble humidifier can be increased by heating the water. A typical reservoir has a volume of 300 ml.

Advantages
- Compact.
- Cheaper than other active humidifiers.
- Produces a higher absolute humidity than passive humidifiers.

Disadvantages
- Risk of bacterial growth and colonization in the water bath.
- Water aerosols can lead to transmission of infection into the patient's respiratory tract.

- Increases resistance to flow in the inspiratory limb of the breathing circuit because the fresh gas flow is bubbled through water.
- As water vapour cools, it may condense and build up within the oxygen tubing (rain-out).
- Mineral build-up along capillary network can cause occlusions to oxygen inlet.
- There is a risk of overheating and airway burns if the thermostat fails. If the water is not heated, a bubble humidifier's efficiency may be less than that of a HME.

 Safety

Some bubble humidifiers incorporate a high-pressure alarm that triggers at 4–6 p.s.i. with an automatic pressure relief valve. Newer designs also include baffle systems to prevent liquid water entering the oxygen tubing.

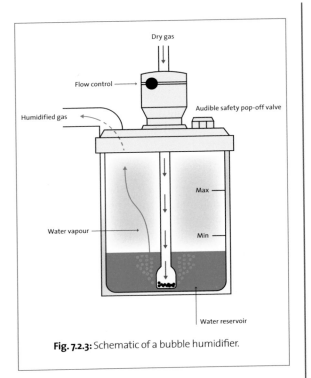

Fig. 7.2.3: Schematic of a bubble humidifier.

Nebulized humidifiers

A gas-driven nebulizer passes a high velocity stream of gas across the end of a tube that is positioned in a reservoir of water. The fast moving gas generates a negative pressure around the nozzle and draws water into the tube as a result of the Venturi effect (see *Section 1.12: Venturi masks*). The impact of the high velocity gas causes the water to break up into tiny droplets, which are carried by the gas flow to the patient. Droplets of water may be broken up further by colliding with an anvil.

Spinning disc nebulizers comprise a porous spinning disc partially immersed in a water bath. As the disc spins, it draws

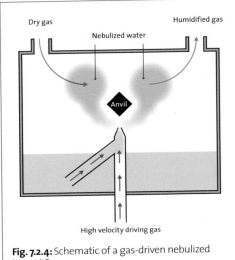

Fig. 7.2.4: Schematic of a gas-driven nebulized humidifier.

water up from the bath and releases it as small droplets through small holes into the path of the FGF. The absolute humidity generated may be augmented by heating the water reservoir.

Ultrasonic nebulizers apply a 2–3 MHz vibration to a plate that is positioned in a water reservoir. The vibrational force is transmitted to the water surface and can produce water droplets as small as 1 μm in size. These water droplets are entrained with fresh gas that flows through the nebulizer chamber. Over-humidification of gases with an ultrasonic humidifier is a risk and may result in pulmonary oedema. Close monitoring of the patient is therefore mandatory.

Advantages
- Produce higher absolute humidities compared to passive HMEs.
- There is no added dead space.
- Less likely to occlude.
- Decreased resistance to breathing when compared to HMEs.

Specific disadvantages
- Risk of over-humidifying patient leading to pulmonary oedema or altered fluid balance through absorption.
- Provide a route for bacterial and viral infection.
- Expensive.
- Require an electrical power supply.
- Bulky and noisy when compared to other humidifiers.
- Require a sterile water supply.

Porous surface contact humidifiers

A porous polyethylene fibre block is positioned on top of a heated water bath and fresh gas flows over and through it. Water is drawn up by capillary action along the fibres, creating a three-fold increase in the surface area for humidification, when compared to traditional chamber-type humidification systems. The Hummax humidification system (Metran) is capable of humidifying gases at flows of 3–30 ml.h^{-1}. The pore size of its fibre block is as small as 0.1 μm.

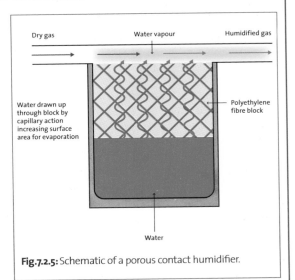

Fig.7.2.5: Schematic of a porous contact humidifier.

Advantages
- 0.1 μm pore size can theoretically filter bacteria.
- Efficient humidification is possible because of the increased water/gas contact surface area.

Disadvantage
- Calcification of the porous surface over time reduces efficiency.

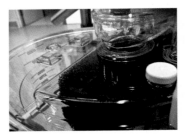

Fig. 7.3.1: A Medtronic cardiotomy blood reservoir filter that forms part of a cardiopulmonary bypass circuit.

Overview

Filtration is the process by which particles are removed from streams of fluid or gas by a semi-permeable membrane. Various types of filter play an important role in anaesthesia and critical care. These may be classified into screen and depth filters. In screen filters, all the pores rest in the same plane. Depth filters possess multiple layers of pores that force the fluid through a tortuous path that increases the likelihood of particle impaction. This classification is controversial, not least because screen filters exhibit depth when observed microscopically.

Uses

Examples of commonly encountered filters include breathing system filters, epidural filters, IV infusion filters, blood filters, platelet filters, filter needles and haemofilters.

How it works

The principle mechanisms of filtration are:

- direct interception
- diffusional interception
- inertial impaction
- electrostatic deposition.

The degree to which each of these mechanisms plays a role in a given filter depends on the physical properties of the particles being filtered, whether they are suspended in a liquid or a gas, and the properties of the filter itself.

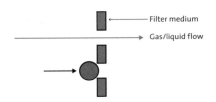

Fig. 7.3.2: Direct interception.

Direct interception
Particles that are larger than the pore size of the filter will be trapped (or intercepted) by it.

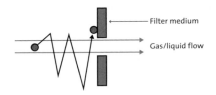

Fig. 7.3.3: Diffusional interception.

Diffusional interception
One might expect that particles that are smaller than the pores in a filter would pass freely. However, separation of these small particles can still occur because their random (Brownian) movement within the gas or liquid make them 'appear' larger than they are. These random movements (caused by multiple collisions with other molecules) mean that these particles deviate away from the line of fluid flow and are therefore more likely to impact filter fibres.

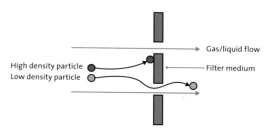

Fig. 7.3.4: Inertial impaction.

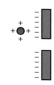

Fig. 7.3.5: Electrostatic deposition.

Inertial impaction

Inertial impaction affects particles that are denser than the fluid in which they are travelling. Less dense particles can change direction quickly to follow the fluid flow around the solid fibres of the filter medium. However, higher density molecules are unable to change direction as readily because of their inertia (the tendency of a body to resist changes in its speed or direction, which is dependent on its mass). These particles therefore tend to continue in a linear trajectory and impact the filter.

Electrostatic deposition

This is the process by which weakly charged particles are attracted towards opposite weak charges on the filter material. These weak electrostatic forces are also known as van der Waals forces.

Filter efficacy

Both inertial and diffusional impaction work best when filtering solid particles from a gas rather than a liquid. This is in part because the difference in density between a solid particle and a gas is far greater than between a solid particle and a liquid.

The efficacy of a filter can be measured by its removal rating. Many manufacturers quote a 'nominal filter rating', which gives a percentage rating for the efficacy of a filter for particles of a given size. It is calculated by introducing a contaminant of known size upstream of the filter and then microscopically analysing the downstream filtrate; a nominal rating of 99% at 0.2 μm means that 99% of contaminants equal to or greater than 0.2 μm have been successfully removed by the filter. This rating can be misleading because under certain circumstances, larger particles can pass through the filter, e.g. due to high upstream pressures.

⊕ Advantages

- Reduce contamination, particularly of a patient's body by solid contaminants.
- Reduce risk of bacterial transmission.

⊖ Disadvantages

- Increase resistance to the flow of fluids.
- Add bulk and weight to equipment.
- Limited lifespan due to clogging.
- Efficacy falls under extremes of pressure and temperature, which can alter the physical characteristics of the filter material.
- Filter media may trigger inflammatory reactions such as the activation of complement or leukocytes.
- Filters are not effective at protecting against most viruses.

Specific types of filter

Heat and moisture exchange filters and haemofilters are covered in separate dedicated sections within the book (*Sections 7.1 and 9.10*, respectively).

Epidural filters

Epidural filters are used to prevent the injection of contaminants that have the potential to induce CNS infection or inflammation. They are low volume hydrophilic filters, used for two-way in-line filtration of aqueous solutions. The average volume of an epidural filter is 0.45 ml. One end attaches to an epidural catheter and the other has a Luer or, more recently, non-Luer connector (see *Section 8.7*) that attaches to syringes or epidural giving sets. Most epidural filters have a strong acrylic casing that has a flat profile to improve patient comfort and is transparent to aid the identification of blood during aspiration.

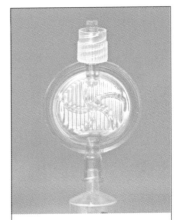

Fig. 7.3.6: An epidural filter.

Most epidural filters quote filtration efficacy for a particle size of 0.2 μm over a filter surface area of 4 cm². This should be effective in removing the majority of bacteria. Modern epidural filters have been engineered to minimize drug binding, withstand pressures of up to 7 bar, retain bacteria and endotoxin effectively for up to 96 hours and eliminate injected air bubbles.

The filter adds significant resistance to injection. Whilst all epidural filters vary in their resistance, a typical water flow through a 0.2 μm filter is 15 ml.min⁻¹ when a pressure of 80 cmH₂O is applied.

Specific advantages

- Effective filter of particulate matter and bacteria down to 0.2 μm.
- Able to maintain efficacy up to burst pressures of 7 bar.
- Transparent so that blood in the filter can be identified quickly.
- Allows two-way filtration.

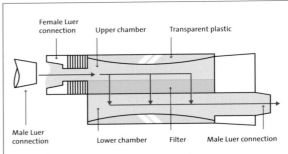

Fig. 7.3.7: Schematic of an epidural filter.

Specific disadvantages

- Has a residual volume of approximately 0.45 ml.
- Adds bulk to the end of an epidural catheter.
- Commonly used epidural filters have standard Luer locks which increase the risk of inadvertent injection of harmful drugs into the epidural space.
- Effective for approximately 96 hours.

Blood (giving set) filters

With the exception of human albumin, immunoglobulin and stem cells which require a 15 μm filter (found on standard intravenous giving sets), all blood products must be given through a blood giving set with a 170–200 μm filter to filter particulate matter and thrombi from donor blood products during infusion.

A standard blood giving set has a compressible double-chambered reservoir with an in-line mesh filter (170–200 μm pore size). This removes large clots and aggregates and is used for transfusions of fresh frozen plasma (FFP), cryoprecipitate, platelets and leucocyte-depleted red cells. The tubing is usually 150 cm long, with a Luer lock fitting at its distal end.

Blood and platelets in the UK are now leucodepleted pre-storage in an effort to reduce the transmission of vCJD and transfusion reactions. A specific bedside leucodepletion filter to remove white cells (20–50 μm pore size) is therefore no longer required. Platelets must, however, still be administered through a giving set with a 170–200 μm filter. This can either be through a standard blood giving set or a specific platelet giving set

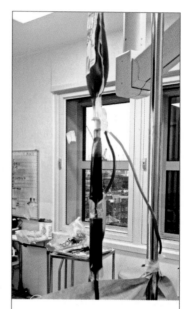

Fig. 7.3.8: Blood giving set.

with a 200 μm filter (e.g. the Baxter platelet administration set). The only real advantage of a specific platelet giving set is that it has a lower prime / deadspace volume, which reduces platelet wastage. If a standard blood giving set is used to administer platelets, it is important that a fresh giving set is used, because platelets may be wasted by getting caught up in red blood cell fragments within the filter.

There has been some interest about the role of pieces of debris that develop in blood products during storage which are too small to be filtered by standard blood giving set filters (microaggregates). These can in theory act as micro-emboli which mediate both mechanical obstruction of capillary beds and adverse immune reactions. However, the evidence is limited for the use of specific microaggregate filters and their small pore size (20–40 μm) may impair flow rates. Microaggregate filter pore sizes are also similar to those of leucocyte depletion filters, so the filter may trap a proportion of the platelets. For these reasons, microaggregate filters aren't used often.

Table 7.3.1: The administration of blood products.

Component	Filter pore size required (μm)	Speed of transfusion	Storage
Packed red cells (leucodepleted)	170–200	Complete within 4 h of issue	At 4°C for up to 42 days
Platelets (leucodepleted)	170–200	Should be administered within 30 min of issue	5 days in a platelet agitator at room temperature
Fresh frozen plasma	170–200	Usually administered over 30 min	Frozen (−30°C): 1 year Once thawed, it should ideally be given immediately, but can be stored for up to 24 h at 4°C or 4 h at 22°C
Cryoprecipitate	170–200	Usually administered over 30 min	Frozen (−30°C): 1 year Once thawed, it should ideally be given immediately, but can be stored for up to 24 h at 4°C
Human albumin solution (HAS)	15 – vented filter set (standard IV admin. set)	Usually administered over 30 min	3 years at less than 25°C and 5 years at temperatures between 2 and 8°C

Advantages
- Reduces the infusion of blood clots and aggregates.

Disadvantages
- Requires changing when flow rate is compromised or at least 12 hourly.
- Increased resistance to flow leads to increased transfusion times.

Standard IV giving sets and burette filters

Standard IV fluid infusion sets and burettes are used for the administration of all IV fluids except blood products, although it should be noted that specialist burettes incorporating a blood filter are available for paediatric transfusion.

A standard infusion set or burette usually incorporates a 15 μm filter. Standard IV infusion sets have a drip factor of 20 drops/ml (i.e. for every 20 drops that enter the drip chamber, 1 ml of fluid is infused under standardized conditions).

Burette sets are used, particularly in paediatrics, for more accurate and controlled delivery of IV fluids and drugs. The dependent end of the burette's chamber empties

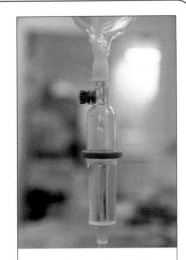

Fig. 7.3.9: A standard IV fluid giving set.

into a drip chamber through a 'microdropper' that delivers 60 drops/ml of fluid. Most burettes also incorporate a floating ball valve that prevents entrainment of air from the empty burette chamber into the drip chamber.

Advantages
- Simple.
- Accurate.
- Kink resistant tubing.
- Can be used with infusion pumps.

Disadvantages
- Need to be changed at least every 72 hours.
- Unsuitable for the transfusion of blood products.
- Rapid infusion is not possible due to high resistance to flow.

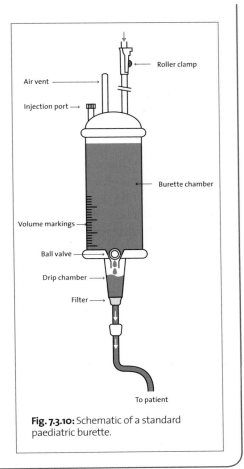

Fig. 7.3.10: Schematic of a standard paediatric burette.

Filter needles

Filter needles are used to prevent the inadvertent injection of particulate contaminants into the body. These can include small shards of glass from vials, plastic, rubber and undissolved or precipitated drugs. Studies have shown that particles as small as 6 µm can cause occlusion of the micro-circulation and phlebitis. Injected glass particles have also been reported to induce fibrotic reactions in the lungs, liver and gastrointestinal system. Current guidelines recommend that filter needles used for drawing up drugs have a maximum pore size of 5 µm, which can effectively filter particles from 10 to 1000 µm in diameter. Smaller pore filters (e.g. 0.22 µm) are also effective at removing bacterial contaminants.

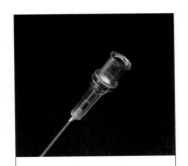

Fig. 7.3.11: A filter needle.

Advantages

- Prevent drawing up and injection of particulate matter from glass vials.
- Smaller (0.22 µm) filters are also effective at filtering bacteria.

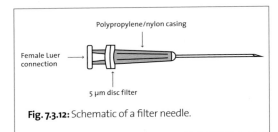

Polypropylene/nylon casing

Female Luer connection

5 µm disc filter

Fig. 7.3.12: Schematic of a filter needle.

Disadvantages

- Need to change to a standard needle before patient is injected.
- Increase resistance when drawing up drugs.
- Single use only.
- Not all drawing up needles incorporate a filter. The difference is not always clear.

Chapter 8
Regional anaesthesia

8.1 Nerve stimulators

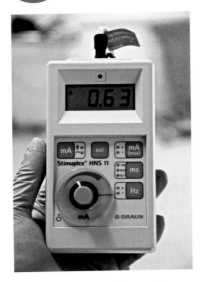

Fig. 8.1.1: A nerve stimulator used in regional anaesthesia.

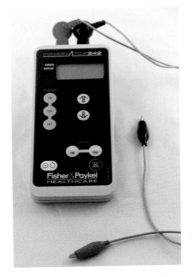

Fig. 8.1.2: A nerve stimulator used for monitoring neuromuscular blockade.

Overview

Nerve stimulators produce direct current of specific amplitude, duration and frequency to produce depolarization of peripheral nerves.

Uses

Two types of nerve stimulator are commonly used by anaesthetists. One is used for the localization of nerves during the insertion of regional nerve blocks. The other is used to monitor neuromuscular blockade. A further type of nerve stimulator may be used by surgeons operating in close proximity to important nerves to identify their course.

The principles of how nerve stimulators work are the same, regardless of their application.

How it works

The physiology of nerve stimulation
If the electrical energy delivered by a nerve stimulator is sufficient to cause a rise in the membrane potential of a nerve, such that it exceeds its threshold potential, depolarization will occur and an action potential will propagate. There are five main variables that can be manipulated in order to achieve depolarization of a nerve: the amplitude of the current, the duration and frequency of the stimulus, the proximity of the electrode to the nerve, and its polarity. The energy delivered to the nerve per stimulus is the product of the current amplitude and the duration of the stimulus.

Amplitude
A supra-maximal stimulus is one with sufficient current amplitude to cause 100% of motor neurons within the nerve to be depolarized. Supra-maximal stimuli are required during monitoring of neuromuscular blockade so that any variation in the twitch characteristics (for example, fade) must be due to a factor other than the number of neurons recruited during repeated stimulation.

Duration

For a given current amplitude, shorter impulse durations will preferentially stimulate large fibres. Therefore action potentials can be stimulated in motor fibres (which have a larger mean diameter than sensory fibres) by the application of current for approximately 0.1 msec. Conversely, stimulation of the smallest pain transmitting C-fibres requires stimuli of a significantly greater duration (e.g. 0.4 msec). Shorter impulses deliver insufficient energy to stimulate motor fibres, whereas longer impulses are more likely to cause pain and to directly stimulate adjacent muscle fibres.

Polarity

Interestingly, significantly less energy is needed to stimulate a nerve that is adjacent to the *cathode* than one adjacent to the *anode*. Therefore the negative terminal should be connected to the electrode closest to the target nerve or the stimulator needle.

Proximity

The relationship between the energy required to depolarize a neuron and the distance between the neuron and electrode obeys the inverse square law, meaning that four times the energy is required if the distance is doubled.

Electrical components of a nerve stimulator

Nerve stimulators incorporate the following components:

- power source
- constant current generator
- oscillator – this is a key component of a nerve stimulator; based on the control settings, a microprocessor interrupts the constant current generator and influences the frequency and duration of the stimulus
- display and controls
- anode and cathode:
  - for regional anaesthesia, the anode (a standard ECG electrode) is placed on the skin surface to complete an electrical circuit with the block needle cathode.
  - during monitoring of neuromuscular blockade there are two skin electrodes.

RHEOBASE and CHRONAXIE

If you are doing well in a physiology or physics viva, you may be asked about *rheobase* and *chronaxie*. The terms are not as complicated as they sound. They are mathematical terms coined by the French physiologist Louis Lapicque over 100 years ago, to quantify and compare the electrical excitability of nerves and muscle fibres. To understand these terms, remember the basic principle that the ability of an electrical stimulus to produce depolarization of a nerve depends on the energy delivered, which for a square wave stimulus, is the product of the <u>current</u> applied and its <u>duration</u>.

Rheobase: is the minimum *current* amplitude of indefinite duration that results in an action potential.

Chronaxie: is the minimum *time* over which a current that is at twice the rheobase, should flow in order to stimulate an action potential.

Types of stimulation pattern

Regional anaesthesia

A typical starting current is 1 mA. The current duration is usually set to 0.2 msec and the frequency of the stimuli is usually set at 2 Hz (one every 0.5 seconds). If a low frequency is set and the needle is moved quickly, there is a risk that the needle will contact the nerve before the next muscle twitch is seen. Nerve damage is therefore a risk of using a frequency that is too low and/or moving the needle too quickly. Conversely, if the frequency is set too high it can be painful and cause tetany. A frequency of 2 Hz is a compromise that allows faster and more natural manipulation of the needle with good visual feedback for the operator.

A nerve stimulator needle is appropriately positioned when a twitch (e.g. patellar twitch for a femoral nerve block) can be elicited by a current of 0.3–0.5 mA. A higher current implies that the needle is too far from the nerve for an effective block, whereas a lower current implies that the needle may be within the nerve, risking nerve rupture during injection.

There should be a loss of twitch on the injection of 1 ml of local anaesthetic as the nerve is pushed away from the needle tip by the anaesthetic and there should be minimal resistance to injection using a 20 ml syringe. High resistance, or persistence of the twitch, implies intraneural positioning and no further injection should take place until the needle is withdrawn.

Neuromuscular blockade monitoring

The activity of neuromuscular blocking agents should be monitored in order to produce optimum muscle relaxation and to guide the timing of its reversal. Different patterns of nerve stimulation can be used to alter the sensitivity of the monitoring. The skin has a high resistance so currents of 40–60 mA are required.

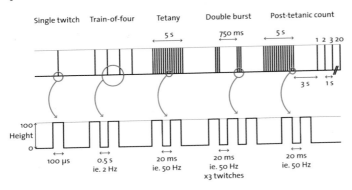

Fig. 8.1.3: Patterns of nerve stimulation.

Single twitch
A single square wave of current lasting 0.1–0.2 msec is applied to the nerve. The muscle twitch amplitude begins to fall when >70% of acetylcholine receptors are occupied.

Train-of-four
Four single twitches are applied at a frequency of 2 Hz. The ratio of the fourth twitch amplitude to the first twitch amplitude provides a more sensitive indicator of the level of neuromuscular blockade than a single twitch.

Table. 8.1.1: Interpretation of the number of twitches seen during train-of-four nerve stimulation. Note that even when four twitches are seen, up to 75% of receptors at the neuromuscular junction may be blocked and the patient's respiratory effort may still be insufficient for safe extubation. It is therefore prudent to give neostigmine (and glycopyrolate) at this point, prior to weaning and extubation.

Number of twitches seen	Nicotinic acetylcholine receptors blocked at the neuromuscular junction (%)
4	<75
3	75
2	80
1	90
0	100

Tetanic, double burst and post-tetanic count patterns of stimulation are used when there is intense neuromuscular blockade because there may be no visible twitches to a train-of-four stimulus in these circumstances. They are all variations of tetanic stimulation and rely on the principle that high frequency stimulation of nerves leads to the mobilization of pre-synaptic acetylcholine, which will briefly overcome the neuromuscular blockade and cause visible muscle contractions.

Tetanic stimulation

A 50 Hz stimulation applied for 5 seconds will cause a sustained (tetanic) contraction of the muscle. If a neuromuscular blocker is present at a high concentration at the neuromuscular junction, the sustained contraction will fade over the period of the stimulus.

Double burst stimulation

This comprises two bursts of tetanic stimulation separated by a pause. The exact number of stimuli and the length of the pause can vary, but a typical setting is three tetanic pulses at 50 Hz then a pause of 750 msec followed by another three pulses at 50 Hz. The fade that occurs between the two bursts is easier to see than with a single tetanic stimulus alone.

Post-tetanic count

This pattern involves a 5 second tetanic stimulation at 50 Hz, followed by a pause of 3 seconds and then 20 pulses at 1 Hz. The number of twitches that are observed in response to the 20 pulses are counted and can be used to predict how long neuromuscular blockade will last. A post-tetanic count of 12–15 suggests that the return of a train-of-four twitch is imminent.

Methods of assessing responses to stimulation

(1) Observing or palpating twitches. This is highly subjective.
(2) Mechanical force transducers: the force generated during the isometric contraction of the muscle can be measured using a strain gauge.
(3) Accelerometers: a piezoelectric crystal transducer attached to the finger measures the acceleration of the finger during stimulation. Piezoelectric crystals have the interesting property of generating an electric current when pressure is applied to them. The acceleration is proportional to the force of contraction.
(4) Integrated electromyography: This detects the electrical potential caused by muscle cells as action potentials are generated.

Advantages

- Inexpensive.
- Portable.
- Simple to use.
- Sensitive.
- In regional anaesthesia, the risk of nerve damage is lower than using the obsolete technique of eliciting paraesthesia with a needle.
- Easier technique to learn than using real-time ultrasound for regional anaesthesia.

Disadvantages

- Regional anaesthesia should usually be performed when the patient is conscious, and the muscle contraction elicited by a 2 Hz stimulus may be unacceptably uncomfortable for some patients. It may also be inappropriate for patients with painful conditions such as fractures.
- Arguably, regional anaesthesia performed with a nerve stimulator is still a blind technique and so the risk of intraneural and intravascular injection may be significant.
- Interpretation of muscle twitches when monitoring neuromuscular blockade is largely subjective. Techniques for objectifying their use such as mechanical force transducers can be cumbersome and expensive.

8.2 Nerve stimulator needles

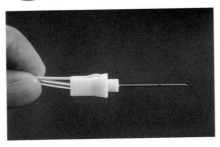

Fig. 8.2.1: A nerve stimulator needle.

Overview

Stimulator needles are used in conjunction with nerve stimulators. They are short-bevelled, hollow needles with a Luer connector for attachment to a syringe and metal shaft that forms the cathode of a nerve stimulator. A separate skin electrode forms the anode and completes the circuit.

Uses

Used for the localization of nerves during regional anaesthesia, and deposition of local anaesthetic.

How it works

The physics and physiology of nerve stimulation are discussed in *Section 8.1*. Nerve stimulator needles usually have a 30° short bevel, come in a variety of lengths (25–150 mm) and diameters (20–25G), and have depth markings along their surface.

Most needles are electrically insulated, except at the tip where the current is needed. This allows a smaller current to be used because less electrical power is dissipated into the surrounding tissue along the shaft of the needle. It also allows more accurate determination of the position of the target nerve relative to the tip of the needle.

⊕ Advantages

- The short bevel provides superior tactile feedback compared to sharper, long-bevelled needles.
- Modified Tuohy needles are available to facilitate the insertion of continuous nerve block catheters.

⊖ Disadvantages

- Intra-neural needle placement and injection is a recognized complication.
- Often requires an assistant to help adjust the nerve stimulator and inject the drug whilst the operator manipulates and steadies the needle. This is especially true if real-time ultrasound is also being used.

ⓘ Safety

Nerve blocks should be carried out with a nerve stimulator that has a disconnection alarm to reduce the risk of inadvertent neural injury.

It is increasingly accepted that regional anaesthesia is safest when performed on a conscious or lightly sedated patient.

Newer needles also have echogenic coatings so that they can easily be visualized with ultrasound, allowing nerve stimulation and ultrasound imaging at the same time. It is not conclusive whether this technique is inherently safer than using ultrasound alone.

Pencil point nerve stimulator needles are now available. In theory, they are less likely to cause neural damage because of their blunt tip, but inserting it through the skin can be difficult for this very reason.

8.3 Spinal needles

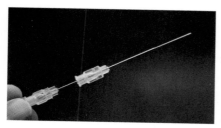

Fig. 8.3.1: A spinal needle.

Overview

Spinal anaesthesia was first performed by Leonard Corning in 1885 when he accidentally breached the dura whilst investigating the effects of cocaine on the spinal nerves of dogs. Soon after, Quincke described a lumbar puncture technique to treat the symptoms of raised intracranial pressure using a sharp, bevelled needle that cut through the dura. It was Augustus Bier though, in 1898, who first experimented with spinal anaesthesia using cocaine on humans through what he described as a 'Quincke needle'.

Uses

- Spinal anaesthesia.
- Lumbar puncture for diagnostic sampling of CSF.
- Therapeutic drainage of CSF.
- Intrathecal chemotherapy.

How it works

Since the time of Bier's first successful spinal anaesthetic, the design of the spinal needle has seen many variations. All comprise a hollow metal needle with a metal or plastic hub that attaches to a syringe. Various sizes are available, but the use of smaller (e.g. 27G) needles has been shown to produce a lower incidence of post-dural puncture headache (PDPH). The needle has a tip designed to aid penetration through soft tissue and a stylet is often used to prevent coring and to improve rigidity.

The evolution of spinal needle design

Over the years the material used, the shape and sharpness of the bevel, the diameter and tapering of the needle, the position of the distal aperture, the number of apertures and the use of introducers are areas of spinal needle design that have been refined, tested and debated.

At the turn of the twentieth century the association between the size of the hole made in the dura, the magnitude of the subsequent CSF leak and the incidence and severity of PDPHs was noted. This led to the introduction of wider bore introducer needles to aid penetration of skin and ligaments and much finer cutting spinal needles were inserted. Even with these changes, PDPH rates remained as high as 10%.

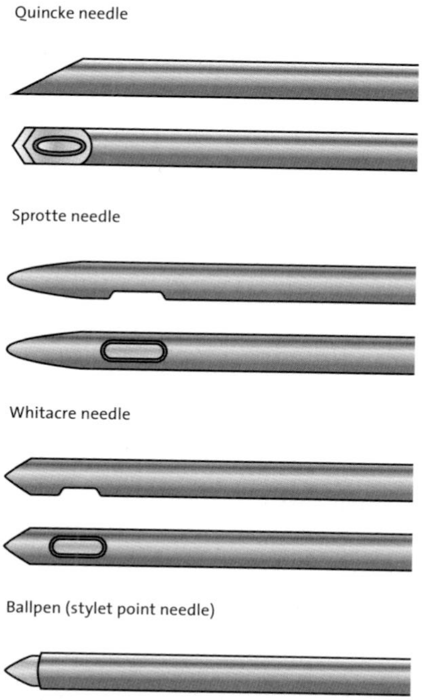

Quincke needle

Sprotte needle

Whitacre needle

Ballpen (stylet point needle)

Fig. 8.3.2: Comparison of spinal needles.

Work by early pioneers of spinal anaesthesia, such as Labat and Greene in the 1920s, led to the discovery that round-tipped bevelled needles produced smaller holes in the dura and therefore significantly reduced PDPH rates to 4–5%. The Greene atraumatic spinal needle subsequently became very popular throughout the mid-twentieth century.

Whitacre made the next major advance in spinal needle design through his pencil-point design in 1951. Instead of a terminal eye at the end of the needle, Whitacre designed a needle with a solid conical tip and a proximal aperture on the side of the needle. The Whitacre needle separates, rather than cuts dural fibres as it enters the subarachnoid space. Once the needle is removed, the uncut dural fibres close again, thus reducing CSF leakage. An added benefit is that the blunt pencil-point design produces a noticeable 'click' as it passes through the dura, giving the operator tactile feedback of the needle's entry into the subarachnoid space. The Whitacre needle produces a PDPH rate as low as 2–3% and it quickly superseded the Greene spinal needle in popularity. In 1987, Sprotte introduced a modified Whitacre needle. The Sprotte modifications included a larger aperture to aid aspiration of CSF and injection of drugs. It also featured a longer tip, improving the atraumatic separation of dural fibres compared to the original Whitacre needle and therefore led to further reduction in PDPH rates. Newer spinal needle designs continue to be developed and stylet-point needles have also been marketed recently.

Quincke spinal needle (cutting)

The Quincke needle has a diamond-shaped cutting bevel and an opening at the tip.

Advantages
- Cuts through tissue and ligaments, making insertion easier.
- The aperture is at the tip of the needle, so it is less likely to straddle the dural membrane, reducing the risk of failed spinals.

Disadvantages
- Higher incidence of PDPH (8% vs. 3% for a 25G Whitacre needle).
- The cutting tip potentially increases the risk of nerve damage.
- Less tactile feedback (in terms of a 'dural click') as it passes through the dura.
- Risk of tissue coring and aperture occlusion as no stylet is used.

Whitacre spinal needle (atraumatic pencil-point)

The Whitacre needle was designed in 1951 and has a solid conical blunt tip and a lateral rectangular aperture just proximal to it. It is the most commonly used needle for spinal anaesthesia in the UK.

Advantages
- Causes less dural trauma because its tip separates the longitudinal fibres of the dura without cutting them, hence reducing CSF leakage and PDPH rates.
- Blunt tip generates a more convincing 'dural click' on breaching the dura when compared to a cutting needle like the Quincke.

Disadvantages
- Small lateral orifice increases resistance to CSF aspiration and anaesthetic injection.
- The orifice sits proximal to the tip, and may straddle the dural membrane, increasing the risk of spinal failure by inadvertent injection into the epidural space.

Sprotte spinal needle (modified atraumatic pencil-point)

In 1987, Sprotte modified the Whitacre needle to improve dural fibre separation. It retains a conical blunt tip but the lateral aperture is larger, oval shaped and sits further from the tip.

Advantages
- Larger aperture for faster backflow of CSF into the hub on entering the subarachnoid space.
- Less resistance to injection and aspiration.
- Tapered tip allows gradual and less traumatic separation of dural fibres, reducing PDPH rates compared to Whitacre needles.

Disadvantages
- The lateral aperture is larger and a greater distance from the tip compared to the Whitacre needle, increasing the risk of straddling the subarachnoid and epidural space at the time of injection and raising the likelihood of a failed or partial block.

Ballpen (stylet point needle)

The Ballpen (Rusch) is a stylet point spinal needle. It comprises a sharp stylet within the lumen of the hollow spinal cannula. Unlike other stylets, it protrudes 2–3 mm from the distal end of the spinal cannula with a smooth junction between the two. When the sharp stylet is removed, the hollow spinal needle remains within the subarachnoid space.

Advantages

- The tip of the spinal cannula remains within the subdural space on removal of the stylet.
- No problems with coring of tissue or blockage of the aperture.
- Opens at the distal tip of the needle, reducing the risk of injecting into the epidural space, as sometimes occurs with side aperture devices such as the Whitacre or Sprotte needles.
- The distance the needle tip needs to move into the subarachnoid space before CSF is seen is less, theoretically reducing the risk of neurological damage compared to Whitacre and Sprotte needles.
- The pencil-point stylet aids atraumatic insertion through the dural membrane, giving a PDPH rate comparable to the Whitacre and Sprotte needles.

Disadvantages

- Withdrawal of the stylet may dislodge the hollow cannula from the subarachnoid space.
- If the needle is advanced so that only the very tip of the stylet enters the subarachnoid space, the cannula may be left in the epidural space when the stylet is removed.

8.4 Epidural needles

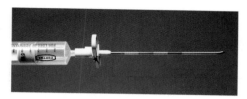

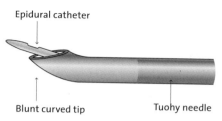

Epidural catheter

Blunt curved tip

Tuohy needle

Fig. 8.4.1: A Tuohy needle.

Fig. 8.4.2: The curved tip of a Tuohy needle.

Overview

Epidural anaesthesia has its origins at the turn of the twentieth century when Sicard and Cathelin described injecting cocaine through the sacral hiatus to treat sciatica. It was, however, Pagés who first described a lumbar approach to the epidural space in 1921. His work was built on by Dogliotti in the 1930s who described how the epidural space could be identified using a loss of resistance syringe. Continuous epidural anaesthesia in labouring women was subsequently pioneered by the Romanian obstetrician Aburel in 1930s Europe and, simultaneously, by Hingson in America who modified continuous spinal anaesthesia techniques for this purpose.

Modern epidural needles are routinely referred to as 'Tuohy needles' after Edward B. Tuohy, a prominent American anaesthesiologist and an early proponent of neuraxial anaesthesia. He modified a Huber needle for the purposes of continuous spinal (but not initially epidural) anaesthesia. Huber was a dentist who had invented a revolutionary new hypodermic needle in the 1940s, whose long, sharp, curved tip reduced coring of tissue and pain on insertion through the skin. Tuohy exploited the Huber needle's curved tip to direct the insertion of a spinal catheter into the subarachnoid space and introduced a stylet to further reduce tissue coring. However, it was his Cuban colleague, Curbello, who first used the directional tip on Tuohy's needle to feed a silk catheter into the lumbar epidural space and deliver continuous epidural anaesthesia.

Tuohy's modification of the Huber needle has continued to evolve over the years. In the 1950s, Hustead blunted the tip of the curved epidural needle and smoothed the heel of the needle's bevel to reduce inadvertent shearing of the catheter. Weiss is accredited with adding wings to aid gripping and manipulation of the needle and Lee added depth markings at 1 cm intervals. Other proposed modifications, such as Sprotte's pencil-point epidural, were less successful.

Uses

- The insertion of epidural catheters to provide continuous anaesthesia and analgesia in peri-operative and obstetric settings.
- Single-shot injections for the treatment of chronic pain.
- For combined spinal epidural (CSE) anaesthesia in combination with an extra-long spinal needle.
- Placement of intrathecal catheters, pleural catheters and other peripheral nerve block catheters.

How it works

An epidural needle is hollow and has a curved tip that is designed to reduce the risk of dural puncture, to prevent coring of soft tissues and to allow directional placement of epidural catheters.

Markings, that usually start 3 cm from the tip of the needle, denote 1 cm spacings. At the proximal end of the Tuohy needle, there is a hub to which a loss of resistance syringe can be attached. A detachable wing perpendicular to the needle facilitates grip and the controlled application of force along the shaft of the needle.

Standard epidural needles are normally 8 cm long and 16–18G in diameter, but longer and wider needles are available. A wider bore epidural needle provides better tactile feedback as it passes through soft tissue and ligaments, but requires a greater force on insertion and potentially risks a more severe PDPH. Some designs of epidural needle have a hub that locks a spinal needle in place. The CSEcure system comprises a 27G spinal needle with a locking collar that enables the spinal and epidural needle relationship to be fixed when injecting the spinal anaesthetic during a CSE.

Advantages

- Tactile feedback as it passes through tissues and ligaments.
- Blunt, curved tip reduces the incidence of dural puncture.
- The curved tip also facilitates directional placement of the catheter.

Disadvantages

- Dural puncture almost invariably leads to a PDPH due to its wide bore.
- Some have suggested that shearing of the epidural catheter may occur as it moves past the tip of the needle, particularly if withdrawn with the needle *in situ*.

Epidural catheters

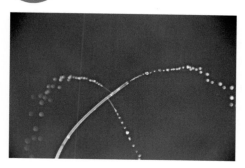

Fig. 8.5.1: An epidural catheter.

Overview

Early epidural techniques usually relied on individual injections of anaesthetic into the epidural space. However, the development of epidural catheters made continuous epidural anaesthesia and analgesia possible.

Uses

- Continuous perioperative analgesia and anaesthesia.
- Continuous labour analgesia.
- Continuous nerve blockade.

How it works

Adult epidural catheters range from 18 to 20G in diameter and up to 915 mm in length. They are made of transparent polymers such as nylon, Teflon, polyurethane or silicone because of their tensile properties and resistance to kinking and shearing forces. Transparency also aids the rapid identification of blood within the catheter. Some epidural catheters are designed to be radio-opaque. Catheters often incorporate a flexible tip that reduces tissue damage on insertion, and it is often distinctively coloured so that it is easy to confirm that the catheter is intact when it is removed. It has 1 cm markings along its length and it is recommended that no more than 4–5 cm is left in the epidural space, to reduce the risk of knotting or migration of the catheter.

Studies have shown that catheters with a single opening at the distal end are less efficacious because injected anaesthetic does not spread over a large area and consequently only produces a narrow band of anaesthesia. Catheters with three lateral holes at their distal end produce enhanced distribution of anaesthetic and have demonstrated superior analgesia and reduced need for catheter manipulation during labour.

Once the catheter has been placed and the needle removed, a Luer-lock connector is commonly clamped in position to connect the catheter to an epidural filter. However, non-Luer connectors have been developed following a recent mandate from the National Patient Safety Agency (NPSA) and these are expected to become commonplace in the near future.

⊕ Advantages

- Facilitates continuous analgesia and anaesthesia.
- Can remain *in situ* for up to 5 days post-operatively.
- Allows titration of analgesia and anaesthesia more gently compared to a single-shot spinal or single-shot epidural technique.

⊖ Disadvantages

- The presence of a catheter increases the risk of an epidural abscess or haematoma compared with single-shot techniques.
- The catheter is small enough to enter a vein within the epidural space, increasing the risk of intravascular local anaesthetic injection.
- Catheter migration, kinking or knotting may occur and breakage is possible.
- Standard Luer connectors increase the risk of injecting incompatible drugs into the epidural space.

8.6 Loss of resistance syringe

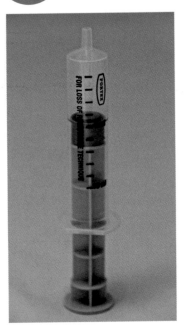

Fig. 8.6.1: A loss of resistance syringe.

Overview

The loss of resistance (LOR) technique for identifying the epidural space requires sustained pressure applied to the plunger of a syringe filled with saline or air on the end of a needle. It was first described by the Italian surgeon, Achille Mario Dogliotti in 1933. His LOR technique remains popular today and is therefore sometimes referred to as *Dogliotti's principle*.

Uses

Facilitates identification of the epidural space using a Tuohy needle.

How it works

A LOR syringe is a low friction syringe that attaches to the proximal end of a Tuohy needle via a Luer (or more recently a non-Luer) connection. Its internal surfaces are lubricated and a minimal contact interface between the syringe plunger and barrel reduces friction further and facilitates a smooth plunger movement that yields a high degree of tactile feedback for the operator. It is usually made from a clear plastic such as polypropylene. LOR syringes typically hold 7 ml of fluid.

A constant pressure should be applied to the plunger of a LOR syringe as the Tuohy needle is inserted through the spinal ligaments. The resistance to plunger movement will initially be high as the needle passes through dense ligamentous tissue. When the tip of the Tuohy needle breaches the ligamentum flavum and enters the epidural space, there is a sudden loss of resistance and the plunger advances crisply and empties the saline in the syringe into the epidural space. This provides tactile and visual confirmation that the epidural space has been successfully located.

Advantages

- Provides tactile and visual feedback that the tip of the Tuohy needle has entered the epidural space.
- Injection of saline into the epidural space expands its volume locally. This may reduce the risk of dural puncture and also facilitates threading of an epidural catheter.

Disadvantages

- There are case reports of LOR syringes sticking, which increases the risk of a dural puncture.
- The presence of a LOR syringe on the end of the Tuohy needle may be cumbersome for the operator.

8.7 Luer and non-Luer connectors

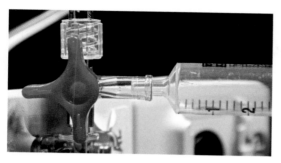

Fig. 8.7.1: A standard Luer slip connection (horizontal) and Luer lock connection (vertical).

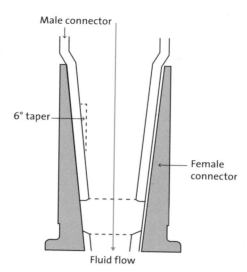

Fig. 8.7.2: Schematic of a Luer slip connection.

Overview

Luer connections were developed in the late nineteenth century by Hermann Luer, initially as small bottle stoppers. Their simplicity and ease of use led to them becoming ubiquitous in tubing and syringes used to deliver everything from enteral feed to epidural medication. Unfortunately this has led to several fatal wrong-route drug administration errors, including IV chemotherapeutic agents being given intrathecally, and the injection of bupivacaine intravenously instead of into the epidural space.

These tragedies led both the European Standards Organization and the UK's National Patient Safety Agency (NPSA) to call for the development of a series of non-Luer connectors, so that each type of device would have its own system. For example, it should only be possible to connect epidural tubing to epidural equipment, and impossible to connect it to an IV cannula.

Uses

Used for the interconnection of medical tubing, syringes and other fluid delivery equipment.

How it works

A Luer connection comprises a conical male connector with a 6% taper and a matching female receptor. Devices such as syringes and needle hubs can be connected quickly and securely through a Luer connection with a 'push and twist' mechanism. Later a jacket and screw thread were added to lock the connection in place and this is referred to as a Luer lock.

Many different designs of non-Luer connection have been patented and tested as a result of the NPSA mandate. The focus to date has mainly centred on neuraxial anaesthesia equipment and enteral feeding tubes. NHS procurers will therefore soon face a bewildering range of safe connection devices. Examples include the following systems: Neurax (B-Link), Safeconnect (B Braun Medical), Spinalok (Intervene) and Correct Inject (Smiths Medical).

The Neurax system (SureScreen Diagnostics) is similar to a standard Luer system with a male conical connector inserting into a distal female connector. However, the taper and diameter of the cone are different. In the Spinalok system, the polarity of the male and female connection is completely reversed, i.e. a female connection is found on the syringe and male connection on the epidural filter.

Advantages

- It is hoped that non-Luer connectors will reduce the incidence of wrong-route drug administration.

Disadvantages

- Some of the early non-Luer designs were able to cross-connect with standard Luer connections.
- The usability of some of the new devices has been rated below that of standard Luer equipment in recent clinical (simulator-based) testing.
- There are several manufacturers of non-Luer connection devices. Each is unique and is incompatible with devices that have been designed for the same purpose by other manufacturers. At present, there is no universally accepted non-Luer connection for neuraxial or enteral feeding equipment.

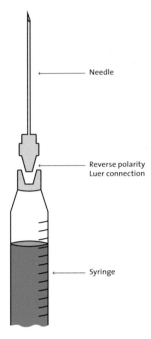

Needle

Reverse polarity Luer connection

Syringe

Fig. 8.7.3: Schematic of a reverse polarity Luer connection.

8.8 Sub-Tenon's set

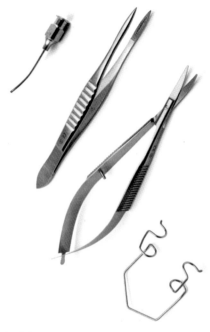

Fig. 8.8.1: The instruments required for sub-Tenon's anaesthesia – a sub-Tenon's cannula, Moorfield's forceps, Westcott spring scissors and a sprung wire speculum.

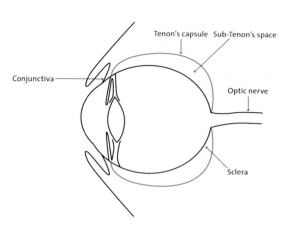

Fig. 8.8.2: Anatomy of sub-Tenon's space.

Overview

The sub-Tenon's block is a method of delivering regional anaesthesia to the orbit. It has become increasingly popular because serious complications are rare. Most importantly, the sub-Tenon's technique has a significantly reduced incidence of globe perforation compared with sharp needle blocks (retrobulbar and peribulbar).

Uses

The sub-Tenon's set is a collection of instruments used to perform a sub-Tenon's block.

How it works

The set contains Moorfield's forceps, Westcott spring scissors, a sprung wire speculum and a curved sub-Tenon's cannula. To carry out the block on a suitably assessed and consented patient:

- Apply topical anaesthesia to the conjunctiva, e.g. proxymetacaine.
- Clean the conjunctiva with iodine solution.
- Insert the eyelid speculum to hold the eye open.
- Ask the patient to look superolaterally, in order to access the inferomedial quadrant.
- Using the Moorfield's forceps, grasp the conjunctiva and the underlying Tenon's capsule together around 7–10 mm from the inferonasal limbus. The forceps are blunt and non-toothed to prevent trauma.
- Make a small incision with the Westcott scissors.
- Pass the curved, sub-Tenon's cannula posteriorly around the globe; the cannula should pass easily without force. Stevens first described a metal cannula that is 19G and 25 mm long and these remain common, though flexible plastic cannulae have also been used.
- Up to 3–5 ml of local anaesthetic mix is injected. A mixture of 2.5 ml 2% lignocaine, 2.5 ml 0.5% bupivicaine with 150 IU hyaluronidase is one example of the many mixes in use. Hyaluronidase is an enzyme which breaks down connective tissue and therefore improves the spread of the local anaesthetic.

- Gentle globe massage improves the distribution of the local anaesthetic. The onset time is around 5–10 minutes and the block can be expected to last around an hour. It may be topped up by the surgeon.

⊕ Advantages

- There are few serious complications.
- Sub-Tenon's provides reliable anaesthesia in experienced hands.
- The block has been administered safely to patients on warfarin, aspirin and clopidogrel.

⊖ Disadvantages

- Complete globe akinesia is not always possible.
- Chemosis (sub-conjunctival oedema) is common, but improves with gentle pressure and is short-lived.
- Some surgeons do not like sub-Tenon's anaesthesia for glaucoma surgery because of the theoretical risk of raised intraorbital pressures.

Chapter 9
Critical care

9.1 Intravenous cannulae

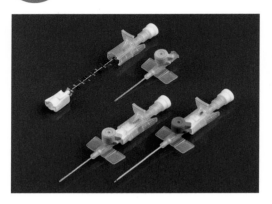

Fig. 9.1.1: The Venflon Pro Safety range of IV cannulae. Image reproduced with permission from BD UK Ltd.

Overview

Intravenous cannulae are available in a wide variety of shapes and sizes.

Uses

They are inserted into a peripheral vein and can be used to deliver fluid therapy or IV drugs to the patient.

In rare circumstances a cannula may be used for an alternative purpose, such as the initial emergency treatment of a tension pneumothorax.

How it works

Although many different designs are available, all IV cannulae consist of a needle within a plastic tube. The tip of the needle is exposed at one end of the tube and this is inserted through the skin into a vein. The plastic cannula can then slide off the needle into the lumen of the vein before the needle is removed and discarded. The cannula has a connection port that stays outside the body and can be connected to an infusion.

Cannulas are sized according to standard wire gauge (SWG). This is an old-fashioned method of measuring the cross-sectional area. It refers to the number of wires of the same size as the cannula that could pass through a hole of a standard size in parallel. The bigger the wires, the fewer could fit through the hole, and therefore larger cannulae have a smaller gauge number.

The maximum flow rate through a cannula depends most on the fourth power of its radius (from the Hagen–Poiseuille equation). The maximum flows quoted by manufacturers are determined by running distilled water through the cannulae under standardized conditions (*Table 9.1.1*). The maximum flow rate through a cannula is important because it dictates the speed at which fluid can be given.

Table 9.1.1: Cannula sizes, colour codes and maximum flows for the BD Venflon Pro IV cannula.

Cannula size (SWG)	Colour	Approximate maximum flow (ml.min^{-1})
14	Orange	270
16	Grey	236
18	Green	103
20	Pink	67
22	Blue	42

Flow was measured using deionized water at 22°C with a pressure gradient of 10 kPa through 110 cm of tubing with an internal diameter of 4 mm. 24G cannulae (yellow) also exist with flows of 13–22 ml.min^{-1} depending on manufacturer.

⊕ Advantages

- Usually easy to insert quickly.

Disadvantages

- May provide a route for infectious agents to reach the bloodstream or subcutaneous tissues. Cannulae are often removed or replaced after 72 hours if possible.
- Have a short functional lifespan, with a tendency to migrate into subcutaneous tissues or become occluded if they are not well cared for.

Safety

- Safety cannulae are available which have a clip at the end of the needle that activates as it is withdrawn. The clip covers the tip of the needle and is therefore said to reduce the risk of sharps injury. As part of the EU Directive to prevent injuries and infections to healthcare workers from needle stick injuries, safety cannulae must be available in UK hospitals from May 2013.

Other notes

Not many people talk about standard wire gauge these days, although anaesthetists and guitarists are two groups who may still be found discussing the subject: both cannulae and guitar strings are measured in SWG. The strings E, A, D, G, B and E on a standard six string electric guitar may be 9, 11, 16, 26, 36, and 46 gauge, respectively.

9.2 Central venous catheters

Overview

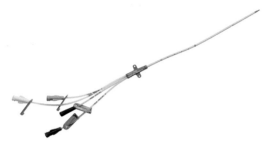

Fig. 9.2.1: An adult quad-lumen central venous catheter. Image reproduced with permission from Teleflex Incorporated. ©2013 Teleflex Incorporated. All rights reserved.

Central venous catheters are inserted into the internal jugular, subclavian or femoral veins. Lines with up to five lumens are available in typical adult lengths of 16 or 20 cm. The lines are available in a variety of diameters (measured in French gauge). The lumens within them are measured in standard wire gauge (*Table 9.2.1*).

Table 9.2.1: Table of sizes of lumens in typical central venous catheters of different sizes. Single and double lumen catheters are also available with a variety of different lumen sizes.

Three lumen (7F)	Four lumen (8.5F)	Five lumen (8.5F)
2 × 18G	2 × 18G	3 × 18G
1 × 16G	1 × 16G	1 × 16G
	1 × 14G	1 × 14G

Uses

A standard central venous catheter may be required for several reasons, with the most common including:

- administration of drugs that cause phlebitis in smaller peripheral veins
- infusion of potent vasoactive drugs that require guaranteed uniform mixing throughout the blood volume
- measurement of central venous pressure
- where peripheral venous access is difficult
- occasionally for regular sampling of blood in a patient who is difficult to take blood from peripherally.

Other indications for central venous cannulation also exist, but the equipment used is different:

- renal replacement therapy (see *Section 9.10*)
- transvenous pacing
- pulmonary artery catheters (see *Section 9.6*)
- for long term administration of IV drugs (for example, antibiotics or chemotherapy) or total parenteral nutrition using a tunnelled line such as a Hickman.

How it works

Central lines are inserted using the Seldinger technique under strict aseptic conditions. The target vein is cannulated, and a guide wire is passed through the cannula. The cannula is then removed leaving the wire *in situ*. After dilation, the central line is passed over the wire and into the vein. The guide wire is then removed before the line is sutured into place and covered with a transparent sterile dressing.

Initial cannulation of the vein can be performed with live two-dimensional ultrasound guidance and NICE recommended this technique in 2002. Evidence suggests that the use of ultrasound makes location of the vein easier and reduces the incidence of accidental arterial puncture and other complications, for internal jugular lines in particular.

There has been a move away from the routine removal or replacement of central lines after a fixed time period in an attempt to reduce the incidence of line-related sepsis, because evidence suggests it makes no difference. Other steps that can be taken to reduce the risk include the following.

- The use of full aseptic technique during insertion, including hand washing, the use of sterile gloves, gown, hat, mask and drape.
- Skin preparation using 2% chlorhexidine rather than 10% povidone–iodine appears to be more effective. The antiseptic should be allowed to dry.
- Some evidence suggests that lines inserted into the femoral vein have a higher incidence of infection, therefore avoidance of this site may reduce infection rates. There is also some evidence that central lines placed in the femoral vein may be associated with higher rates of deep vein thrombosis (DVT).
- The use of a line with the minimum number of lumens necessary.
- The use of a line made of Teflon or polyurethane (these seem to suffer with a lower incidence of infection than lines made from other materials).
- The use of a line impregnated with an antimicrobial agent such as silver sulphadiazine or chlorhexidine. The former will degrade on exposure to light, which is why central lines are often protected by an opaque plastic sheath in their packaging. Other catheters are coated with antibiotics such as rifampicin and minocycline. Impregnated lines are especially recommended if they are to remain in place for longer than 5 days.
- Using a dressing that is transparent, so that changes in skin colour or signs of local infection can easily be seen.
- At least daily review of the on-going need for the line.

Central venous pressure measurement is achieved by the connection of one lumen of the central line to a transducer via a continuous saline column in the same manner as an arterial line is used to measure arterial pressure.

⊕ Advantages

- Can be used for both measurement of central venous pressure and administration of drugs and fluids.
- Venous blood samples can be taken from the line.

⊖ Disadvantages

The disadvantages of central venous lines are mostly related to possible complications, including:

- bleeding, haematoma, accidental puncture or cannulation of arteries
- infection and line sepsis
- venous thrombosis
- pneumothorax or haemothorax if cannulating the internal jugular or subclavian veins; chylothorax is also possible on the left
- incorrect line positioning
- embolism of air or the guide wire into the circulation
- arrhythmias may be provoked if the guide wire or line is inserted further than necessary.

Other notes

Typical central venous catheters have three, four or five lumens. The sizes of each lumen are shown in *Table 9.2.1*.

9.3 Other vascular access devices

Short term venous access is usually achieved using a standard peripheral cannula and, in most circumstances, these are adequate. However, they have several disadvantages such as a short functional lifespan, a tendency to migrate from the vein into subcutaneous tissue or become occluded, and a risk of infection or line sepsis. Central venous catheters are used in circumstances when central venous pressure (CVP) monitoring is required, or when vasoactive or irritant drugs are to be infused, but these catheters suffer from some of the same disadvantages as peripheral cannulae, and also have their own problems.

Many other vascular access devices are available. They are generally more complicated to insert and have their own disadvantages, but they are able to overcome some of the limitations of standard devices. They are often used to administer chemotherapeutic agents, total parenteral nutrition (TPN) and prolonged courses of antibiotics. Several other designs are available for renal replacement therapy (RRT; *Section 9.10*).

Some of these lines are tunnelled. This means that the line passes 10–15 cm subcutaneously between the site where it pierces the skin to where it enters the blood vessel. Many tunnelled lines also have cuffs made of a material such as Dacron. These are positioned in the tunnel between the skin and the vessel and encourage the deposition of fibrin and collagen. The cuff therefore seals the tunnel and may help prevent the introduction of pathogenic organisms to the bloodstream. However, some evidence also suggests that micro-organisms gain access to the circulation via the catheter lumen rather than via the external surface.

Anaesthetists are likely to encounter patients who already have these lines *in situ* for a variety of reasons. However, it is not often appropriate for patients to have them inserted acutely while they are on intensive care due to the prevalence of sepsis in this population.

Long-term general vascular access lines

Broviac and Hickman

The Broviac catheter was developed in 1973 for the administration of TPN. It was an early design of tunnelled central venous catheter and required venous cut-down to insert. It was 90 cm in length and made from a newly developed silicone elastomer called Silastic. The internal and external diameters were 1.0 and 2.2 mm, respectively. In 1979, the Broviac design was modified by Hickman, who increased the calibre of the catheter so that the internal and external diameters were 1.6 and 3.2 mm, respectively. This allowed blood to be withdrawn and drugs to be infused more easily. Both types of catheter are cuffed.

Today, Broviac lines are available with one or two lumens and in a range of sizes. They are generally smaller than Hickman lines and are most commonly used in paediatric practice. Hickman lines have up to three lumens and are larger, being used in adult patients.

Advantages
- Can be used to administer drugs such as antibiotics, TPN, and chemotherapy.
- Blood can be taken, saving the patient multiple venepuncture attempts.

Disadvantages

- Silastic is a soft material and collapses if highly negative pressure is applied. This fact, along with the relatively small calibre of the lumens means these catheters are not suitable for RRT or taking large quantities of blood.
- Requires regular flushes with heparinized saline when not in use in order to maintain patency.
- It is not uncommon for patients to require sedation or general anaesthesia for the insertion and removal of these lines.

Groshong

The Groshong catheter is also made of Silastic and has a valve at the tip of each lumen. It is a simple pressure-sensitive slit valve that opens intra-luminally when suction is applied so that blood can be taken, and extra-luminally when positive pressure is applied, so that fluid can be infused. When there is no pressure application the slit is closed. This helps prevent blood reflux and occlusion of the lumen by thrombus.

The Groshong valve is available as a tunnelled line similar to the Hickman, and as a peripherally inserted central catheter (PICC).

Advantages

- Less susceptible to occlusion by thrombi and only requires weekly flushing with saline when not in use.
- If a lumen is not closed or clamped, there is a reduced risk of bleeding through it.
- Some Groshong catheters can be repaired relatively easily if the external portion is damaged.

Disadvantages

- Made of thin Silastic, and is said to tear and kink more easily than some other designs.
- Patients may require sedation or general anaesthesia for insertion and removal.

Peripherally inserted central catheters

The PICC line is not tunnelled but inserted into a peripheral vein. It is much longer than a standard cannula and reaches proximally into the great veins. Adult PICCs are 60 cm in length. This allows drugs to be given centrally without some of the disadvantages of a central line. They are usually made of silicone or polyurethane and are available with one, two or three lumens.

PICC lines are used when the duration of a course of a particular drug is long. They have been shown in several

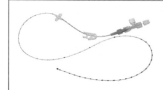

Fig. 9.3.1: The Lifecath PICC line. Images provided by Vygon (UK) Ltd; © Vygon (UK) Ltd 2013.

studies to be associated with a lower risk of blood-borne infection than standard peripheral cannulae, especially when they are used on an outpatient basis. The reasons for this are not well defined, although it may be that they are often cared for by dedicated vascular access teams who perform regular dressing changes and use a non-touch technique when handling them. They are also usually sited into relatively proximal veins (e.g. between the axilla and the antecubital fossa) compared with standard cannulae, which allows them to be fixed in position more reliably. This may also contribute to the lower risk of infection.

During insertion, the distance between the insertion site and the medial border of the ipsilateral clavicle is measured. Using an aseptic technique, the vein is cannulated in the same way as for a normal cannula. The tourniquet is then released and the PICC line is threaded into the vein using sterile forceps until the measured distance is reached. The tip should then be positioned in the superior vena cava. The cannula is secured, dressed and wrapped to keep it clean.

A chest X-ray is often performed to ensure the tip of the cannula is correctly positioned.

⊕ Advantages
- Easy to insert under local anaesthetic.
- Provide central venous access without some of the disadvantages of a central line.
- Useful for long-term treatment – can often be left *in situ* for up to 12 weeks.
- Patient is not subjected to multiple cannulation attempts.
- Can be used for taking blood samples as well as giving drugs.

⊖ Disadvantages
- Provide a route for infection into the central circulation.
- Requires good peripheral veins for insertion. More difficult to insert than normal cannula.
- It is not possible to administer resuscitation fluids rapidly, because the length increases the resistance to flow (see Hagen–Poiseuille equation in *Fig. 6.3.3*).
- May become blocked, especially by blood clots if the line is used to take blood samples and is then not properly flushed.
- The line may be in an inconvenient place for the patient when it is not being used.
- Cannot be used for taking blood for antibiotic levels if the line has been used to administer the antibiotic in the first place, because there is a risk of contamination of the sample and an artificially high result. This goes for all intravenous access devices.
- It can be difficult to pass a PICC line around the acute angle at the axilla. Fluoroscopic guidance is sometimes needed.

Implantable ports

Catheter ports provide a means of easily accessing the circulation without the need for a permanent transcutaneous line. There are many different trade names, including Port-A-Cath (Smiths Medical), SmartPort (Angiodynamics), Bardport (Bard Access Systems), and others.

These systems consist of a tunnelled silicone or polyurethane catheter similar to a Hickman line, with one end positioned in the superior vena cava. However, instead of the other end being external it is attached to a port and implanted beneath the skin. Therefore, once the device has been inserted there are no transcutaneous or external parts.

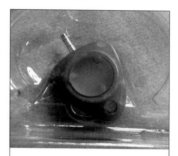

Fig. 9.3.2: Ported lines have a port like this one implanted subcutaneously.

The port consists of a disc-shaped reservoir, often made of titanium and typically 2.5–4 cm in diameter, covered by a soft silicone membrane. When access is required the skin over the port is cleaned and local anaesthetic cream is applied. A Huber needle is then inserted through the skin and the silicone membrane into the reservoir and can be used to take a blood sample or infuse a drug.

Advantages
- Can remain *in situ* for months or even years.
- Only needs to be flushed with heparinized saline once a month when not in use.
- More aesthetically acceptable to some patients than catheters with external parts.

Disadvantages
- Patients may require sedation or general anaesthesia during insertion and removal.
- Some discomfort may be felt during access because a hypodermic needle must be used. Skin changes may occur if used very regularly for a long period.

Renal replacement therapy lines

Acute renal replacement lines

These are probably the type of line most frequently encountered by anaesthetists for RRT because they are often used in intensive care. Like all lines in this category, they are a type of central venous catheter. They have two large calibre lumens (each allowing a flow of at least 300 ml.min^{-1}) and sometimes a third smaller lumen. Like standard central lines, they are available with adult lengths of 16 or 20 cm and they are placed in the internal jugular, subclavian or femoral veins using the Seldinger technique. They are made from polyurethane or silicone.

The distal ends of the two large lumens are separated, with one opening at the tip of the line and the other opening more proximally through a side channel.

Both lumens on the line are then connected to an RRT machine. This aspirates blood from the patient via the first lumen for filtration or dialysis. After this has occurred, the blood is re-infused into the patient via the second lumen. The separation between the distal openings of the two lumens helps prevent recirculation (when the machine aspirates blood that it has only just re-infused).

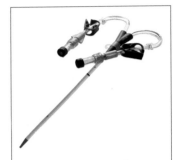

Fig. 9.3.3: An acute renal replacement access line. Image reproduced with permission from Teleflex.

Advantages
- Inserted using the same technique as a standard central line and can be used immediately.
- The third smaller lumen that is present on some of these lines can be used as a standard central line lumen to infuse drugs or measure CVP.
- Blood samples can be taken from the line.
- Some designs allow the line to be rotated within its housing while it is sutured in place. This provides a method of stopping the line abutting vessel walls and becoming occluded.

Disadvantages
- Disadvantages of these lines relate to their complications, which are similar to those for standard central lines, though the larger diameter increases the risk of bleeding.
- Lumens may become blocked or partially occluded by thrombus, or by abutting the vessel wall so that they do not allow sufficient flow for RRT.

Tesio

Many catheters consist of a single line with several lumens running within it. The Tesio system is different in that it has two separate 10F lines that are independently placed by a surgeon or an interventional radiologist into the right atrium and superior vena cava. Both lines are then tunnelled under the skin and each has a Dacron cuff. The lines are joined when they emerge from the skin by the attachment of a hub.

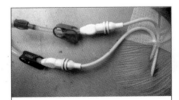

Fig. 9.3.4: A Tesio line.

Advantages
- The detachable hub allows each line to be placed independently and this allows more precise positioning of the catheter.
- The hub can also easily be replaced if it becomes damaged, without the need to insert a whole new catheter. Furthermore, this design allows the external part of the catheter to be cut and shortened should it become occluded or damaged. A new hub can then be connected to the shortened ends.

Disadvantages
- It is not uncommon for patients to require sedation or general anaesthesia for the insertion of these lines.
- Insertion carries similar risks as other central venous catheters.

Catheter sheaths

Pulmonary artery catheter sheaths

A pulmonary artery catheter (PAC) sheath is a type of central venous catheter. It has a single wide-bore lumen that is continuous with both a side port and the insertion point for the PAC. Sheaths are available in a variety of sizes from 7.5 to 15 cm in length and 4 to 9F in diameter. They are usually inserted into the subclavian or internal jugular veins.

The sheath's primary purpose is to aid the introduction of a PAC (although they can also be used to allow introduction of an intra-aortic balloon pump). This passes through the sheath, and into the central vein. From here it can pass into the pulmonary artery via the right heart. The portion of the PAC that is outside the body is kept inside a clear plastic cover that connects to the sheath and keeps the PAC sterile.

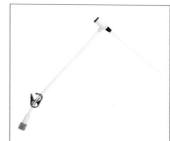

Fig. 9.3.5: The percutaneous pulmonary artery catheter introducer sheath. Image reproduced with permission from Teleflex.

The sheath has a purpose in its own right, even if a PAC is not being used. Due to its relatively large calibre and short length, the sheath provides an excellent means of rapidly infusing large volumes of fluid or blood products during resuscitation.

PAC sheaths are inserted using the Seldinger technique in a similar manner to other central venous lines. One difference is that the dilator is loaded into the sheath and the two are inserted over the guide wire together, instead of the dilator being passed and removed and then the sheath being inserted. The dilator is only inserted a short distance into the vessel before the sheath is advanced forward. The dilator and the guide wire are then removed together.

Advantages
- Can be used for insertion of PAC or for fluid resuscitation.

Disadvantages
- Disadvantages of sheaths relate to their complications, which are identical to those for standard central lines.

9.4 Incentive spirometry

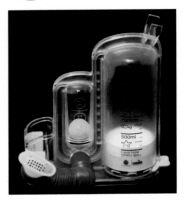

Fig. 9.4.1: An incentive spirometer.

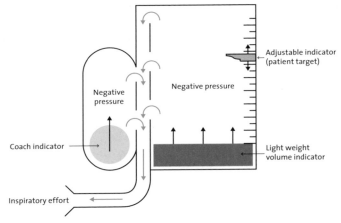

Adjustable indicator (patient target)

Negative pressure

Negative pressure

Coach indicator

Light weight volume indicator

Inspiratory effort

Fig. 9.4.2: Schematic of the inner workings of an incentive spirometer.

Overview

Following his observations of soldiers wounded during the First World War, MacMahon first suggested that deep breathing exercises could help reduce the risk of post-operative respiratory complications in 1915. By the late 1950s and 60s it was clear that, in spite of major advances in surgery and anaesthetics, a significant proportion of patients were still suffering from respiratory complications related to lung atelectasis.

The original incentive spirometer was invented in 1970 by RH Bartlett and was an electronic bedside device that encouraged patients to take deep breaths. A light indicated that the appropriate tidal volume had been achieved.

Modern incentive spirometers are simple, disposable devices. However, their function is similar to that of Bartlett's spirometer; they prevent and treat atelectasis in post-operative patients by encouraging sustained maximal inspiratory efforts through visual feedback.

Uses

Incentive spirometers are used to help prevent and treat atelectasis and lower respiratory tract infections in hospitalized patients, often post-operatively.

How it works

Modern spirometers are available for use with adults and children. They comprise a mouthpiece connected to a chamber which the patient holds. The patient is encouraged to make a steady and sustained inspiratory effort through the mouthpiece until a target volume (initially set at approximately 1250 ml in adults) is reached. Visual feedback is provided during the breath in two forms. Firstly, a ball floats in a flowmeter (also known as a coach indicator) and the patient tries to maintain it at a particular vertical height. This ensures that the patient does not breathe faster or slower than the desired rate. Secondly, a piston floats upwards within a cylindrical chamber and indicates the inspired volume. The patient tries to achieve a target volume that has been set using an external sliding marker.

The patient is encouraged to inspire the target volume, and then hold this for 3–5 seconds before exhaling. Patients should try to use incentive spirometry for 10 minutes per hour that they are awake. After using the device, they are encouraged to cough and expectorate any secretions. This process is believed to open up collapsed alveoli.

⊕ Advantages

- Reduces the incidence of post-operative atelectasis and its complications.
- Simple to use.
- Visual feedback and goal-setting encourage its use by patients.
- Adult and paediatric forms available.
- Adaptors available for tracheostomy patients.

⊖ Disadvantages

- Patients must be able to take a deep breath before they can use the device (vital capacity should be >10 ml.kg^{-1}).
- Success depends on patient motivation and good analgesia.

9.5 Doppler cardiac output monitors

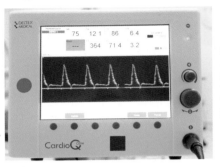

Fig. 9.5.1: A CardioQ-ODM oesophageal Doppler monitor.

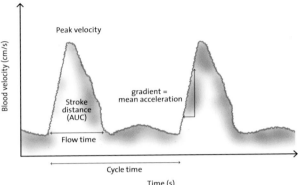

Fig. 9.5.2: The trace obtained from an oesophageal Doppler monitor.

Overview

The Doppler effect is the apparent change in wave frequency that occurs when the source of the wave is in motion relative to the receiver. It applies equally to sound waves and electromagnetic radiation, and it can be used to calculate blood flow and cardiac output using ultrasound.

Doppler ultrasound monitoring is considered to be one of the least invasive methods of measuring cardiac output, although a probe must be inserted into the oesophagus and therefore the method is not often suitable for patients who are fully conscious.

Several different oesophageal Doppler monitors may be encountered by anaesthetists. These include older systems such as the Hemosonic and the Medicina (neither of which is still in production), and the CardioQ-ODM system (Deltex Medical). The latter is commonly used and consists of a single-use, latex-free ultrasound transducer mounted at a 45° angle at the tip of a 90 cm insulated and flexible probe that is connected to a computer and monitor (see *Fig. 9.5.1*). The probe has length markings at 35, 40 and 45 cm to guide correct positioning.

Uses

Cardiac output monitoring is used during surgery and in critical care to guide administration of fluids and inotropes.

In particular, Doppler monitoring has been used in enhanced recovery programmes. Improved outcome (including shorter hospital stay and lower complication rates) following major abdominal, cardiac, orthopaedic and other types of surgery has been demonstrated in randomized trials when intra-operative fluid management has been guided using Doppler cardiac output monitoring.

In 2011, NICE recommended that use of the CardioQ-ODM monitor be considered for patients undergoing major or high-risk surgery, or in patients where the clinician would consider using invasive cardiovascular monitoring.

How it works

The probe is inserted into the oesophagus of a patient, via the oro- or nasopharynx. The probe is inserted to between 35 and 40 cm if placed orally and between 40 and 45 cm if placed nasally, although this will vary between patients. The aim is to position the probe in the oesophagus where it runs posterior to, and parallel with, the descending aorta (at roughly the level of T5 to T6). The probe is then connected to the monitor and the computer prompts the user to enter the patient's details such as age, weight and height.

Ultrasound is emitted from the probe at 4–5 MHz (depending on the monitor) and passes through the oesophageal and aortic walls before being reflected by the red blood cells and returning to the probe. Due to the Doppler effect, the frequency will decrease if the cells are travelling away from the probe and increase if they are travelling towards the probe. The faster the cells travel, the greater the shift in frequency. Therefore, the change in frequency can be used to calculate the velocity of the blood as it flows through the aorta, using the following equation:

$$V = \frac{(f_s \times c)}{(2 \times f_o \times cos\theta)}$$

where V is the blood velocity, f_o and f_s are the original and shifted frequency of the ultrasound waves, respectively, c is the speed that ultrasound waves travel through tissue (approximately 1540 m.s^{-1}) and θ is the angle of the ultrasound waves relative to the blood flow.

The monitor displays a waveform of blood velocity against time, and the probe is adjusted until this becomes clear and undistorted. Different monitors then use different methods to calculate the cardiac output.

Some systems use the data that were entered about the patient to calculate the cross-sectional area of the descending aorta using a nomogram (e.g. the Medicina). Other systems directly measure the aortic diameter using M-mode ultrasound (e.g. the Hemosonic). Blood velocity is plotted against time, producing a curve for each cardiac cycle. The area under this curve represents the distance travelled by the blood per cardiac cycle. Multiplying this distance by the estimated cross-sectional area of the aorta gives the volume of blood moving per cardiac cycle, which is therefore the uncorrected stroke volume. Uncorrected cardiac output is then calculated by multiplying by the heart rate. A correction to these volumes must then be made, because only approximately 70% of cardiac output passes into the descending aorta (the rest passing into the head, upper limbs and coronary circulation).

The CardioQ-ODM monitor works in a slightly different way. During its development, a diverse group of patients had their cardiac output measured using the thermodilution technique with a pulmonary artery catheter (PAC). At the same time, an oesophageal Doppler was used to measure the stroke distance (the distance blood moves per cardiac cycle) in the descending aorta. This allowed the development of a mathematical algorithm that predicts what the stroke volume would be (according to the PAC) given a particular stroke distance (measured by Doppler ultrasound) in a particular patient. Therefore, the CardioQ-ODM does not measure or calculate the aortic cross-sectional area at all. This method means that no extra correction is required in order to account for the blood that does not pass into the descending aorta or the variations in the aortic diameter caused by elastic changes during the cardiac cycle.

All systems display haemodynamic data such as cardiac output, stroke volume and heart rate. Systemic vascular resistance can also be calculated by dividing the arteriovenous pressure gradient (mean arterial pressure minus central venous pressure) by the cardiac output. The units are then converted into dynes.s.cm^{-5}. Other information that can be obtained includes the flow time (the time taken for the stroke volume to be ejected), and the peak blood velocity. *Table 9.5.1* shows some of the measurements made by the CardioQ-ODM monitor and their normal values.

Table 9.5.1: Some variables measured by the CardioQ-ODM oesophageal Doppler monitor.

Variable	Reference range	Description
Cardiac index (CI)	2.5–4.0 l.min^{-1}.m^{-2}	The cardiac output is the volume of blood ejected by the left ventricle in one minute. The CI is the cardiac output corrected for body size. CI is equal to cardiac output divided by body surface area.
Stroke volume index (SVI)	35–65 ml.beat^{-1}.m^{-2}	The SVI is the volume of blood ejected by the left ventricle during one cardiac cycle. The SVI is the stroke volume corrected for body size.
Stroke distance (SD)	*	The SD is the distance in centimetres that the blood moves along the aorta during one cardiac cycle.
Corrected flow time (FTc)	330–360 ms	The flow time is the time taken for the stroke volume to pass a fixed point in the aorta. This is then corrected for heart rate by dividing by the square root of the time taken for one cardiac cycle.
Peak velocity (PV)	50–120 cm.s^{-1}*	The PV is the highest blood velocity detected during one cardiac cycle.
Systemic vascular resistance index (SVRI)	1970–2390 dynes.s.cm^{-5}.m^{-2}	The systemic vascular resistance is the arterio-venous pressure difference (MAP – CVP) divided by the cardiac output. The units are also converted into dynes.sec.cm^{-5} and the value is then corrected for body size to produce the SVRI.

*Reference range varies depending on the patient's age and other parameters.

⊕ Advantages

- Easy to use and easy to learn the technique.
- Response to fluid challenges can be rapidly assessed. May help to avoid under- or over-filling the vascular space during surgery.
- Probes are easy to position.
- Probes can be left *in situ* for some time, provided the patient is sedated or anaesthetized.
- The probe will usually work properly in the presence of diathermy due to its insulation.
- Probes can be passed into the oesophagus via the nose or mouth.
- Avoids the possible complications of more invasive techniques of cardiac output monitoring.

⊖ Disadvantages

- Systems using a nomogram to calculate the aortic cross-sectional area may be inaccurate because nomograms are based on averaging data from a population of patients. An individual's actual aortic calibre may differ from the average. This is also a problem with systems that use nomograms to correct for other factors, such as the proportion of cardiac output that passes into the descending aorta. The impact of this problem is likely to be more marked with absolute values, rather than trends.

- The percentage of cardiac output that flows through the descending aorta is unlikely to be fixed – especially in the critically unwell. Therefore systems that use fixed corrections may be less accurate.
- Due to the pulsatile nature of aortic blood flow and the elasticity of the aortic wall, the calibre of the descending aorta is not constant, although systems that depend on its cross-sectional area assume that it is for the purposes of calculating flow. This may also lead to inaccuracies.
- The algorithm used by the CardioQ-ODM monitor is based on data from measurements taken from a population of patients with a PAC. It is therefore theoretically possible that its accuracy will be affected because the system assumes the patient being monitored obeys the algorithm. However, the algorithm has been validated many times and no modifications have been required since it was first used over 20 years ago.
- The presence of turbulent flow in the aorta (particularly caused by co-arctation) may cause velocity calculations based on Doppler shifts to be inaccurate.
- Different probe positions and orientations within the oesophagus may give different readings of cardiac output. It can be difficult to know which is the most accurate, and Doppler monitors have been said to be operator dependent because of this. It is also possible for the probe to move during surgery, leading to a variation in measurements.
- It can be difficult to use this technique in patients who are not sedated or anaesthetized.
- Doppler probes have been used with laryngeal mask airways (particularly those with gastric ports), however, they may be more difficult to insert and manipulate than if used with an endotracheal tube.

⊘ Safety

There are few contraindications to the use of the oesophageal probe. Those that do exist include:

- severe facial trauma or carcinoma of the pharynx, larynx or oesophagus
- concurrent use of intra-aortic balloon pumps
- thoracic aortic aneurysm
- tissue necrosis of the oesophagus or nasal passages or the presence of oesophageal varices
- the close proximity of surgical lasers.

Other notes

A new device, the CardioQ-ODM+ combines oesophageal Doppler monitoring with pulse pressure wave analysis (PPWA) to give haemodynamic data based on analysis of both the ultrasound signal and the arterial pressure wave.

9.6 Pulmonary artery catheters

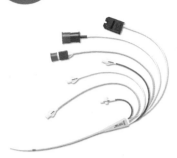

Fig. 9.6.1: The Swan–Ganz catheter. Image reproduced with permission from Edwards Lifesciences.

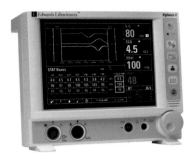

Fig. 9.6.2: The Vigilance II monitor. Image reproduced with permission from Edwards Lifesciences.

Overview

The pulmonary artery catheter (PAC) was invented in the early 1970s by Jeremy Swan and William Ganz, and was the commonest method of measuring cardiac output and right-sided cardiac pressures for many years. The PAC has fallen out of favour in recent times due to several factors. These include the complications that have been shown to occur as a result of their insertion, the emergence of less invasive devices for estimation of cardiac output and the finding that the data obtained from PACs do not necessarily improve outcome. Despite this, the PAC is still considered the gold standard method of determining cardiac output and other haemodynamic data in the operating theatre and in critical care.

PACs are long central venous catheters, made of an antimicrobial coated non-latex polymer. They are 110 cm in length with markings every 10 cm. They are available in sizes from 5 to 8F. The number of lumens is variable, but four to five is typical, with different lumens opening at different places along the length of the catheter.

In order to insert a PAC, a sheath needs to be inserted into a central vein first. The PAC is then introduced through this in an aseptic fashion. PACs have a protective plastic cover that is continuous with the sheath so that the catheter can be handled without risk of infection. The distal lumen of the PAC opens into a balloon. This is inflated with up to 1.5 ml of air during insertion to float the catheter into its correct position. The balloon is also used during measurement of pulmonary artery wedge pressure.

Uses

General indications for the insertion of a PAC include the assessment of circulating volume status and cardiac function in the critically ill patient. However, because there are several other methods of assessing these variables and there are significant risks associated with the insertion of a PAC, the indications are more specific, including:

- differentiating between cardiogenic and non-cardiogenic pulmonary oedema
- guiding the administration of inotropes and vasopressors in conditions such as pulmonary hypertension or ventricular failure
- closely assessing haemodynamic parameters when medical conditions that affect them co-exist (e.g. severe sepsis with renal and left ventricular impairment).

How it works

Pressure measurements

The PAC is flushed with saline before insertion through the *in situ* PAC sheath. A pressure transducer is connected to the distal lumen and the pressure trace is used to determine the location of the tip of the catheter. *Figure 9.6.3* shows a schematic of the pressure waveforms encountered as the catheter is advanced.

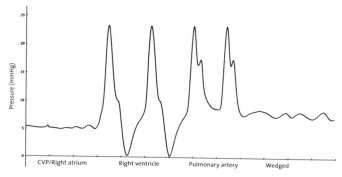

Figure 9.6.3: The pressure waveform seen as the tip of the pulmonary artery catheter passes through the right heart and pulmonary vessels.

The balloon is inflated and floats in the blood stream. Initially the pressure trace will show the CVP but as the PAC is advanced it passes through the right atrium and tricuspid valve into the right ventricle. The trace at this point changes so that the systolic pressure is approximately 20–25 mmHg and the diastolic pressure is almost zero. As the PAC continues to advance it passes through the pulmonary valve and into the pulmonary artery. Here, the systolic pressure will be almost identical to that in the ventricle, but the diastolic pressure will rise to approximately 10 mmHg. A dicrotic notch is also often present on the down-stroke of the wave that indicates the closure of the pulmonary valve at the end of systole.

The PAC is then advanced further until the artery becomes too small to allow passage of the inflated balloon. Here, there is a continuous column of blood between the tip of the catheter and the left atrium, and the catheter is said to be wedged. The pulmonary capillary wedge pressure (PCWP) is a reflection of left atrial filling pressure and can be used to guide fluid therapy in patients with left ventricular impairment.

The balloon must be deflated after measurement of the PCWP, but can be re-inflated if another measurement is necessary. A balloon left inflated may lead to erosion of the wall of the pulmonary artery, and eventually to its rupture. The balloon must also always be deflated if the PAC is to be withdrawn, to prevent damage to heart valves.

All of the pressures described so far are measured through a distal lumen as it moves through the heart during insertion of the PAC. However, once it has been properly positioned, the lumen approximately 30 cm proximal to the catheter tip can be transduced simultaneously. When correctly positioned, this will open into a central vein or right atrium and can therefore be used to measure the CVP without the need for a separate central venous catheter.

Cardiac output measurements

PACs can be used to measure cardiac output either intermittently or semi-continuously. Measured and calculated variables, along with graphical representations, are displayed on a monitor.

In the intermittent method, a bolus of fluid that has been chilled to between 0 and 12°C is rapidly injected into the proximal lumen of the PAC. The opening of this lumen is approximately 30 cm from the tip of the catheter, and lies in or proximal to, the right atrium. The temperature of the blood falls as the cold bolus is injected and this is detected by a thermistor at the distal end of the PAC as the blood passes through the pulmonary artery. The graph of the magnitude of temperature change against time rises and then falls back towards baseline in an exponential fashion and therefore a semi-logarithmic plot of the same data is linear. The area under the latter graph is calculated by integration and is inversely proportional to the flow in the pulmonary artery. The modified Stewart–Hamilton equation is used to calculate the actual cardiac output (see *Fig. 9.6.4*).

$$CO = \frac{V(T_o - T_i).K}{\int_{t_1}^{t_2} \Delta T \, dt}$$

Fig. 9.6.4: The modified Stewart–Hamilton equation used to calculate cardiac output using thermodilution. CO = cardiac output, V = volume of cold bolus, T_o = starting blood temperature, T_i = cold bolus temperature, K = a constant to account for density and the specific heat of the bolus fluid, $\Delta T \, dt$ = temperature change detected by the thermistor over a specified period of time (between t_1 and t_2).

Note that the cardiac output is inversely proportional to the transit time of the cooled blood and the mean temperature depression. The average of three separate measurements is taken to improve accuracy, and the cardiac output is often corrected for body size by dividing it by body surface area to give cardiac index. Other variables such as stroke volume can also be corrected in this way. *Table 9.6.1* shows variables that can be measured or derived using a PAC.

Table 9.6.1: What can you measure with a PAC?

Variable	Normal adult range
Directly measured variables	
Central venous pressure (CVP)	0–8 mmHg
Right atrial pressure (RAP)	0– 8 mmHg
Right ventricular pressure (RVP)	15–30 / 0–8 mmHg
Pulmonary artery pressure (PAP)	15– 30 / 4–12 mmHg
Pulmonary capillary wedge pressure (PCWP)	2–12 mmHg
Cardiac output (Q)	4.5– 6.0 l.min^{-1*}
Mixed venous oxygen saturation (SvO_2)	75%
Heart rate (HR)	70–100 beats.min^{-1*}
Derived variables	
Cardiac index (CI)	2.5–4.0 l.min^{-1}.m^{-2*}
Stroke volume (SV)	60– 80 ml.beat^{-1*}
Stroke volume index (SVI)	35– 65 ml.beat^{-1}.m^{-2*}
Systemic vascular resistance (SVR)	1000–1200 dyne.s.cm^{-5}
Systemic vascular resistance index (SVRI)	1600–2400 dyne.s.cm^{-5}.m^{-2}
Pulmonary vascular resistance (PVR)	60–120 dyne.s.cm^{-5}
Pulmonary vascular resistance index (PVRI)	250–340 dyne.s.cm^{-5}.m^{-2}
Arterial oxygen content (CaO_2)	180 ml.l^{-1}
Mixed venous oxygen content (CvO_2)	130 ml.l^{-1}
Oxygen delivery (DO_2)	850–1050 ml.min^{-1*}
Oxygen consumption (VO_2)	180–300 ml.min^{-1*}

*Reference range varies depending on the patient.

PACs are also available that can semi-continuously monitor cardiac output, and provide a measurement approximately every minute. These work in a similar fashion to those described above, except that the catheter incorporates a coil that intermittently heats and increases the temperature of the blood in the right ventricle, in place of the cold bolus injected into the right atrium. The change in temperature is measured by the thermistor at the distal end of the PAC as above, and cardiac output is calculated using the same method. The heating of the coil occurs at pseudo-random time intervals and power settings to improve the signal to noise ratio.

Other measurements and functions

A PAC can be used for several other purposes, including the following.

- The distal lumen can be used to sample blood from the pulmonary artery, allowing measurement of mixed venous oxygen saturation (SvO_2). Some PACs have a fibreoptic probe at the distal end that allows continuous measurement of SvO_2 using the same principles as a jugular venous bulb probe.
- Temporary pacing wires can be passed through the proximal port of the PAC, allowing pacing from the right ventricle.
- Values for haemoglobin concentration and arterial oxygenation can be combined with measurements from the PAC, allowing calculation of oxygen consumption (VO_2) and oxygen delivery (DO_2) and estimation of the shunt fraction.
- Other derived parameters include pulmonary and systemic vascular resistances (*Table 9.6.1*).

⊕ Advantages

- A wide range of haemodynamic variables can be measured or calculated and trends or response to intervention can be observed.
- Continuous or semi-continuous measurement of some variables is possible.
- No potentially toxic indicator dyes are required to perform measurements.
- Allows rationalization of drug and fluid therapy for critically ill patients.
- Extra lumens allow the PAC to be used to infuse drugs into the central venous circulation in the same way as a standard central line.

⊖ Disadvantages

- No study has convincingly demonstrated that clinical outcome is improved as a result of the insertion of a PAC.
- Considerable practice is required to float the tip of the PAC into the correct position.
- Data obtained from the PAC have been shown to be regularly misinterpreted by clinicians, leading to incorrect management.
- Several factors may make the data obtained from a PAC inaccurate.
  - If the volume of cold bolus injected is too large or too small, the cardiac output may be under- or over-estimated, respectively. Similarly, if the bolus is the wrong temperature, errors will be introduced.
  - A sudden bolus of ice-cold fluid directly into the atrium may result in a drop in heart rate and therefore the measuring technique artificially reduces the variable being measured.
  - Measurements from the PAC should be made at end-expiration to avoid inaccuracies due to the effect of respiration on intra-thoracic pressure.
  - Intra-cardiac shunting will result in the cold bolus either being diluted by blood shunted from the left heart, or itself being shunted to the left. Either will cause inaccuracy in measurements.

- Significant complications are associated with insertion and use of PACs over and above those associated with standard central venous cannulation, and morbidity resulting from their insertion is of the order of 4 in every 1000 patients. Possible complications include:
  - ventricular arrhythmia and/or conduction defects
  - knotting of the catheter within the heart during insertion
  - balloon rupture
  - pulmonary infarction if the balloon is left inflated
  - pulmonary artery rupture – this has a mortality rate of approximately 30%
  - thromboembolism – the risk of this is reduced if heparin-coated PACs are used
  - endocarditis
  - pulmonary or tricuspid valve regurgitation
  - air embolism.

9.7 Other cardiac output monitors

Cardiac output monitors are used in the critical care unit and in theatre. They are particularly helpful in guiding the use of inotropic and vasopressor drugs and also in the administration of IV fluid therapy. Examples of conditions when their use may be considered include the recovery from major surgery, acute cardiac failure or renal failure (particularly when the two co-exist), sepsis, severe dehydration, and many others.

Historically, and arguably, the gold standard technique for measuring cardiac output involves using a pulmonary artery catheter (PAC). However, it is a fairly invasive process and the incidence of serious complications after the use of PACs is relatively high. In recent years, measurement of cardiac output using an oesophageal ultrasound probe has become popular but it also has its own set of disadvantages.

There are several other ways of measuring cardiac output and as technology has improved, an increasing number of sophisticated and relatively non-invasive cardiac output monitors have appeared on the market.

The Fick principle and partial gas rebreathing

In 1870 Adolf Fick described a method of estimating blood flow through an organ based on the principle of conservation of mass: the uptake of a substance by an organ is equal to the blood flow through it multiplied by the arteriovenous concentration difference. If the organ in question is the lungs and the substance being measured is oxygen, then this equation can be rearranged to give the Fick equation shown in *Figure 9.7.1a*. Flow through the lungs is equal to cardiac output.

One method of using the Fick principle to calculate cardiac output requires a PAC. The VO_2 is measured by spirometry and the CaO_2 is calculated using an arterial blood gas sample and the haemoglobin concentration. The CvO_2 must be calculated using the mixed venous blood from the pulmonary artery.

The accurate measurement of VO_2 is laborious and the insertion of a PAC carries significant risks. Therefore, the equation can be altered so that carbon dioxide can be used to calculate cardiac output instead of oxygen. This equation is shown in *Figure 9.7.1b*. The VCO_2 can be calculated by multiplying the mixed expiratory CO_2 concentration by the minute volume. The $CaCO_2$ can be calculated using the measured $PaCO_2$ from an arterial blood gas sample or end-tidal CO_2.

The need to measure $CvCO_2$ can be removed using a partial rebreathing technique as follows. During a short period of rebreathing (up to 50 seconds), the end-tidal PCO_2 rises in proportion to the cardiac output, as does the $CaCO_2$. However, the $CvCO_2$ does not rise significantly over this duration. This allows the end-tidal CO_2 and the $CaCO_2$ before and after rebreathing to be substituted into the modified Fick equation. The cardiac output is therefore derived by comparing the change in end-tidal CO_2 with the change in $CaCO_2$ during the rebreathing period (see *Fig. 9.7.1c*). The NICO (Philips Respironics) cardiac output monitor uses this technique.

$$Q = \frac{VO_2}{CaO_2 - CvO_2}$$

Fig. 9.7.1: (a) The Fick equation for calculating flow through an organ using oxygen. Q = flow, VO_2 = oxygen consumption, CaO_2 = arterial oxygen content, CvO_2 = venous oxygen content.

$$CO = \frac{VCO_2}{CvCO_2 - CaCO_2}$$

(b) The modified Fick equation for calculation of cardiac output using the partial rebreathing method. CO = cardiac output, VCO_2 = carbon dioxide production, $CvCO_2$ = venous carbon dioxide content, $CaCO_2$ = arterial carbon dioxide content.

$$CO = \frac{\Delta VCO_2}{\Delta CaCO_2}$$

(c) Substitution of the change in CO_2 production and arterial CO_2 content during a rebreathing period allows calculation of cardiac output without the need to measure the venous CO_2 content ($CvCO_2$).

Advantages
- Non-invasive.
- Easy to use.

Disadvantages
- Inaccurate unless the patient is intubated because respiratory gases must be collected and analysed accurately.
- Ventilator settings must be fixed and all breaths during the measurement must be mandatory and therefore of equal tidal volume.
- This method also becomes inaccurate if there is a large V/Q mismatch, shunt, dead space volume, or barrier to diffusion of CO_2, meaning its usefulness is limited in critically ill patients.
- Gives no information regarding stroke volume, systemic vascular resistance, or other cardiovascular indices.

Pulse pressure waveform analysis

Several products are available that estimate cardiac output by analysing the arterial pulse pressure waveform. This method is attractive because invasive arterial blood pressure monitoring is commonly performed and has few complications.

Because the pressure wave is generated by the ejection of the stroke volume into the arterial vasculature, analysis of the wave can be used to estimate the volume that caused it. In order to perform this calculation information is required regarding the aortic compliance, aortic capacitance and vascular resistance. These variables can be estimated from population data based on the age, sex and body surface area of the patient, or they can be inferred from a calibration measurement of cardiac output using a different method (e.g. indicator dilution).

PiCCO$_2$

PiCCO$_2$ (Pulsion Medical Systems) calculates cardiac output using pulse contour analysis. This method calculates the area under the systolic portion of the arterial pressure waveform in order to estimate stroke volume. A proximally placed arterial cannula (femoral, brachial or axillary) is therefore required so that the dicrotic notch is reliably seen in the waveform, allowing the end of systole to be accurately determined. The system relies on a high-fidelity transduction of the arterial pulse waveform, therefore anything affecting the shape of the wave (e.g. over- or under-damping) may affect the measurement. The cardiac output is given by multiplying the stroke volume by the heart rate.

PiCCO$_2$ is calibrated using a thermodilution method similar to that used by the PAC to calculate cardiac output: a 15 ml bolus of isotonic saline at approximately 8°C is rapidly injected into a central venous catheter and a thermistor incorporated into the arterial cannula detects the temperature drop. Therefore, in contrast to the PAC, the cold bolus passes through the entire right side circulation and is ejected from the left ventricle before being detected. Cardiac output calculations based on transpulmonary thermodilution techniques such as this have been shown to compare favourably with pulmonary artery thermodilution. In both cases, the cardiac output calculation is based on the modified Stewart–Hamilton equation (*Fig. 9.7.2*).

$$CO = \frac{m}{\int_{t_1}^{t_2} [i]\, dt}$$

Fig. 9.7.2: The modified Stewart–Hamilton equation for use with indicator dilution techniques. CO = cardiac output, m = mass of indicator, $[i]dt$ = indicator concentration detected over a specified time period (between t_1 and t_2).

The work of Stewart and Hamilton established that the volume of distribution of an indicator can be calculated from the product of flow and the mean circulation time. A consequence of using transpulmonary thermodilution is therefore the ability to calculate the volume of distribution of the cold bolus within the thorax. This is done by multiplying the cardiac output by the mean transit time of the bolus from the injection site to the detection site. The volume is known as the intrathoracic thermal volume (ITTV).

Other work by Newman in 1951 showed experimentally that the time taken for an indicator to wash out of a series of linked chambers of different sizes was dependent on the volume of the largest chamber. Therefore, the downward gradient of the indicator washout exponential can be used to calculate the volume of the largest chamber. In the case of transpulmonary thermodilution, the lungs represent the largest chamber and so the pulmonary thermal volume (PTV) can be calculated using the gradient of the washout curve detected at the arterial thermistor.

Further variables can then be derived:
- the global end diastolic volume (GEDV) is equal to the ITTV minus the PTV; the GEDV gives an indication of preload based on the volume of all four cardiac chambers
- the intrathoracic blood volume (ITBV) is the sum of the volume of blood in the heart and the volume of blood in the pulmonary vascular tree; the ITBV has been shown to hold a consistent relationship with the GEDV, being 25% higher and so it is therefore simply the GEDV multiplied by 1.25

- the extravascular lung water (EVLW) is equal to the ITTV minus the ITBV and it gives an index of the volume of water in the lungs that is not in the vascular space (it does not include water in pleural fluid); it can therefore be used to help judge whether pulmonary oedema is present.

Table 9.7.1: Some variables measured or calculated by PiCCO$_2$. Variables with an asterisk are commonly divided by the patient's body surface area to convert them to an index (e.g. cardiac index, CI, instead of cardiac output).

Variable	Explanation
Cardiac output (CO)*	Volume of blood ejected by left ventricle per minute.
Stroke volume (SV)*	Volume of blood ejected by left ventricle per beat.
Stroke volume variation (SVV)	The percentage variation in stroke volume over the preceding half a minute.
Global end diastolic volume (GEDV)*	The total volume of blood remaining in the heart (the sum of all four chambers) at the end of diastole.
Intrathoracic blood volume (ITBV)*	The volume of blood in the lungs added to the GEDV.
Extravascular lung water (EVLW)*	A measure of the permeability of the pulmonary vasculature.
Cardiac function index (CFI)	Indication of cardiac function independent of preload. Equal to CO/GEDV.
Systemic vascular resistance (SVR)*	Resistance to blood flow offered by the systemic arterial vasculature.
Left ventricular contractility (DP/dt)	Maximum generation of pressure per unit time by the left ventricle.

Advantages
- Good correlation with PAC thermodilution.
- Does not require a PAC.
- Able to derive variables not possible with most other cardiac output monitors.
- Can be used in children over 2 kg.

Disadvantages
- Requires a central venous catheter and a proximal arterial line, so still relatively invasive.
- Requires regular recalibration.
- Requires very accurate arterial pressure transduction, as the system is sensitive to damping.
- Unable to provide valid continuous measurements using pulse-contour analysis if an intra-aortic balloon pump is present.

LiDCO

LiDCO Group manufacture two variations of the LiDCO device, the LiDCO-plus and the LiDCO-rapid. The former is calibrated using an indicator dilution technique and is more accurate than the latter, which does not require indicator calibration and is only intended for intraoperative monitoring.

The LiDCO-plus is calibrated in a similar way to the PiCCO$_2$ monitor, except it uses an injection of a small amount of lithium chloride (2–4 µmol.kg^{-1}) instead of cold saline. The lithium is injected into a central or peripheral vein (a central venous catheter is not a requirement) and subsequently circulates through the heart and lungs before being detected at an arterial line that samples blood at a rate of 4.5 ml.min^{-1}. The detector consists of a modified PVC membrane that only allows lithium ions to pass, resulting in the development of a voltage across the membrane that is proportional to the plasma lithium concentration. The lithium concentration–time curve is used to calculate cardiac output using a modified Stewart–Hamilton equation.

The LiDCO-plus may be rendered less accurate in the presence of some non-depolarizing muscle relaxants under certain conditions. This is because molecules that contain a quaternary ammonium group are detected by the lithium sensor. Drugs that are especially problematic are atracurium and rocuronium. Other muscle relaxants can be used as long as the LiDCO-plus calibration is performed before they are administered or after a sufficient delay. The device also cannot be used with patients who are taking therapeutic lithium.

The LiDCO-rapid is not calibrated using lithium measurement, but uses data obtained from a large post-operative group of patients. The machine prompts the user to enter the age, weight and height of their patient so that the appropriate calibration can be performed.

Both the LiDCO-plus and LiDCO-rapid use an algorithm known as PulseCO to convert the arterial pressure wave into a volume wave and it is this algorithm that is altered by the calibration. PulseCO is based on aortic compliance data obtained from cadavers and uses a method of signal processing called modified auto-covariance to calculate the stroke volume. The calibration scales the result of the algorithm to account for the individual patient's aortic capacitance.

As PulseCO does not depend on the actual shape of the pressure waveform, it is less susceptible to damping. A peripheral arterial line is therefore sufficient for use with LiDCO systems. This method of calculating stroke volume from the pressure waveform is often known as pulse power analysis.

Advantages
- Central venous access is not essential. Relatively non-invasive.
- Good correlation with PAC measurements of cardiac output.
- The LiDCO-rapid does not require manual calibration.
- Less affected by damping in the monitoring system.

Disadvantages
- LiDCO-plus cannot be used with patients who are taking therapeutic lithium and suffers from reduced accuracy in the presence of some non-depolarizing muscle relaxants.
- Lithium is contraindicated in patients who are in early pregnancy or weigh less than 40 kg.
- The LiDCO-plus requires regular recalibration.
- The LiDCO-rapid uses population data to calibrate its algorithm.
- Cannot be used with patients who have aortic regurgitation or in those with an intra-aortic balloon pump *in situ*.

FloTrac Vigileo

The FloTrac Vigileo (Edwards Lifesciences) works in a similar way to the LiDCO-rapid, insofar as it analyses the arterial pressure wave from a standard arterial line and derives cardiac output using a mathematical algorithm based on the patient's age, sex, weight and height. The arterial line is connected to the FloTrac sensor, a modified pressure transducer.

The algorithm estimates stroke volume by sampling the arterial pressure trace at 100 Hz over 20 seconds. The standard deviation of the resulting 2000 data points for arterial pressure (σAP) is calculated and multiplied by a correction factor (known as χ) that accounts for the compliance and resistance of the arterial tree. χ is estimated from the patient's age, sex, weight and height, and also converts the units of σAP from mmHg into ml.beat^{-1}.

The algorithm has been altered twice, most recently in 2009. The latest version is able to estimate cardiac output more accurately in patients with low systemic vascular resistance and also updates more often than the original version.

This monitor is also able to give a continuous measurement of central venous oxygen saturations ($ScvO_2$) using an oximetry catheter. Although ideally mixed venous oxygen saturation (SvO_2) is used to calculate oxygen consumption (VO_2) this requires the use of a PAC. An acceptable correlation between $ScvO_2$ and SvO_2 has been demonstrated, allowing the Vigileo to estimate VO_2.

Advantages
- Relatively non-invasive. No central venous catheter is required.
- Can measure $ScvO_2$ and therefore estimate VO_2.
- Does not require manual calibration.

Disadvantages
- A high quality arterial line signal is essential because the system is sensitive to damping.
- Accuracy in patients who have arrhythmias or who are haemodynamically unstable has been questioned.
- Cannot be used in the presence of an intra-aortic balloon pump (see *Section 9.19*).
- Uses population data to estimate compliance and resistance of the arterial tree.

Bioimpedance

A fixed amplitude, high frequency alternating current is passed between two electrodes that are placed on opposite sides of the thoracic wall. The voltage across the electrodes is measured and the impedance can be calculated. The impedance varies with factors including the intrathoracic blood volume. If only the pulsatile component of the impedance is analysed, the stroke volume and cardiac output can be derived.

The pulsatile component is only a small proportion of the whole (i.e. there is a small signal to noise ratio), and so accurate detection is difficult. The data obtained using this method have often been shown to be inaccurate, especially in unwell patients.

Advantages
- Completely non-invasive.

Disadvantages
- Interference from nearby electrical equipment (particularly electrosurgical devices) will affect the reading.
- Muscular movement will also cause interference. This limits the use of this device in patients who are not sedated or under anaesthesia.
- Accuracy in haemodynamically unstable patients has been questioned, particularly in earlier models of devices using this technique.

Bioreactance

The non-invasive cardiac output monitor (NICOM, Cheetah Medical) works in a similar way to bioimpedance methods. Electrodes are placed on opposite sides of the thorax and a 75 kHz radiofrequency signal is emitted at one and detected at the other. The signal amplitude is reduced as it passes across the thorax due to impedance. However, there is also a phase shift between the emitted signal and the detected signal due to the capacitative and inductive (reactance) properties of the thorax. Both the reduction in amplitude and the phase shift depend on the intra-thoracic volume, of which the stroke volume is a component. The stroke volume can therefore be calculated using an algorithm that analyses the pulsatile component of the signal.

The use of phase shift as well as amplitude improves the signal to noise ratio significantly compared to monitors that use only impedance to measure stroke volume. The difference can be thought of as similar to that between AM and FM radio.

Advantages
- Completely non-invasive.

Disadvantages
- As with bioimpedance devices, the accuracy of this method in critically ill patients has been questioned. One possible reason that has been suggested is that the accumulation of interstitial oedema may alter the reactance properties of the thorax.

Finapres and Finometer

The Finapres system (Finapres Medical Systems) is a device that utilizes the Penaz principle to provide a continuous non-invasive measurement of blood pressure. The Penaz principle states that if a force acts on a body in one direction, its magnitude may be determined by measuring a second force that is acting in the opposite direction and is sufficient to prevent movement of the body.

A finger is placed within a pneumatic cuff. An LED within the cuff passes light through the finger to a photodetector on the other side. The volume of blood in the finger rises and falls with the cardiac cycle and this causes a cyclical variation in the amount of light that is transmitted through the finger. As the volume in the finger increases, the light transmission decreases, and vice versa. The system attempts to keep the light transmission through the finger constant by varying the pressure in the cuff. As blood arrives at the finger during systole, the cuff pressure increases to keep the volume in the finger constant. During diastole, the cuff pressure falls again. The arterial pressure is therefore derived by measuring the cuff pressure necessary to keep the light transmission through the finger constant.

The Finometer uses an algorithm known as Modelflow to convert the pressure waveform obtained by Finapres into a volume waveform. This allows calculation of stroke volume and cardiac output.

Advantages
- Completely non-invasive.
- Small and lightweight. Can be made portable.

Disadvantages
- Although measurements made by the Penaz technique have been shown to be accurate in people with well-perfused fingers, there has been debate about the validity of this technique in patients who are hypotensive or who have poor peripheral perfusion.

9.8 Intra-abdominal pressure measurement

Overview

The main indication for measuring intra-abdominal pressure is the suspicion of intra-abdominal hypertension or compartment syndrome following surgery or trauma. The former is defined as a pressure of 12 mmHg or more in the abdominal cavity, and the latter as a pressure of 20 mmHg or more with associated organ dysfunction such as acute renal impairment.

How it works

In order to measure the intra-abdominal pressure, the distal end of the measurement set must be placed within the abdomen. This is carried out most frequently by measuring intravesicular pressure via the urinary catheter; ideally at least 25 ml of fluid should be in the bladder to carry this out. Intra-gastric, intra-colonic, and intrauterine techniques have also been used.

The pressure may be measured using a manometer (measuring the height of a column of fluid, which can be as simple as lifting the catheter tubing and measuring with a ruler). Alternatively, and more accurately, specialized manometry kits are available, or a pressure transducer may be attached to a continuous column of pressurized saline using the same method as invasive blood pressure measurement.

The intra-abdominal pressure rises and falls with respiration, and also depends on the posture of the patient. Therefore, the pressure reading is taken at the end of expiration when abdominal wall muscles are relaxed and with the patient in the supine position.

⊕ Advantages

- Very easy to measure, especially in critical care where most patients will already have a urinary catheter.
- This is the only method of formally diagnosing abdominal compartment syndrome, and can lead to decompressive treatments.
- Measurement may be continuous or intermittent depending on the requirement.

⊖ Disadvantages

- Intra-abdominal pressure varies quite significantly between patients, depending on their body mass index, posture, respiratory state and other variables. The measured pressure must be taken with as many of these standardized as possible. Trends may be more significant than single readings.

9.9 Intracranial pressure measurement

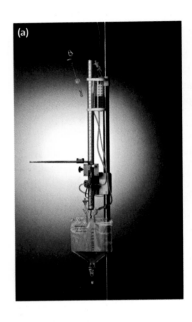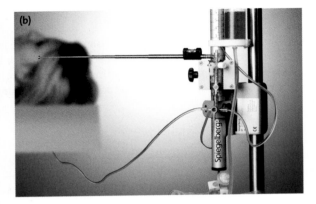

Figure 9.9.1: An external ventricular drain (a) can be used to remove excess cerebrospinal fluid and help maintain the intracerebral pressure at or below a set value (b). Images from Spiegelberg GmbH & Co. KG, Germany.

Overview

There are three main tissues that make up the intracranial volume: blood, brain and cerebrospinal fluid (CSF). Intracranial pressure (ICP) is normally 8–12 mmHg, but can rise rapidly if there is an increase in the volume of one of the intracranial tissues because the skull is a bony vault and cannot allow expansion of one component without reduction in another. This concept is known as the Monro–Kellie doctrine.

Uses

In cases where there has been intracranial haemorrhage, brain tumour or obstruction of CSF drainage, monitoring of ICP may be indicated. A raised ICP may prompt the initiation of a particular treatment or investigation (especially CT scanning), and a knowledge of its value also allows calculation of the cerebral perfusion pressure (CPP = MAP – (ICP + CVP)).

How it works

Schematic diagrams of each type of monitor are shown in *Figure 9.9.2*.

External ventricular drains

The EVD is considered to be the gold standard technique for ICP monitoring. A fine plastic catheter is inserted by a surgeon through a burr hole, and passes through the meninges and brain into the lateral ventricle. The CSF in the catheter forms a continuous fluid column that is connected to a strain gauge transducer that works in the same way as an invasive blood pressure monitor (*Section 6.13*). The ICP may also be read using a simple manometer using the vertical height of the CSF column above a zero calibration point. This zero point is taken to be the patient's mastoid process, external auditory canal, tragus of the ear or other fixed point.

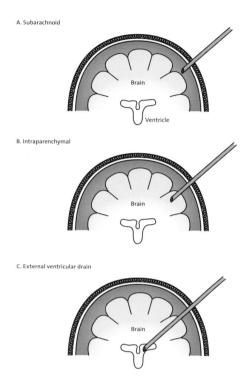

Fig. 9.9.2: The intracranial positions of different intracranial pressure monitors.

As well as monitoring ICP, CSF can be drained via the catheter if necessary, and the equipment can be set up so that CSF will automatically drain if the ICP rises above a set pressure. Surgeons will often instruct that the drain should be 'kept at 15 cm'. This means that the CSF column is allowed to be 15 cm higher than the zero point before it starts to drain, and in theory this should prevent the CSF pressure rising above 15 cmH$_2$O. A modern EVD system is shown in *Figure 9.9.1*.

CSF can also be sampled from the EVD for microbiological or biochemical analysis.

Extraparenchymal monitors

These monitors include extradural, subdural and subarachnoid monitors. They are inserted by a surgeon through the skull, and a fine catheter is placed in the relevant space. Various methods are used to measure the pressure including wire strain gauges and fibreoptic systems. In the former, a small wire strain gauge is mounted on the end of the catheter. The system is arranged so that an increase in pressure causes the wire to be stretched and the electrical resistance through it can be used to calculate the pressure.

Fibreoptic pressure transducers are also small enough to be catheter-mounted. The light from the fibreoptic cable is passed onto a mirror which reflects it onto a detector. The mirror is distorted by an increased pressure, which alters the amount of light reflected onto the detector. The amount of reflection detected is used to calculate the pressure.

Intraparenchymal monitors

These monitors work in the same way as the extraparenchymal ones, except that the transducing catheter is passed through all the meninges and into the brain tissue itself. They are usually positioned approximately 15–20 mm below the surface. They are considered to be more accurate than extraparenchymal devices.

⊕ Advantages

- EVDs are accurate and can be recalibrated at the bedside.
- EVDs can be used to treat raised ICP as well as monitor it by allowing drainage of CSF.
- Extra- and intraparenchymal monitors are relatively easy to insert and do not always require a general anaesthetic.

⊖ Disadvantages

- EVD catheters and intraparenchymal monitors involve piercing brain tissue, which may be dangerous or not possible in some patients (e.g. those with coagulopathy).

- EVD catheters can easily become blocked due to their small calibre. This prevents accurate measurement of ICP and drainage of CSF.
- Extra- and intraparenchymal devices are not as accurate as EVDs and have no facility to allow drainage of CSF.
- Extra- and intraparenchymal devices cannot be recalibrated, and readings are subject to drift. Modern devices suffer with this problem to a lesser degree than older ones.
- All types of ICP monitor are associated with intracranial infection. EVDs have a higher incidence of this than other devices (3–5% vs. 1–2%).

Other notes

If there is a contraindication to inserting an invasive ICP monitoring device, other techniques, such as transcranial Doppler ultrasound can be used to measure surrogate variables like intracerebral blood velocity.

9.10 Renal replacement therapy in critical care

Overview

Renal replacement therapy (RRT) can be used in the acute setting, usually in critical care, or in the longer term management of chronic renal failure. The methods used can differ depending on the setting and indication.

Uses

The indications for RRT include:

- electrolyte imbalance (especially hyperkalaemia)
- metabolic acidosis
- fluid overload (e.g. pulmonary oedema unresponsive to treatment with diuretics)
- uraemia causing symptoms (e.g. urea >35 mmol.l^{-1} with confusion suggesting encephalopathy)
- removal of some drugs or toxins from the blood (see below)
- severe hyperthermia (> 40°C).

How it works

RRT is a cover-all term for several techniques that are used to remove unwanted small molecule solutes and water from the blood using a semi-permeable membrane. It may be intermittent or continuous.

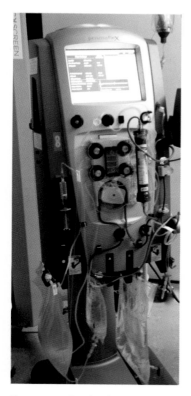

Figure 9.10.1: Renal replacement therapy in progress.

Intermittent techniques are commonly used in the management of chronic renal failure. They include intermittent haemodialysis which is usually performed for 3–4 hours, three times per week and involves the use of a long-term vascular access device such as a Tesio line or the formation of an arteriovenous fistula. In peritoneal dialysis, dialysate is injected into the peritoneal cavity through a catheter in the abdominal wall. It remains there for several hours before being drained. Water and solutes are dialysed through the peritoneum.

Continuous techniques are usually encountered in critical care settings in the UK. Continuous arteriovenous haemofiltration utilizes the patient's arterial blood pressure to circulate the blood but requires the cannulation of both an artery and a vein. The cannulation of arteries large enough to achieve the required blood flow results in a high rate of morbidity and therefore modern continuous RRT is performed using a double lumen catheter in a single vein and mechanical pumps to circulate the blood.

A roller pump takes blood via a pressure sensor into the machine. The pressure sensor can detect occlusions in the vascular access that may be caused by kinks or clots. The filtered blood is then returned to the same vessel that it came from. Sometimes a warmer or a heat exchanger is used to increase or decrease the temperature of the blood.

The three most common modes of continuous RRT are dialysis, filtration or a combination of both. Other modes also exist. Continuous forms of RRT are preferred in critical care because of their more desirable cardiovascular stability profile. *Figure 9.10.2* shows the basic difference between dialysis and filtration.

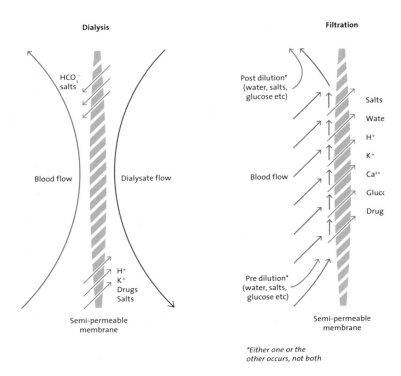

Dialysis

HCO$_3^-$
salts

Blood flow

Dialysate flow

H$^+$
K$^+$
Drugs
Salts

Semi-permeable
membrane

Filtration

Post dilution*
(water, salts,
glucose etc)

Salts

Wate

H$^+$

K$^+$

Blood flow

Ca^{2+}

Gluc

Drug

Pre dilution*
(water, salts,
glucose etc)

Semi-permeable
membrane

*Either one or the
other occurs, not both

Figure 9.10.2: The difference between dialysis and filtration.

Continuous venovenous haemodialysis

Dialysis is the selective removal of solutes from the blood as a result of their different degrees of diffusion through a semi-permeable membrane. It is very effective for molecules smaller than 500 Daltons and also works for molecules between 500 and 5000 Da, although filtration is more efficient for these larger molecules.

In continuous venovenous haemodialysis (CVVHD), blood is taken from the patient and flows against a semi-permeable membrane. On the other side of the membrane, and flowing in the opposite direction, is the dialysate. This is therefore described as countercurrent flow. The blood and dialysate contain solutes at different concentrations, and these move across the semi-permeable membrane down their respective concentration gradients. Some solutes will have a higher concentration in the blood and others will have a higher concentration in the dialysate and therefore not all solutes will move in the same direction. For example, bicarbonate will typically move from the dialysate to the blood whereas potassium and hydrogen ions will move from the blood to the dialysate.

The speed of dialysis of a solute depends on its concentration gradient across the membrane. The countercurrent flow helps to maintain the concentration gradients for different solutes, and leads to more efficient dialysis. After the blood has passed through the dialyser, it is returned directly to the patient and the used dialysate is discarded.

The diffusion of a solute depends on random molecular motion (Brownian motion), the speed of which is inversely proportional to the molecular weight. Large molecules are therefore dialysed less efficiently than small ones, even though the pores in the semipermeable membrane are of a sufficient size to allow their passage.

Technically speaking, it is not possible to remove water from the circulation using dialysis, because dialysis is the diffusion of *solute* across a semi-permeable membrane. RRT machines in CVVHD mode can be set to remove water, however, but this is done by increasing the hydrostatic pressure gradient across the membrane, usually via a reduction in the dialysate pressure. Confusingly, water is therefore removed using filtration (see below), even when the machine is in CVVHD mode.

Continuous venovenous haemofiltration
Filtration is the selective passage of solutes and water in the blood through a semi-permeable membrane as a result of a hydrostatic pressure gradient. It is an effective technique for removing both small and large molecules of up to 50 kDa from the blood and is also capable of removing excess water.

Blood is pumped at a relatively high pressure along the semipermeable membrane. However, there is no dialysate fluid on the opposite side of the membrane in CVVHF. Water and solutes are forced through the membrane by the pressure, and form the ultrafiltrate. This is rapidly removed from the other side of the membrane and discarded, creating a negative pressure which adds to the pressure gradient across the membrane. This high gradient causes water to move quickly and frictional forces make solutes move with it. This is known as solvent drag or convection.

Due to solvent drag, the molecular weight of the solute has less bearing on the speed of movement through the membrane than in dialysis, and larger molecules are filtered just as efficiently as small ones.

The speed of filtration of a solute depends on the magnitude of the pressure gradient across the membrane, as well as other factors such as the flow of blood and how porous the membrane is.

In order to maintain circulating volume, a balanced electrolyte solution is added to the blood before it is returned. If there is euvolaemia, then the volume added is equal to that of the ultrafiltrate. If the patient is fluid overloaded, then the volume of electrolyte solution added back to the blood will be less than that of the ultrafiltrate. It is also possible to return fluid to the patient. The solution can be added before (predilution) or after (postdilution) the blood has been filtered. These approaches each have advantages and disadvantages. Predilution reduces clotting in the filter and protein 'caking' on the membrane occurs to a lesser extent. However, some of the predilution solution will be filtered off, making the method less efficient. In postdilution, the concentration of solutes to be filtered is higher, and so theoretically more convection occurs using this method.

Slow continuous ultrafiltration (SCUF) is a technique used to remove water with little change in solute concentrations. It is essentially CVVHF running at a slow rate without a replacement solution being added back to the blood as it returns to the patient.

Continuous venovenous haemodiafiltration
As the name suggests, CVVHDF is a combination of the two techniques above. Blood is filtered by a hydrostatic pressure gradient at a semi-permeable membrane, but a dialysate fluid is present on the opposite side of the membrane and so diffusion also occurs.

A replacement electrolyte solution is added to the blood before it is returned to the patient, as it is in CVVHF. The volume added is dependent on the fluid status of the patient, but also on the ratio of filtration to dialysis that has occurred.

Anticoagulation
The contact of blood with the synthetic materials that make up the extracorporeal circulation causes activation of the clotting cascade. There are several options to prevent this and therefore stop machine failure due to occlusion by blood clots.

Simple methods of reducing the risk of blood clotting include avoidance of kinking of the tubing, the use of predilution rather than postdilution, and ensuring the blood flow does not drop below approximately 100 ml.h^{-1}. Bubble traps can also be used to prevent the formation of a blood:air interface.

The patient may be systemically anticoagulated. This can be achieved using unfractionated or low molecular weight heparins or prostacyclin (PGI$_2$), which has a short half-life but is expensive. The disadvantage of this is that it puts the patient at a higher risk of bleeding.

Another option is to anticoagulate the extracorporeal circuit only. This has the advantage that the patient's coagulation should not be affected. One method of doing this is to infuse unfractionated heparin as blood is removed from the patient and then reverse the effect with protamine as it is returned. An alternative is the use of citrate, which prevents blood clotting by chelation of calcium ions. It can be added to blood coming into the RRT machine and then its effect can be reversed by the addition of extra calcium as the blood is returned. This provides excellent anticoagulation, but carries the potential risks of hypocalcaemia and metabolic alkalosis, and thus needs to be carefully monitored. An especially prepared dialysate or replacement fluid that contains the right amount of calcium is used.

Semi-permeable membranes

Semi-permeable membranes may be synthetic and made of substances such as polysulphone or polyacrylonitrile, or may be made of naturally occurring materials such as cellulose. In either case, there are several properties of the membrane that affect its function.

- The permeability of the membrane dictates the flow of solutes across it. Different membranes have different properties that make it easier or more difficult for diffusion or filtration to occur. These properties include the number of pores per unit area, the size of the pores, whether the membrane is made of a hydrophobic or hydrophilic material, its pH and whether it has a charge. Pores in membranes used clinically have a diameter of about 5 nm and allow the passage of substances with a molecular weight of up to 50 kDa.
- The biocompatibility is the extent to which inflammatory enzyme cascades (such as the complement system) are activated by the membrane. A higher biocompatibility suggests a lower inflammatory response. Synthetic membranes are engineered to be more biocompatible than naturally occurring ones.
- The thickness of the membrane is also a determinant of diffusion and filtration rate: the thicker the membrane, the slower the rate.
- Membranes with a high surface area are more efficient than those with a low surface area for both diffusion and filtration. Most membranes used clinically have a surface area of between 0.5 and 2 m^2.

While membranes do not allow large molecules to pass, some allow them to adhere in a process known as adsorption (or apheresis). This may be important in removing medium-sized molecules such as cytokines and other inflammatory mediators from the blood. Membranes that have been modified to exploit this property may have a role in the treatment of severe sepsis and septic shock over and above the more usual purpose of supporting patients with renal failure. Examples include polyacrylonitrile membranes that are coated with polyethyleneimine to make them positively charged and therefore encourage negatively charged endotoxin to adhere. Polystyrene divinyl benzene (Cytosorb) is a biocompatible compound that can be included as beads in some haemofilters. Many key cytokines (e.g. interleukin-6) adhere to it and are therefore removed from plasma.

Fluids used in RRT

Fluids used in RRT are either dialysate solutions for CVVHD or replacement solutions for CVVHF. In either case, they are balanced salt solutions, having physiological solute concentrations and pH.

The composition of dialysate fluid varies, but generally has a low potassium concentration (e.g. 1mmol.l^{-1}) and a high bicarbonate concentration (e.g. 35mmol.l^{-1}). Other substances present include sodium, calcium, magnesium, chloride and glucose.

Replacement fluid used in CVVHF is very similar, although the buffer can be either bicarbonate or lactate. The latter is more convenient because it is stable in solution and therefore the fluid has a long shelf life. Lactate is normally metabolized into bicarbonate in the body on an equimolar basis. However, in critically ill patients (particularly those with liver dysfunction or severe hypoperfusion) this may not occur. If lactate-based replacement fluids are used in these situations, acid–base derangement may worsen and therefore bicarbonate-based solutions are used instead. However, these must be made up just prior to use.

Drugs removed by RRT

The extent to which drugs can be removed by RRT depends on several factors that are common to all small molecules. These factors can be divided into those concerning the drug and those concerning the type of RRT. Drug factors include the molecular weight, the extent to which it is bound to plasma proteins, the solubility in water, the charge and the volume of distribution. Factors related to the type of RRT include the size of the pores in the membrane, the material the membrane is made from, its charge, the mode used (CVVHD vs. CVVHF) and the blood and dialysate flow.

The sieving coefficient is a reflection of the above factors and is defined as the ratio of drug (or any solute) concentration in the ultrafiltrate to its concentration in the unfiltered plasma. A high coefficient (approaching 1) implies that the drug is freely removed, whereas a low coefficient implies it is poorly removed. However, these values must be interpreted with caution, because they do not take volume of distribution into account. The classic example of this is digoxin, which has a sieving coefficient of 0.96 but is not removed at all efficiently from the patient by RRT because its volume of distribution is large, at $4–7 \text{l.kg}^{-1}$. By comparison, phenobarbital is removed relatively well by RRT and has a sieving coefficient of 0.86 and a volume of distribution of 0.5l.kg^{-1}.

⊕ Advantages

- RRT in critical care provides a technique for performing the functions of the kidney.
- It is possible that removal of inflammatory mediators by dialysis or filtration in the context of severe sepsis may have an impact on morbidity or mortality. Clinical trials are currently underway.

⊖ Disadvantages

- Disadvantages include those of central venous cannulation.
- The initiation of RRT represents a haemodynamic insult, with fluid shifts, cool priming fluid entering the circulation and cytokine release. It may therefore result in haemodynamic instability.
- Occlusion and clotting of blood in the extracorporeal circulation is a problem even with systemic anticoagulation.
- Thrombocytopenia may occur due to platelet activation and consumption due to roller-pumping, or more rarely as a result of the use of heparin.

- Although RRT has been used for many decades, opinion is still divided over which mode is best, when RRT should be started and what the optimal flows are. Evidence is sparse on these subjects.

⊘ Safety

- Disconnection of lines may lead to rapid exsanguination. Connections must be kept to a minimum and those that do exist should be thoroughly checked. Pressure sensors are incorporated into the extracorporeal circuit and will sound alarms or stop the pumps in the event that a disconnection is detected.

Other notes

There are other forms of RRT less commonly seen in critical care, including the following.

- Haemoperfusion is a technique that allows RRT without the use of a semi-permeable membrane. Blood is perfused over an ion exchange resin or a substance such as activated charcoal. This removes various substances from the blood (up to a molecular weight of 500 Da). It is especially good at removing some drugs. The major disadvantages of this technique are that water cannot be removed and glucose and platelet removal can be excessive, leading to hypoglycaemia and thrombocytopenia.
- Plasma exchange is performed with a membrane that allows the transit of molecules much larger than those allowed by standard dialysis or filtration membranes. Molecules of up to 500 kDa may pass, and therefore whole plasma is removed from the blood. The replacement fluid is a mixture of FFP and albumin. Plasmapheresis is a similar technique that involves the use of a centrifuge to remove plasma rather than a membrane.

Liver replacement therapy, involving passing blood from the patient over a mesh containing animal hepatocytes before returning it, is currently being researched.

9.11 Extracorporeal membrane oxygenation

Overview

While cardiopulmonary bypass (CPB) is used to replace the function of the heart and lungs in the short term during cardiothoracic surgery, extracorporeal membrane oxygenation (ECMO) is used to support or replace cardiac and pulmonary function in the longer term on intensive care.

The technique has been used for some time in paediatrics where it is used to treat neonates with respiratory distress. In recent years, as technology has improved, it has also been used more frequently in adult patients, especially following the H1N1 influenza pandemic in 2009.

Uses

ECMO is indicated where there is severe cardiac or respiratory failure that has a potentially reversible cause, but where the condition is not improving. Specifically it may be considered if a patient is being treated with maximal conventional treatment, and still has one of the following:

- PaO_2 to FiO_2 ratio of less than 13.3 kPa (100 mmHg) despite intubation and an optimal ventilator strategy
- respiratory acidosis with pH less than 7.20
- cardiogenic shock despite maximal inotropic therapy and use of an intra-aortic balloon pump.

ECMO may also be initiated when a patient fails to wean from CPB following surgery, and it can be used as a bridge heart transplant or implantation of a ventricular assist device (VAD). Occasionally it may be used as part of the management of cardiac arrest.

How it works

ECMO has many components in common with CPB. Blood is taken from the body via a cannula and passes through filters, a heat exchanger and an oxygenator before being pumped back into the body. These components are described in more detail in *Section 9.13* on CPB.

The cannulae can be placed using different configurations. If respiratory support alone is required, then a venovenous arrangement is usually used. This means that blood is taken from a vein, oxygenated and pumped at low pressure back into a different vein. Should haemodynamic support be required in addition to this, the return cannula is placed in an artery (often iliac) and blood is pumped back to the patient at arterial pressure, retrograde flow permitting systemic perfusion. This is a venoarterial arrangement.

Cannulae are usually placed percutaneously via the femoral or internal jugular vessels. Alternatively, they may also be placed into vessels within the thorax during surgery.

⊕ Advantages

- Although early trials appeared to show that ECMO did not improve outcome in adults, the availability of better technology used in recent years may have changed this. Although it has been criticized, the CESAR trial in 2009 showed an improved 6-month survival rate in patients with severe respiratory failure referred for ECMO compared with those given standard treatment (63% vs. 47%).
- Allows protective ventilator strategies to be used whilst maintaining gas exchange.
- Haemofiltration can be incorporated into the ECMO circuit if necessary.

Disadvantages

- As with all extracorporeal blood circuits, anticoagulation is required to reduce the risk of thrombosis and pump failure or, in venoarterial ECMO, stroke. In the case of ECMO, unfractionated heparin is usually used to keep the activated partial thromboplastin time ratio greater than 1.5.
- Bleeding is common (either from the cannulation sites or elsewhere) and at least half of patients on ECMO will suffer some sort of haemorrhagic complication.
- Venoarterial ECMO may lead to ischaemia in the limb distal to the arterial cannula due to the retrograde infusion. This can be avoided by the insertion of a second cannula into the artery allowing perfusion distal to the obstruction.
- As with most extracorporeal circuits, inflammatory and coagulation cascades are activated by the foreign surfaces encountered by the blood. Consumptive thrombocytopenia is not uncommon.
- ECMO is expensive and only available in specialist centres.
- Both venous and arterial cannulation sites are susceptible to infection.

Safety

Safety aspects of ECMO relate mostly to ensuring the integrity of the cannulae and the connections between components of the circuit. Due to the high flow through the ECMO machine, disconnection would be catastrophic.

Other notes

ECMO can also be used in an arteriovenous configuration. This requires good native cardiac function, as the patient's own blood pressure is used to drive the machine instead of using a mechanical pump. This allows simpler transfer of patients, because without the pump the machine is smaller and does not require power for oxygenation to occur.

9.12 Novalung iLA membrane ventilator

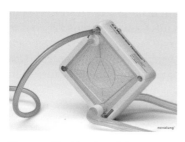

Fig. 9.12.1: The Novalung iLA Membrane Ventilator. Image reproduced with permission from Novalung GmbH.

Overview

The Novalung interventional lung assist membrane ventilator (iLA) is a device first marketed in 2002 that has many parallels with extracorporeal membrane oxygenation (ECMO) and cardiopulmonary bypass (CPB). It is primarily used to reduce the $PaCO_2$ and therefore correct respiratory acidosis in acute or chronic ventilatory failure, although it can also modestly improve oxygenation.

The iLA consists of an extracorporeal blood circuit that allows gas exchange to occur across a semipermeable membrane within the device.

Uses

There are no published randomized controlled clinical trials of iLA at the time of writing, however, it has been used to treat many conditions including acute respiratory distress syndrome (ARDS), acute severe asthma, severe pneumonia, inhalational lung injury, pulmonary hypertension and post-operatively in thoracic surgery patients. In some cases the iLA has been used to support ventilation while the underlying condition is treated and in others it has been used as a bridge to lung transplantation.

Good evidence now exists for low volume, low pressure ventilatory strategies during the management of lung injury (especially ARDS), and the iLA is a device that may make these strategies easier to implement without the need to tolerate hypercapnia.

How it works

13–17F cannulae are used to access two large blood vessels, often the femoral artery and vein. Blood arriving at the iLA through the blood inlet port passes into an initial prechamber that has de-airing ports. Any bubbles or collections of gas can be removed via these ports, particularly during priming of the device. The blood then passes into the main chamber where gas exchange occurs, before passing through the blood outlet port and back into the patient via the second cannula.

The membrane used for gas exchange in the main chamber is made of polymethylpentene and is arranged in an elaborate pattern to maximize surface area ($1.3\,m^2$). The blood side of the membrane is coated with heparin to help prevent clotting. Standard oxygen tubing is connected to the gas inlet port and oxygen flows through the device before being expelled to the atmosphere via the gas outlet port. Blood and gas flow in opposite directions on opposite sides of the membrane and there is no direct mixing.

Maximum blood flow through the iLA is $4.5\,l.min^{-1}$, although the flow is more often around $2\,l.min^{-1}$. The extent to which carbon dioxide is removed from the blood depends on the rate of gas flow through the iLA – the higher the rate, the more CO_2 is removed because the gradient for diffusion is more efficiently maintained. The resulting PCO_2 in the patient therefore depends on the percentage of cardiac output that flows through the device, the rate of gas flow through the device, and the residual function of the patient's lungs.

The iLA is usually used in an arteriovenous configuration. That is, the blood flows through the device from the artery to the vein using the pressure gradient generated by the patient's heart as the driving force. In situations where there is low cardiac output and/or blood pressure, the iLA can be configured in a venovenous arrangement which requires a mechanical pump to move the blood through the device. In situations of mild hypoxia, the iLA may be used to help oxygenate the blood and in these circumstances the device may be used in a venoarterial arrangement. This requires a higher pressure mechanical pump and only modest oxygenation may be achieved in comparison with ECMO.

⊕ Advantages

- Relatively small, only moderately invasive device.
- May be easier to set up and insert than other extracorporeal devices that assist ventilation.
- Effectively removes CO_2 from the blood and allows protective ventilator strategies.
- Small priming volume of 175 ml (cf. ECMO or CPB which may be over 1000 ml).

⊖ Disadvantages

- Risks and complications of the device include:
  - bleeding; the combination of systemic anticoagulation with heparin (required to help prevent clotting of blood within the device) and cannulation of large arteries mean bleeding is not uncommon
  - accidental de-cannulation
  - thrombosis within the device caused by under-anticoagulation may result in its failure
  - air embolism
  - risk of infection.
- Can only achieve modest improvements in oxygenation.

ⓘ Safety

Safety aspects of the iLA relate mostly to ensuring the safety of the cannulae and their connections and the anticoagulation of the patient.

9.13 Cardiopulmonary bypass

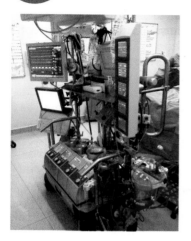

Fig. 9.13.1: A modern cardiopulmonary bypass machine.

Overview

Cardiopulmonary bypass (CPB) is a technique that allows a machine to take over the function of the heart and lungs, usually during surgery.

The first successful operation using CPB was in 1953, when an 18 year old patient underwent surgical repair of an atrial septal defect. The technology has moved on considerably since that time, and although the CPB machine is operated mainly by the perfusionist, anaesthetists should have a good working knowledge of the principles involved because they remain responsible for the patient while bypass is running.

Uses

CPB is used to provide the cardiothoracic surgeon with a motionless and bloodless field in which to operate. Examples of types of surgery that require CPB include valve replacements, congenital cardiac defect repairs, major thoracic aortic surgery and transplants. Coronary artery bypass graft surgery is often performed using CPB, but 'off-pump' graft surgery (i.e. without the use of CPB) is also common.

In rare circumstances, CPB may be used as a resuscitation measure. In cases of cardiac arrest caused by severe hypothermia, CPB can be used to ensure oxygenation and circulation whilst it also slowly warms the patient. Femoro-femoral CPB may also be of use in the management of a patient with an intrathoracic mass in whom ventilation following anaesthesia is impossible.

How it works

Before CPB can be started, anticoagulation must be given to prevent the blood clotting in the machine because this could cause catastrophic failure of CPB and death of the patient. Anticoagulation must therefore be sufficient and is usually achieved by giving 300–400 IU.kg^{-1} unfractionated heparin IV and aiming for an activated clotting time (ACT) of over 400 seconds.

The circuit

Before use, the circuit is primed with fluid, the choice of which varies between crystalloid and blood. The latter may be chosen to help prevent dilutional anaemia, although it may be argued that the former improves blood rheology. Mixtures of blood products and crystalloid solutions may be used, and mannitol or sodium bicarbonate may also be added.

The circuit itself is made of PVC tubing which is coated in biocompatible substances such as heparin to help prevent activation of the clotting and inflammatory systems.

The typical procedure for initiation of CPB for a cardiac case is as follows.

- The aorta is cannulated distal to the planned cross clamp position.
- The venous cannula or cannulae are then inserted. A single cannula may be placed in the right atrium, or alternatively two cannulae may be inserted, one into the superior and one into the inferior vena cava. The method of venous cannulation will depend on the planned surgery and the preference of the surgeon.

- The aortic cannula is always placed first and removed last because in an emergency it is possible to rapidly initiate CPB using prime volume and blood returned from surgical suction while the venous lines are being positioned.
- When bypass begins, venous blood is drained by gravity from the venous cannula into a reservoir. From here it passes through a bubble trap and into the blood pump which sends the blood forward at arterial pressure through a heat exchanger and a gas exchanger. The blood is then filtered before it flows through the aortic cannula distal to the cross clamp. The filters remove small blood clots, fat or other solid material.
- Another cannula is placed in either the aorta proximal to the cross clamp, or in the individual coronary artery ostia. A small amount of blood is diverted from the main circuit after it has passed through the gas exchanger to have cardioplegia solution added to it. A separate pump is then used to send this blood into the coronary arteries. The amount of cardioplegia given and the systemic perfusion are therefore controlled independently. It is also possible to give cardioplegia solution without mixing it with blood. Occasionally the cardioplegia cannula will be placed into the coronary sinus where the cardiac veins open into the right ventricular cavity, so that retrograde perfusion of cardioplegia solution occurs.
- Blood is able to enter the venous reservoir via two suction catheters as well as the main right atrial cannula. One of these is used by the surgeon to remove blood from the surgical field in the same manner as suction is used elsewhere in surgery. The other is referred to as the vent and is placed within the cavity of the left ventricle, where it is used to remove shunted blood from sources such as the thebesian veins and bronchial veins that would otherwise cause the ventricle to distend. The negative pressure on the general suction and on the vent can be controlled independently. The general suction is sometimes separated from the bypass circuit so that instead of suctioned blood being returned to the reservoir, it flows into a cell saver that washes it before isolating the red cells for reinfusion. This method helps prevent fat embolus, and is another way of attempting to reduce the inflammatory response that occurs when blood comes into direct contact with extravascular substances.
- A haemofilter may also be incorporated into the circuit, allowing the machine to take over the function of the kidneys as well as the heart and lungs.

Figure 9.13.2 shows the basic CPB circuit.

Blood pumps
There are two main types of blood pump. Older machines use roller pumps, in which the blood is propelled forward by a roller that rotates, compressing the tubing as it goes round. Although these pumps are cheap and simple, they have some disadvantages.

Roller pumps can cause activation and consumption of platelets, and red cells can be damaged or haemolysed as they are compressed by the roller. Similarly, white cells may be activated by the action of the roller pump which results in the release of proinflammatory and vasoactive substances. Another potential problem with these devices is that they will continue to pump the set flow, regardless of the presence of an occlusion downstream. This can cause a large increase in pressure and risks rupture of the circuit.

More modern CPB machines usually use centrifugal blood pumps. These have a magnetic impeller that rapidly rotates to create a spinning vortex which creates a negative pressure and sucks blood into the pump. The centrifugal force then sends the blood through the outlet and towards the patient under pressure. The magnitude of the pressure is related to the speed of revolution of the impeller. These pumps have been shown to cause less platelet and white cell activation, less haemolysis and reduced release of inflammatory cytokines. However, it is not yet accepted that

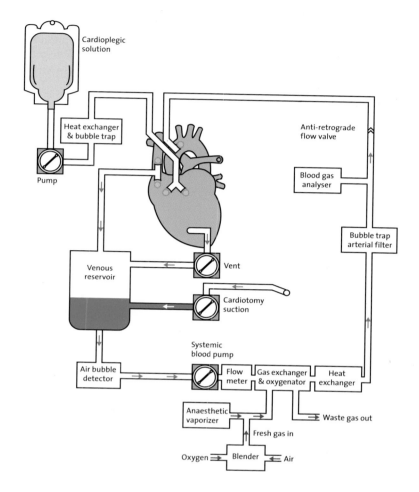

Fig. 9.13.2: A schematic diagram of a CPB circuit.

these advantages definitely translate into an improved outcome. Another advantage of centrifugal pumps over the roller pump is that the presence of a downstream occlusion will not cause a rapid rise in pressure or circuit rupture. This is because the flow of blood is dependent on the afterload on the pump. If the downstream pressure increases significantly, the flow from the pump will fall.

Both roller pumps and centrifugal pumps usually provide non-pulsatile blood flow.

Gas exchanger

The gas exchanger (also known as the oxygenator) adds oxygen to and removes carbon dioxide from the blood.

The original oxygenators bubbled gaseous oxygen directly through the blood. This meant that a blood–gas interface was set up, which caused activation of the clotting cascade and inflammatory enzymes. Therefore, modern oxygenators do not directly mix the blood and oxygen but use a membrane which is between 100 and 200 μm thick and made of polypropylene. They can either be flat sheets or hollow fibres.

On one side of the membrane flows the blood, while on the other side and flowing in the opposite direction is a carrier gas containing oxygen. The oxygen then diffuses through the membrane into the blood and carbon dioxide diffuses in the opposite direction. Other gases, such as volatile anaesthetics, can also be added to the carrier gas and therefore to the blood. The PaO_2 is altered by adjusting the PO_2 in the carrier gas.

The concentration gradient for carbon dioxide diffusing from the blood into the carrier gas depends on flow. A high gas flow means carbon dioxide that has diffused out of the blood is quickly washed away and a high concentration gradient is maintained. This leads to more carbon dioxide being removed and a lower $PaCO_2$. Conversely, if the gas flow is low then the carbon dioxide is not removed from the membrane as quickly and the concentration gradient is lower. Less carbon dioxide is therefore removed from the blood resulting in a higher $PaCO_2$. The $PaCO_2$ can therefore be altered by adjusting the gas flow over the membrane.

⊕ Advantages

- CPB allows open heart surgery and some types of transplant surgery to be performed. It is also commonly used for coronary artery bypass grafting.
- Perfusion pressure, acid–base balance and electrolyte concentrations can be easily monitored and manipulated while on bypass.

⊖ Disadvantages

- High levels of anticoagulation are required, which may lead to post-operative bleeding if it is not adequately reversed.
- Post-operative bleeding may also result from consumption and dilution of platelets and coagulation factors in the bypass circuit.
- Anaemia may be caused by dilution, haemolysis, or bleeding.
- Cannulation of the aorta may lead to dissection, particularly if there is high arterial pressure. Cannulation may also lead to embolism of underlying atherosclerotic plaque which is commonly implicated in stroke following CPB.
- The formation of microscopic blood clots in the bypass circuit may embolize into the patient. Microemboli of this sort can cause cerebral and renal dysfunction post-operatively.
- As with all extracorporeal circulations, air embolism is a possibility, although the reservoir and bubble traps reduce the risk of this.
- Up to 5% of patients will suffer a stroke while on CPB, the neurological severity of which varies.
- Activation of white cells and the complement cascade and release of inflammatory cytokines during CPB has been implicated in causing a variety of undesirable effects post-operatively. These include renal impairment, ARDS and systemic inflammatory response syndrome, all of which prolong recovery time.

⊘ Safety

- Failure of the bypass circuit due to occlusion by thrombus, or failure of the gas exchanger, are extremely rare but theoretical scenarios that would have catastrophic results.
- Heparin must not be reversed until bypass is completely off, and the suction and venous cannulae have been removed. There must be excellent communication between the anaesthetist, perfusionist and surgeon regarding the administration of protamine in particular.

Other notes

Mini-bypass is a technique using a smaller volume circuit that may not incorporate a reservoir. If no reservoir is present, blood is taken from the right atrium via a filter and a bubble trap directly to a centrifugal pump and then into the heat and gas exchangers before returning to the patient.

This reduces the risk of enzyme cascades being activated by a blood–air interface in the reservoir and also means that the tubing length is reduced. This means that the blood is in contact with the foreign surface for a shorter time and a much smaller volume of prime can be used resulting in less haemodilution. Blood that is suctioned or vented is taken to a cell saver rather than the reservoir, and many surgeons perform mini-bypass without using a vent at all.

Research has yet to show a better overall long-term outcome after surgery performed on mini-bypass compared to that on conventional bypass. However, there is some evidence of a reduced incidence of post-operative bleeding with mini-bypass, probably as a result of less dilution and consumption of coagulation factors. On average, there is also a slight improvement in post-operative renal function, which may be a manifestation of fewer microemboli occurring using this technique.

A disadvantage of mini-bypass without a reservoir is an increased risk of air embolism (which would be easily caught by the reservoir in conventional bypass). Another is that if no vent is used, the left ventricle may distend and there may also be bleeding from the coronary arteries as they are being operated on.

9.14 Feeding tubes

Whilst we have grouped them as feeding tubes, there are in fact several other uses for these tubes (particularly the nasogastric tube) which are commonly seen in critical care and in theatre, including the following.

- Administration of enteral nutrition or medications to patients who have a functioning gut but who cannot eat (e.g. those under sedation or anaesthetic; those with severe swallowing difficulties).
- Decompression of the bowel in the perioperative period or as part of conservative management of bowel obstruction. A tube is sometimes an effective treatment for nausea and vomiting in these situations. A nasogastric tube may also be used to decompress the stomach following difficult bag-mask ventilation. This is of particular importance in young children.
- Gastric lavage, or administration of activated charcoal. This is now a very rare indication for a tube, because these procedures are not commonly performed.

Feeding tubes may be passed into the gut via the nasopharynx, or percutaneously through the abdominal wall. The former are often inserted blindly, although an endoscope is commonly used for nasojejunal tubes. Percutaneous tubes are inserted under endoscopic or radiological guidance, or under direct vision during surgery.

The correct position must be confirmed before anything is infused through it. Nasogastric (NG) tubes have been incorrectly placed in a bronchus, resulting in pneumonia and death when feeding was started. Acceptable methods for confirming placement are imaging (usually with a chest X-ray) or a test of the pH of fluid aspirated from the tube. The advantage of the latter test is that it can be performed every time feeding is given, and therefore confirms placement of the tube, whereas the last chest X-ray may have been several days previously. A pH of 4.5 or less is indicative of correct positioning, although the upper pH limit is higher if the patient is being treated with a proton pump inhibitor. Policies vary from one hospital to another about how the position of a tube should be confirmed. The 'whoosh' test, where 50 ml of air are rapidly injected through the tube while the stomach is auscultated with a stethoscope is not specific and is poor at identifying correct placement – it should not be used.

Nasogastric

These tubes may be wide bore (16–18F) or fine bore (6–8F). The latter is used for feeding and giving medications and is usually made of polyurethane, while the former is more commonly used for decompression and is made of PVC. Adult tubes are approximately 1 metre long, and are inserted to a depth of 60–70 cm, although this will vary from one patient to another. The tubes have markings that indicate every 5–10 cm from the distal tip.

Contraindications to NG tubes include strictures or recent surgery in the oesophagus and base of skull fracture or nasal injuries.

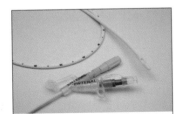

Fig. 9.14.1: A Corflo nasogastric tube. Image reproduced with permission from Corpak MedSystems UK.

These tubes are inserted by sliding the tube into the nose. If the patient is conscious and has some ability to swallow, sipping a small volume of water sometimes helps the tube enter the oesophagus more easily. In sedated and intubated patients blind insertion may work, but the use of a laryngoscope and a well-positioned finger is sometimes the only way to guide the tube into the correct place.

Nasojejunal

Nasojejunal (NJ) tubes are used to overcome some of the problems encountered with NG tubes, which are generally easy to insert, but can be displaced easily. Adequate feeding also depends on good gastric motility, otherwise feed stays in the stomach and cannot be absorbed. Gastroesophageal reflux may also be a problem with NG tubes, as may the aspiration of feed that may result. NJ tubes may be less affected by these issues, because their tip lies distal to the pylorus.

NJ tubes are made of polyurethane or silicone, are approximately 270 cm in length, and are fine bore (6–8F). They are inserted to a depth of approximately 100 cm depending on the patient and the excess tube is cut off and discarded.

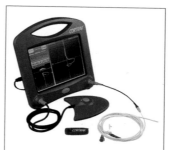

Fig. 9.14.2: The Cortrak Enteral Access System (EAS). Image reproduced with permission from Corpak MedSystems UK.

Insertion is usually performed using an endoscope, although sometimes fluoroscopic techniques are used with a guide wire, or natural peristalsis can be allowed to move the tip of the tube through the gastric pylorus, into the duodenum and then on into the jejunum.

A novel way of inserting these tubes (that can also be used with NG tubes) is the Cortrak Enteral Access System (EAS, Corpak Medsystems UK). This consists of a computer monitor, a receiver unit and a specially designed tube with a transmitter stylet. The monitor receives information about the relative position of the stylet within the gut and displays it as an image. This gives the operator useful information regarding the location of the tip of the stylet and aids insertion of the tube.

Percutaneous endoscopic gastrostomy

While tubes that are passed via the nasopharynx are short-term solutions, percutaneous endoscopic gastrostomy (PEG) tubes are a longer term method of feeding patients. Indications for their use include long-term neurological disability that prevents swallowing (e.g. stroke or multiple sclerosis) and the presence of large head and neck tumours undergoing treatment.

The tubes are inserted using an endoscope. The scope is inserted via the mouth into the stomach and its light can be seen through the skin. It is used as a guide to an appropriate location for the tube to be inserted. A small incision is made in the skin and a guide string is passed via a needle into the stomach lumen. The string can then be caught by the endoscope and brought out through the mouth. The PEG tube is then passed over it and threaded back into the stomach and out through the opening that was made in the abdominal wall. A flange on the inner end of the PEG prevents it from falling out. The tip of the PEG can be visualized and the correct position confirmed using the endoscope.

PEG tubes are more difficult to insert than NG tubes, but are a more permanent solution to feeding problems caused by chronic conditions. They also run the risk of bleeding and infection and the patient may still be at risk of gastroesophageal reflux.

An alternative in patients in whom gastroscopy is contraindicated (such as those with head and neck tumours) is a radiologically inserted gastrostomy (RIG). Similar tubes may also be inserted at the time of surgery.

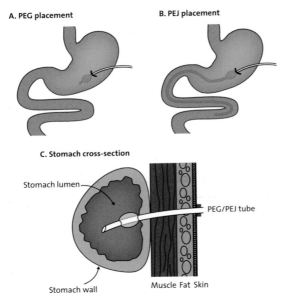

A. PEG placement

B. PEJ placement

C. Stomach cross-section

Stomach lumen

PEG/PEJ tube

Stomach wall

Muscle Fat Skin

Fig. 9.14.3: The internal position of PEG and PEJ tubes.

Percutaneous endoscopic jejunostomy

A percutaneous endoscopic jejunostomy (PEJ) tube is an extension of a PEG. The PEJ is passed through a standard PEG and the distal end is directed through the gastric pylorus and duodenum and into the jejunum. Alternatively, a PEJ may be placed surgically during laparotomy.

The indications for PEJ are similar to those for NJ tube placement, although the PEJ is a better long-term solution than an NJ.

9.15 Infusion pumps

Volumetric pumps

Volumetric pumps are commonly used to control fluid infusions via drips. The drip tubing passes from the fluid bag, through the pump and then connects to the patient's venous access device. The pumps run on mains or battery power and the volumes delivered are accurate to within 5–10%.

Volumetric pumps incorporate pressure transducers and alarms to detect upstream or downstream occlusions. These pumps also stop and sound an alarm should air be detected in the tubing.

Many different pumps are available, and a variety of pumping mechanisms exist, including peristaltic rollers and piston cassettes.

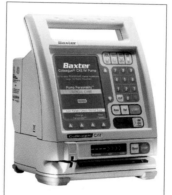

Fig. 9.15.1: The Colleague CXE IV volumetric infusion pump. Image reproduced with permission from Baxter Healthcare Ltd.

Syringe drivers

Syringe drivers use a motor to turn a screw that progressively pushes the plunger of a syringe mounted in the pump. They are generally used for smaller volumes than volumetric pumps and also in situations where the infusion rate needs to be more accurately controlled (e.g. the infusion of vasoactive drugs in critical care). These devices are accurate to within 2–5%.

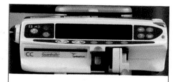

Fig. 9.15.2: An Alaris syringe driver.

Many syringe drivers have safety mechanisms to prevent a bolus being infused following the sudden removal of an obstruction in the infusion tubing. Air and occlusion alarms are also incorporated into these pumps.

Care must be taken to avoid syphoning from syringe pumps (i.e. flow from the syringe to the patient without actively pumping – often due to gravity). Precautions include keeping the pump at or below the level of the patient and the use of anti-syphoning valves.

Target-controlled infusions

TCI pumps are described in *Section 5.12*.

Patient-controlled analgesia

PCA pumps vary in design. Some are volumetric pumps and others use a syringe driver, but all have a control button that the patient can press when they require analgesia.

The pumps allow programming of a bolus dose (given when the patient presses the request button), and a lockout period. The bolus dose cannot be repeated until the time specified in the lockout period has expired.

Most pumps also allow a loading dose of the drug to be given when the pump is first set up, and a background rate of infusion to be programmed. Some pumps allow extra bolus doses to be given by a healthcare professional after a key or password has been entered.

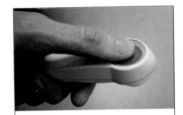

Fig. 9.15.3: A PCA button. The patient can press the button to deliver a dose of IV analgesia.

Elastomeric pumps

These pumps consist of a balloon inflated with the drug to be infused. Over time, the elastic balloon deflates and infuses the drug into the patient. No external power is required. Different pumps are available that infuse over different periods of time (from 30 minutes to 1 week). The flow is accurate to within 10–15%. Balloon volumes of up to 300 ml are available and the pumps can be used for infusion of analgesic agents, chemotherapeutic drugs, antibiotics and other substances.

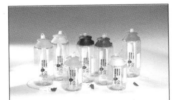

Fig. 9.15.4: Elastomeric infusion pumps. Image reproduced with permission from Baxter Healthcare Ltd.

9.16 Rigid neck collars

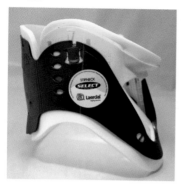

Fig. 9.16.1: An adjustable rigid cervical collar.

Overview

Rigid neck collars are used to help immobilize and stabilize the cervical spine and to support the head in patients with suspected or confirmed cervical spine injuries. They are usually used in combination with sandbags and tape, and it should be emphasized that a rigid neck collar alone will not provide adequate cervical spine immobilization.

Uses

In patients with potentially unstable cervical spines as a result of trauma or degenerative conditions.

How it works

When sited correctly, the collar rests on top of the shoulders with the head supported by a chin rest. There are openings anteriorly that allow access to the front of the neck and these can be used for pulse checks and cricothyroidotomy. Newer designs also have a posterior opening that allows palpation of the cervical spine and openings around the ears to make hearing and communication easier.

The collar folds open so that it can be positioned whilst manual inline immobilization of the cervical spine is maintained. Velcro straps along one side secure the collar. It is essential that the correct size collar is chosen. A pin on the side of the collar corresponds to the position of the angle of the mandible. A collar should be chosen such that the distance between this pin and the lower lateral edge of the collar is the same as the distance between the angle of the mandible and the top of the trapezius muscle. Some collars are adjustable, but the same method is used to size them correctly.

⊕ Advantages

- Aids immobilization of the cervical spine.
- Supports the head.
- MRI compatible.

⊖ Disadvantages

- Uncomfortable to wear for long periods and predispose to pressure sores.
- Restricts mouth opening for instrumentation of the airway.
- Restricts physical examination of the cervical spine.

9.17 Rapid fluid infusers

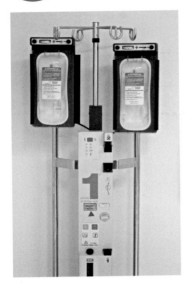

Fig. 9.17.1: The Level 1 rapid infuser.

Overview

Rapid infusers are designed to deliver large volumes of warmed fluid to a patient over a short period of time. The infuser incorporates a heat exchanger, a control panel, and a length of single-use tubing that connects to the patient's intravenous access device. Some models also include an air detector.

Uses

The rapid infuser is usually used to infuse blood products while treating a major haemorrhage. However, it may also be used to deliver other fluids. The fluid delivered to the patient is warmed by the heat exchanger to body temperature and therefore the infuser can also be used in certain situations when treating hypothermia.

How it works

Intravenous access is established with the widest bore cannula possible. When the system is switched on, the fluid is infused into the patient via the tubing, heat exchanger and IV access. The Level 1 infuser (Smiths Medical) achieves this by compressing the fluid bag to a constant pressure of 300 mmHg (regardless of the volume of fluid remaining), whereas the Belmont infuser (Belmont Instrument Corporation) uses roller pumps. Theoretically, flows of up to 1400 ml.min⁻¹ or more can be achieved using these devices. However, in practice the actual infusion rate is limited by the calibre of the IV access device being used.

⊕ Advantages

- Allows rapid simultaneous warming and infusion of resuscitation fluids.
- Once the machine is set up, it is easy to use and quick to connect new fluid bags.
- Most models allow more than one fluid bag to be connected at a time so that while one bag is being infused, a second can be prepared.

⊖ Disadvantages

- It takes time to set the system up and prime the tubing; staff require specific training.
- The manufacturers recommend that these devices are not used to infuse platelets, cryoprecipitate or granulocytes. There is some evidence that warming these products prior to infusion may result in their inactivation.
- It can be easy to cause haemodilution, resulting in anaemia and/or coagulopathy if fluids other than blood products are used. Fluid overload may also occur.

ⓘ Safety

- All fluid or blood bags must be completely emptied of air prior to connection to the rapid infuser. Failure to ensure this may result in air embolism.
- Intravenous access must be reliable, because fluid infused under pressure through a 'tissued' cannula may result in compartment syndrome.

9.18 Defibrillators

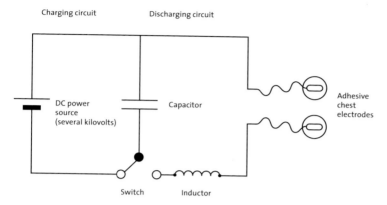

Fig. 9.18.1: A simple defibrillator circuit diagram.

Overview

The use of an electric current to first induce and subsequently cardiovert ventricular fibrillation (VF) was demonstrated in dogs by Jean-Louis Prévost and Frédéric Batelli in 1899. A machine designed specifically to deliver shocks to the myocardium was developed by William Kouwenhoven in 1932 and was used during experiments with the canine heart.

The first recorded occasion when a defibrillator was deliberately used to treat VF in a human was on a 14 year old boy undergoing thoracic surgery in 1947 by Claude Beck, although there are also reports of collapsed patients (with unknown heart rhythms) being revived by electric shocks as early as 1774. Until the 1950s, defibrillators were large, heavy, used alternating current, and it was only possible to defibrillate the heart if the chest was open (i.e. during surgery). This changed when external defibrillators were developed in 1956. Direct current was first used in 1959.

Today, defibrillation is the primary treatment for VF and pulseless ventricular tachycardia (VT), and many different models of defibrillator are available.

Uses

Defibrillators are used to convert abnormal cardiac rhythms back to sinus rhythm.

External defibrillators are used in the management of cardiac arrest both in and out of hospital. They may be automated or manual. External defibrillators can also be used to cardiovert less dangerous rhythms such as atrial fibrillation (AF) and some supraventricular tachycardias (SVT). Some machines can also be used for temporary external pacing.

Internal defibrillators are used in cardiothoracic surgery when the chest is open. Implantable cardiovertor defibrillators (ICDs) are also available.

How it works

A defibrillator consists of two similar circuits. The first consists of a power source, and a capacitor. If the power is supplied by mains electricity, then a diode is included in the circuit that rectifies the AC current to DC. A transformer is also included to step-up the battery or mains voltage to a much higher voltage. The power source is then used to charge the capacitor using this circuit.

The second circuit consists of the same capacitor, the defibrillator electrodes (attached to the patient) and an inductor. The shock is therefore delivered to the patient using this circuit.

The electrodes are incorporated into paddles or adherent pads that are attached to the patient's chest (or to the heart if internal defibrillation is being performed). These plug into the defibrillator machine and can be used to detect the ECG as well as deliver the shock. The operator selects the energy required (unless an automated external defibrillator is being used), and charges the capacitor by pressing a button. When the charge on the capacitor is sufficient to deliver the selected energy, an audible tone sounds and the shock button can be pressed. This discharges the capacitor and administers the shock to the patient. A basic circuit diagram is shown in *Figure 9.18.1*.

Capacitor charging
When the charge button is pressed, a switch in the first circuit described above is closed. The power source then begins to add charge to the capacitor. Electrons are passed from the negative terminal on the power source to one capacitor plate and this plate therefore becomes negatively charged. At the same time, electrons flow from the other capacitor plate to the positive terminal on the power source. This plate therefore becomes positively charged. A potential difference is therefore produced between the capacitor plates.

Because like charges repel and unlike charges attract, it becomes more difficult to remove electrons from the positive capacitor plate and add them to the negative one. Therefore, the rate at which potential difference builds up on the capacitor slows down during charging. When the potential difference on the capacitor equals that at the power source, no further charging of the capacitor can occur. The graph of the development of this potential difference against time is therefore a build-up exponential (wash-in) curve and has the equation:

$$V = V_{max}(1 - e^{-t/RC})$$

where V is the voltage on the capacitor, V_{max} is the voltage on the power source that is charging the capacitor, t is time in seconds and RC is the time constant, which is specific to the capacitor and the characteristics of the first circuit.

If the defibrillator has a 200 µF (microFarad) capacitor and the voltage used to charge it is 1500 V, then when fully charged there will be 300 mC available. The energy that can be delivered is then 225 J. *Section 12.1* which introduces electricity and electrical safety describes the relevant equations.

The amount of energy available for defibrillation is varied by altering the period of time used for charging the capacitor. The capacitor will charge to 63% of its maximum in one time constant, and will be more than 99% charged after five time constants.

Capacitor discharging
When the shock button is pressed, the switch changes to connect the capacitor to the second circuit. Current flows as electrons move from the negatively charged capacitor plate around the circuit via the electrodes and the patient to the positive plate. The shock is therefore delivered to the patient. In the process, the potential difference on the capacitor falls to zero as the electrons re-equilibrate between the plates – this is capacitor discharge.

As the potential difference falls, the magnitude of the positive charge on the capacitor plate becomes lower. The strength of attraction of the electrons to the positive plate is reduced and so the current also falls. The graph of the potential difference on the capacitor against time during discharge is therefore an exponential decay curve and has the equation:

$$V = V_o e^{-t/RC}$$

where V is the voltage on the capacitor, V_o is the starting voltage (which may or may not be the same as V_{max} in the charging equation, depending on whether the maximum charge was used), *t* is time in seconds and RC is the time constant, which is specific to the capacitor and the characteristics of the second circuit.

The probability of a successful defibrillation or cardioversion is greatly increased if the flow of current is sustained for a longer period of time. The second circuit therefore includes an inductor, which prolongs the time before the current falls to zero by a number of milliseconds. However, the current should not flow for longer than 20 ms, because this has been associated with causing refibrillation.

Monophasic vs. biphasic waveforms

The electrical energy delivered by a defibrillator can be represented as a graph of current against time and different manufacturers configure their machines so that a specific shape is produced on this graph – this is known as the shock waveform. Monophasic defibrillators send all of the shock energy in one direction across the heart, from one electrode to the other. However, the graph can either appear as a damped sine wave or look more like a square wave (such as the monophasic truncated exponential); *Figure 9.18.2* shows examples.

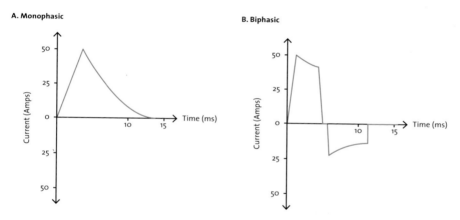

Fig. 9.18.2: Monophasic and biphasic defibrillator shock waveforms.

Modern defibrillators use more sophisticated circuitry to produce a biphasic shock waveform. The current is initially delivered in one direction, before the polarity is reversed and the rest of the current is delivered in the opposite direction.

Biphasic waveforms have been shown to be more likely to convert VF to sinus rhythm than monophasic, and use a lower energy to do so. This is reflected in resuscitation guidelines that recommend the first two monophasic shocks be delivered at an energy of 200 J and the third at 360 J. However, with a biphasic defibrillator all shocks are delivered at 150 J. A lower energy is thought to be advantageous because it may cause less tissue damage.

Some biphasic defibrillators are also able to measure the impedance produced by the patient between the two electrodes and then alter their waveform to the optimum shape to ensure that energy delivery is as efficient as possible.

⊕ Advantages

- Survival of VF and VT has significantly increased since use of defibrillators became common.
- The machine can show a simple ECG tracing that is acquired via the pads, so extra monitors are not immediately required.

- Many defibrillators in hospital can also be used as temporary external pacemakers when haemodynamic compromise is caused by bradycardia. This is unpleasant for conscious patients and so sedation is required.
- Defibrillators in automated mode are very simple to use and can be found out of hospital in the community. They are capable of accurate rhythm recognition, and give the user spoken stepwise instructions in their use.
- Some defibrillators can record audio, which is sometimes useful for audit and research purposes when analysing the performance of cardiac arrest teams.

Disadvantages

- Defibrillators are still seen by many lay people as complex pieces of medical equipment. Campaigns exist to promote the training and use of these machines by lay people because early defibrillation is the key to survival of cardiac arrest.

Safety

- Because external defibrillation uses such high voltages, there is a risk of a shock to personnel who come into contact with the patient at the time the shock is delivered. This risk is increased if the patient is in contact with conducting objects or electrolyte-rich solutions that may have been spilt.
- Sparking occasionally occurs during defibrillation and therefore flammable, explosive or combustible gases such as oxygen should be removed. This is very uncommon using modern adhesive pads.

9.19 Intra-aortic balloon pumps

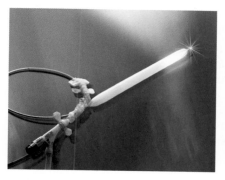

Fig. 9.19.1: An intra-aortic balloon catheter with balloon inflated. Image reproduced with permission from Teleflex.

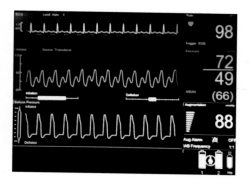

Fig. 9.19.2: An intra-aortic balloon pump monitor showing ECG (top trace, green), arterial pressure with diastolic augmentation (middle trace, red), and balloon inflation pressure (bottom trace, blue).

Overview

The intra-aortic balloon pump (IABP) was introduced in the early 1960s as a treatment for severe cardiac failure and cardiogenic shock. It remains a common method of treating these conditions in critical and coronary care units.

Uses

The indications for the insertion of an IABP include:

- cardiac failure, cardiogenic shock or unstable angina due to severe ischaemia while awaiting a revascularization procedure (either angioplasty or CABG); however, see note below regarding the outcome of the recent SHOCK II trial
- development of arrhythmias caused by ischaemia
- difficulty weaning from cardiopulmonary bypass during cardiac surgery
- any cause of reversible myocardial impairment
- support of cardiac function while awaiting cardiac transplantation.

How it works

An 8–10F coaxial double lumen catheter is inserted into the femoral artery. The inner lumen opens at the tip of the catheter and is used to measure the aortic pressure in the same way as other invasive blood pressure monitors. The outer lumen opens into the balloon just proximal to the catheter tip, and has a volume of between 30 and 50 ml depending on the size of the patient. Ideally the balloon should occupy 80–90% of the diameter of the aorta when inflated, and should be positioned just distal to the origin of the left subclavian artery. A balloon that is too large may damage the aortic wall, whereas one that is too small may not cause sufficient haemodynamic effect. The catheter is connected to the pump machine, which has a computer and carries a gas cylinder. The machine monitors the cardiac cycle using the aortic pressure waveform and a standard three-lead ECG, and these are both displayed on its user interface.

Modern IABP machines use helium for balloon inflation, although air and CO_2 were used previously (see below). The balloon is inflated in early diastole, just after aortic valve closure – at the peak of the T-wave on the ECG or at the dicrotic notch on the aortic pressure waveform. It remains inflated until just before the aortic valve re-opens, and deflates as late as possible in diastole. Example pressure traces are shown in *Figures 9.19.2* and *9.19.3*. The displacement of blood by the balloon has two main effects.

i.   Inflation during diastole leads to a higher early diastolic blood pressure because the volume of the aorta has effectively been reduced by the balloon. This results in improved end-organ perfusion, especially to the heart because coronary perfusion occurs principally during diastole. This effect is known as diastolic augmentation.

ii. Deflation of the balloon as late as possible results in a reduced end-diastolic pressure in the aorta. This results in a reduced afterload (and therefore lower systolic pressure) and consequently reduced myocardial oxygen demand and consumption.

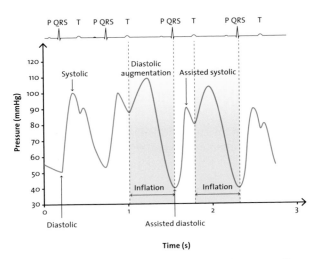

Fig. 9.19.3: A stylized ECG trace showing changes that occur with an IABP.

The machine can be set to inflate the balloon every time the heart beats (a 1:1 ratio), or every other beat (1:2) or every third beat (1:3), etc. This is therefore a method of weaning a patient off the pump as their condition improves by slowly reducing the number of beats that are supported. The machine can also be set to trigger balloon inflation and deflation using either the ECG or the aortic pressure trace. Therefore, should one system fail there is always a back-up. In the event that the patient suffers a cardiac arrest, the IABP should be set to trigger based on the aortic pressure so that it will inflate and deflate during cardiopulmonary resuscitation.

Balloon inflation gases

In older IABP machines, the gas used to inflate the balloon was either CO_2 or air. The advantage of these was that they are non-toxic and dissolve relatively easily in blood. Therefore, in the event of a balloon rupture the gas will dissolve quickly and is less likely to embolize and cause distal ischaemic complications. Unfortunately, it is more difficult to move air or CO_2 rapidly into and out of the balloon.

Modern IABP machines therefore commonly use helium as the inflation gas. This is less soluble in blood and therefore the risk of gas embolus in the event of balloon rupture is slightly higher. However, helium has a very low density compared with air or CO_2 (0.16 kg.m^{-3} compared with 1.18 kg.m^{-3} and 1.81 kg.m^{-3}, respectively) and this confers the following three advantages.

● The Reynolds number predicts whether gas flow will be laminar or turbulent, with values below 2000 indicating that flow is likely to be laminar. Because density is one of the numerators in the Reynolds equation, gases with lower densities will have lower Reynolds numbers and are therefore (if all other factors are equal) more likely to flow in a laminar fashion. Laminar flow is proportional to the driving pressure gradient, whereas turbulent flow is proportional to its square root. Therefore, under laminar conditions flow is higher than it would be under turbulent conditions with the same driving pressure.

- It is possible that the Reynolds number may remain high due to gas moving very rapidly or the use of a wide diameter tube. Flow would then still be turbulent. However, turbulent flow is inversely proportional to the gas density and so helium still has a higher flow than air or CO_2 under these conditions.
- Flow through a narrow aperture or tube is also partially determined by Graham's law of diffusion which states that the diffusion rate of the gas is inversely proportional to the square root of its density.

Advantages

- Some evidence exists that mortality rates following high risk cardiac surgery may be improved if IABP is used.
- Provides a mechanical and non-pharmacological method of supporting a patient with a failing heart while definitive treatment is arranged.

Disadvantages

- Insertion needs to be performed with image intensifier guidance and fluoroscopy.
- Several complications of IABP are possible.
  - Limb ischaemia. This is caused by either thromboembolism or mechanical obstruction of an artery by the balloon. Prophylactic heparin is often given to reduce the risk of the former. The latter should be prevented by correct positioning of the balloon when it is inserted.
  - Haemorrhage. This can be at the insertion site in the femoral artery or elsewhere due to thrombocytopenia caused by the balloon. Heparin may also contribute to this.
  - Infection.
  - Balloon rupture. This may lead to ischaemia in many places due to occlusion of small vessels by helium bubbles.
- Use of the IABP is contraindicated if there is severe aortic regurgitation, aortic dissection, severe peripheral vascular disease (particularly if femoral artery surgery has been performed), severe coagulopathy, and sepsis.

Safety

Safety aspects of the IABP relate mostly to correct insertion and positioning. Failure to position the balloon properly may result in lack of desirable haemodynamic effects and the development of limb ischaemia.

Other notes

The SHOCK II trial published at the end of 2012 studied 600 patients who were admitted to different centres suffering an acute myocardial infarction complicated by cardiogenic shock. An early revascularization strategy was planned for all patients in the study. Two randomized groups were then compared: half of the patients were treated with an intra-aortic balloon pump and half were not. The study did not find any difference in 30 day mortality between the two groups.

9.20 Ventricular assist devices

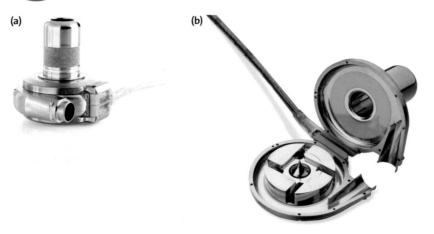

Figure 9.20.1: (a) The HVAD pump and (b) showing impeller and internal workings. Images reproduced with permission from Heartware.

Overview

A ventricular assist device (VAD) is a surgically implanted mechanical pump that takes over all or part of the function of the left (LVAD), right (RVAD) or both (BiVAD) ventricles in patients with severe ventricular failure. The LVAD is the most commonly required type. VADs are not completely internal and have transdermal wires that connect the pump to a controller and power source outside the body. Some VADs have an extracorporeal blood circuit, although these are usually used only in the short term.

Some examples of VADs include the Thoratec Heartmate series, the Heartware HVAD and MVAD, and the Jarvik Heart 2000. Other devices are also available.

Anaesthetists will not routinely encounter these devices unless they work in a specialist cardiothoracic centre, but a working knowledge of them is useful because patients may occasionally present to other hospitals.

Uses

VADs are used to offload the failing ventricle and increase peripheral or pulmonary perfusion. There are three main indications for their use.

- A bridge to heart transplantation. This group make up the majority of patients with VADs. They are eligible for a transplant, but are too unwell to wait for a suitable heart to become available. The VAD is therefore used to assist or take over cardiac function while they are on the waiting list, and is removed when transplant eventually takes place.
- Temporary support of a failing ventricle that has a good chance of recovery, for example, those with severe viral myocarditis.
- Destination therapy. This means that the VAD is implanted as a permanent solution to cardiac failure in patients who are ineligible for heart transplant.

How it works

VADs are typically implanted by a cardiothoracic surgeon through a sternotomy while the patient is under general anaesthetic and on a cardiopulmonary bypass machine. The inflow cannula is inserted through the wall of the ventricle to drain blood from the heart and the outflow cannula is inserted into the aorta in the case of an LVAD or the pulmonary artery in the case of an RVAD (see *Fig. 9.20.2*).

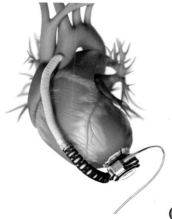

Fig. 9.20.2: The HVAD pump *in situ.* Image reproduced with permission from Heartware.

Older VADs pumped blood in a pulsatile fashion using electric or pneumatic pumps that contained many moving parts and valves. In the second generation of VADs, these were replaced with smaller rotational pumps in which the only moving part is the magnet-driven impeller. They are quieter, easier to implant and last longer than the older VADs.

Wires pass through the skin on the right side of the upper abdomen to the control unit and power pack that is carried by the patient. The controller displays information regarding blood flow through the VAD, the number of revolutions per minute (r.p.m.) that the impeller is making, the remaining battery life and other information.

Advantages

- VADs increase life expectancy of patients with heart failure and allow a good quality of life, often allowing them to return home or to work.
- VADs increase the chance of a patient surviving until a donor heart becomes available for transplant.

Disadvantages

- Long-term systemic anticoagulation, usually with warfarin and an antiplatelet agent, is required while the VAD is *in situ.*
- Bleeding can be a problem both peri-operatively and after hospital discharge.
- Patients often develop hypertension after LVAD implantation, which must be properly controlled to reduce the risk of stroke.
- Other complications of VADs include infection, stroke and thromboembolism, right heart failure following LVAD implantation and VAD malfunction or failure.

Other notes

VADs are compatible with most permanent pacemakers, although some alteration to their programming may be required.

Patients with a VAD often do not have a pulse due to the continuous flow generated by the pump. Therefore, mean arterial pressure is estimated using ultrasonic or invasive techniques.

Chapter 10
Surgical equipment relevant to anaesthetists

10.1 Diathermy

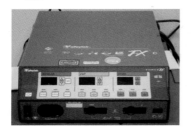

Fig. 10.1.1: A diathermy machine.

Overview

Diathermy uses an electric current to cause localized heating, permitting cutting of tissue and coagulation of blood. It may be unipolar or bipolar, the former having several settings depending on which function is required.

Uses

Diathermy is used to perform incisions and stop bleeding from small vessels during surgery.

How it works

Diathermy produces localized heating so that the temperature rises to over 1000°C. This is achieved by passing an alternating current through the tissue. The heat energy produced is proportional to the electrical power dissipated (the square of the current multiplied by the electrical resistance through the tissue, I^2R).

Alternating current frequency

Alternating current is capable of stimulating excitable tissues. For this reason it can be very dangerous, as is the case if a shock is received from the mains.

Mains electricity is supplied at 50 Hz, which is coincidentally the frequency at which electricity is most likely to stimulate excitable tissues leading to muscle spasm or VF.

The relationship between electrical frequency and the probability of stimulating biological tissues is a curve. As the frequency increases towards 50 Hz, the likelihood of causing VF increases. After 50 Hz, the likelihood begins to decrease again until it passes approximately 100 kHz, when it is negligible.

The frequencies used in diathermy are between 300 kHz and 2 MHz, and so are considerably above those that are likely to cause harm. These high frequency currents can be passed through the patient without the risk of inducing VF or causing electric shock.

The relationship between heat production and frequency does not follow the same curve, and so very high frequencies used in diathermy can still be used to generate large amounts of heat energy.

Current density

The heat energy produced is proportional to the square of the power. The electrical resistance encountered by the current as it passes from the diathermy probe into the patient is a function of the area through which it flows. A small area connecting the probe to the tissue will offer a higher resistance to current than a large area.

The amount of heat energy produced is therefore also proportional to the current density, which is defined as the current divided by the area. If a large current flows through a small area then the current density will be high and the local amount of heat produced will also be high.

Unipolar diathermy

In unipolar diathermy, the surgeon uses a probe (or active electrode) to incise tissues. A large current passes from the diathermy machine, through this probe into the patient. The contact point with the tissue is less than 1–2 mm^2 and therefore the current density at the active electrode

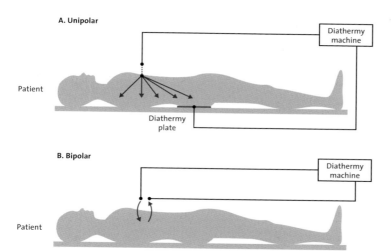

Fig. 10.1.2: The path of current in unipolar and bipolar diathermy.

is high and a large amount of heat energy is produced. The small contact point also allows precise surgical tasks to be performed.

In order to complete the circuit, the current passes back to the diathermy machine via a diathermy plate. This is similar to a defibrillator plate: a sheet of metal foil encased in a plastic coating on one side with an adhesive conducting gel on the other. This is stuck to the patient's skin, usually over the thigh or back. The measurements of the diathermy plate are approximately 10 cm × 10 cm, making the area much larger than the active electrode. The current therefore causes insignificant heating at the plate. The diathermy plate is variously known as the indifferent electrode, the dispersive electrode, the return electrode, the grounding pad and the neutral plate (see *Fig. 10.1.2*).

Different modes are available for use with unipolar diathermy. The output from the diathermy machine in cut mode is a high current in the shape of a continuous sine wave. It uses a relatively low voltage (250 V). In contrast, coag(ulate) mode uses a high voltage (9000 V) in the form of an interrupted sine wave. The interrupted wave is sometimes referred to as damped. Blended modes describe those that have properties somewhere on the spectrum between cut and coag (see *Fig. 10.1.3*). Terms such as desiccation and fulguration describe the effects of the different modes on different tissues.

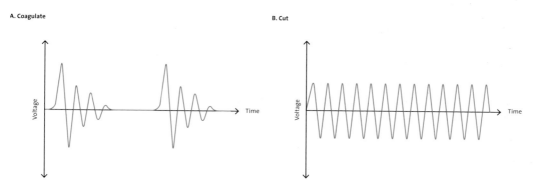

Fig. 10.1.3: Cut and coagulate diathermy waveforms.

Bipolar diathermy

In bipolar diathermy, the probe resembles a pair of forceps. The current passes down one side of the forceps, across the tissue, and up the other side of the forceps. It is therefore very localized and the rest of the patient does not form part of the circuit. No diathermy plate is required. Due to the forceps arrangement, bipolar diathermy is used mostly for coagulating bleeding vessels and is not usually suitable for cutting.

⊕ Advantages

- Allows surgery to proceed with better haemostatic control than using sharp instruments.
- Different modes can be used to achieve different effects on different tissues.

⊖ Disadvantages

- High currents used in diathermy equipment cause induction in cables used for other purposes. This results in interference in the ECG and other monitors when diathermy is in use.
- Cannot be used on end arteries due to the risk of ischaemia. Diathermy also cannot be used on structures supplied by a vascular pedicle such as the testes, because current may concentrate in the pedicle.

⚠ Safety

- If unipolar diathermy is being used, the plate must be properly adhered to the patient. A plate that has become partially removed may allow a higher current density to occur and burns may result. If the plate is removed altogether, current could leave the patient via other routes such as ECG electrodes and cause burns there. In practice, modern diathermy machines have a device (e.g. the contact quality monitor) to ensure the plate is properly adhered to the patient. The machine also uses a floating circuit or isolating capacitor to reduce the risk of current flowing to ground from the patient.
- Pacemakers may interpret the interference from diathermy as cardiac depolarizations. Pacemakers in negative feedback modes (e.g. VVI and DDD) may stop pacing. Pacemakers with defibrillator functions (ICDs) may interpret the interference from diathermy as VF and deliver a shock to the heart. Unipolar diathermy is more problematic than bipolar in this regard, but neither should be considered completely safe to use with a pacemaker. If unipolar diathermy is used in a patient with a pacemaker, the diathermy plate should be positioned as far from it as possible. Safety aspects of surgery in patients with pacemakers is discussed in *Section 12.3*.
- Diathermy smoke has been shown to be hazardous. It may contain viable cells that could potentially pass pathology from the patient to staff; intact human papilloma virus (HPV) has been detected in diathermy smoke. It has also been shown to contain more than 80 chemicals, including benzene which is carcinogenic. Animal studies have shown permanent damage to the respiratory tract caused by these chemicals. Diathermy smoke should be suctioned away from staff and filtered.

Other notes

During the Second World War, German radar beams were used to guide bombers to British targets. The British only knew that radar was being used because of the information obtained by decoding Enigma, which was top secret. The radar beams were therefore given the codename 'headache'. Modified surgical diathermy machines were used in 1940 by the British to transmit interference to block the German radar. They were given the codename 'aspirin'.

10.2 Chest drains

Overview

Chest drains are usually made of PVC and are inserted through an intercostal space using blunt dissection under local anaesthetic, or during cardiac or thoracic surgery. Smaller chest drains are also available that can be inserted using the Seldinger technique under local anaesthesia.

Chest drains are measured in French gauge and are divided into small bore (8–14F), which are usually inserted using the Seldinger technique, medium bore (16–24F), which can be inserted using Seldinger technique or blunt dissection, and large bore (>24F), which are usually inserted using blunt dissection or under direct vision during surgery.

Most drains have side holes in addition to the opening at the tip to help prevent them becoming blocked.

An airtight seal is used to prevent air being drawn up the drain and into the chest during the negative pressure of inspiration. An underwater seal is most common, but flutter valves are also used.

Uses

Chest drains are usually used to drain intrapleural fluid collections or pneumothoraces; however, they may also be placed into the mediastinum or pericardium, especially after surgery.

How it works

Insertion

Guidelines referring to the insertion and management of chest drains have been published by the British Thoracic Society (BTS).

Chest drains for pneumothoraces or fluid collections are commonly inserted into the mid-axillary line in the 'safe triangle', so called because it has few significant blood vessels or nerves. The triangle has its apex just below the axilla, its base formed by a line drawn at the horizontal level of the nipple, and its sides formed by the lateral border of the pectoralis major muscle anteriorly and the anterior border of the latissimus dorsi muscle posteriorly. The use of live ultrasound during insertion of drains is also recommended in many situations in order to identify a safe insertion site.

If the patient is at risk of bleeding, it is recommended that the prothrombin time and platelet count are checked prior to insertion. Non-urgent chest drains should not be inserted until the coagulation is normal, including an INR of less than 1.5. Strict aseptic technique is used throughout the procedure and it should be possible to aspirate air or fluid easily from the pleural space using a narrow bore needle at the time of infiltration with local anaesthetic. If this is not possible, further imaging should be obtained prior to drain insertion.

After infiltration with local anaesthetic and using strict aseptic technique, an incision large enough to accommodate the drain tube is made through the skin. Blunt dissecting forceps are used to divide the muscle until a pop is felt as the parietal pleura is breached – trocars are dangerous and are no longer used. The chest drain is gently inserted through the hole using forceps. It is directed towards the apex for pneumothorax or towards the base for fluid. The drain is then sutured in place and connected via plastic tubing to an underwater seal. Purse string sutures are not recommended.

Seldinger drains are inserted using a guide wire, and are preferred where possible because their smaller size has been associated with reduced length of stay in hospital. After infiltration with local anaesthetic, a needle is inserted through the skin and muscle layers until it passes into the pleural space. The guide wire is then passed through the needle and the needle is removed. After dilation, the chest drain is passed over the wire and into the pleural space and the guide wire is removed. The drain is then sutured in place and connected via plastic tubing to an underwater seal.

A chest X-ray should be obtained following insertion or removal of a drain.

Underwater seals
An underwater seal acts as a valve to allow air or fluid out of the chest while preventing its return. There are two configurations commonly used: either a one bottle or three bottle system (see *Fig. 10.2.1*).

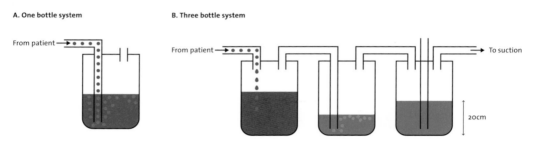

A. One bottle system

From patient ➔

B. Three bottle system

From patient ➔

To suction

20cm

Fig. 10.2.1: The single bottle and three bottle chest drain systems.

One bottle system
The one bottle system is simplest. It is primed with a volume of water not less than 50% of the patient's vital capacity, and the chest drain tubing is connected so that its opening is 2–4 cm below the surface of the water. Air from the chest can then bubble out, but room air cannot be entrained into the drain tubing because water obstructs its entry. Similarly, fluid from the chest can drain out, but air cannot be entrained to replace it. The lung must therefore re-expand.

In some situations air and fluid may both need to be drained (e.g. from a haemopneumothorax). If a one bottle system is used, the amount of fluid in the bottle increases, causing the opening of the drain tubing to become deeper and further from the surface. Due to the higher resistance that this creates, higher intrapleural pressures are required to drain air, and in some cases a tension pneumothorax could develop. Applying suction to the chest drain bottle may help, but the three bottle system is more appropriate.

The three bottle system
In the three bottle system, the chest drain tubing is connected to the top of bottle 1. This bottle has no water prime and the drain tubing connects to its top, allowing fluid from the chest to collect. Air from the chest passes via another tube into bottle 2, which does have a water prime. The tube entering bottle 2 terminates 2–4 cm below the surface of the water prime, and therefore provides the underwater seal in the same way as the one bottle system.

The third bottle is not always necessary. It exists in order to provide and control suction to the chest drain system. It has three tubes on its top. One connects to bottle 2, one connects to the suction pump, and the third connects to the outside environment. This tube passes through the top of the bottle into the water prime. Suction is applied, which causes the pressure in bottle 3 to fall. As it becomes more negative, air is entrained through the third tube and bubbling is seen in the water. The magnitude of the negative pressure exerted on the system is limited by the depth of this tube in the water prime. If it is set up so that the tube is submerged by 20 cm, then it is not possible to apply more than -20 cmH$_2$O pressure to the system because beyond this, air is entrained into the bottle, causing the pressure to re-equilibrate. It should therefore be appreciated that the amount of negative pressure applied to the chest using this system is dictated by the depth that this tube is submerged, and not by the vacuum dial on the suction apparatus.

A version of the three bottle system that is contained within a single unit is commercially available, and less bulky.

Chest drain tubing
The tubing between the chest and the bottle should be long enough to allow the bottle to be kept at least 80–100 cm below the patient. This prevents entrainment of water from the seal into the chest during maximum inspiration. Negative pressures of 50–80 cmH$_2$O can be generated with maximal effort in some people.

The volume of the tubing is also important, and should be at least 50% of the patient's vital capacity. This also helps to prevent water being drawn back from the bottle to the pleural cavity.

Advantages

Advantages of surgical chest drains
- Less prone to blockage.
- Finger sweep permits clearance of pleura, avoiding lung trauma.

Advantages of Seldinger chest drains
- Better seal.
- Familiar Seldinger technique.
- Improved patient comfort and recovery time.

Disadvantages

Disadvantages of surgical chest drains
- Basic surgical kit required for dissection.
- More painful on insertion, and whilst *in situ*.

Disadvantages of Seldinger chest drains
- Narrow lumen is prone to blockage.

Safety

- Chest drain bottles must be kept below the level of the chest. Lifting them higher than this risks siphoning of fluid from the bottle back into the pleural space.
- Suction should only be applied to a chest drain on the advice of a respiratory physician or thoracic surgeon and should not be used routinely.
- Clamping of chest drains is regarded as risky, and it should not be done unless there is a good reason. A chest drain that continues to bubble should never be clamped because tension pneumothorax may result. During the drainage of very large chronic fluid collections, it is recommended that no more than 1.5 litres of fluid is drained in the first hour after insertion to prevent rapid lung expansion and reduce the risk of re-expansion pulmonary oedema. In order to prevent very large volumes of fluid draining in a short time, the drain may be clamped.
- If a patient with a clamped chest drain becomes breathless, the clamp should be removed immediately.
- Drain tubing should be observed carefully, because debris or blood clots may cause blockages and re-accumulation of fluid or air in the chest.

10.3 Lasers

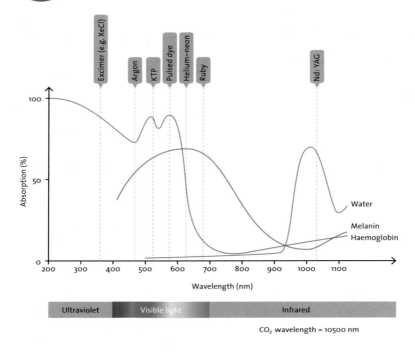

Fig. 10.3.1: The wavelengths of various different lasers, and the absorption spectra of water, melanin and haemoglobin.

Overview

Laser is an acronym for light amplification by stimulated emission of radiation. A laser beam is a non-divergent (all photons moving in parallel – a property also known as collimation), coherent (all photons in phase with each other), monochromatic (single wavelength) beam of light.

Lasers are used in theatre for surgery and in some other pieces of equipment. The anaesthetist must therefore have an understanding of how they work and the safety issues that surround them.

Uses

Lasers are capable of making precise incisions of a defined depth in very small areas with excellent haemostasis. They are used in ENT surgery, thoracic surgery, neurosurgery, dermatology, ophthalmology and many other fields.

Lasers are commonly used for their photothermal effect: absorption of laser light by water results in localized heating and vaporization. Sudden expansion of water in a tissue causes separation and death of cells and the ability to cut through tissues.

Lasers are also used in several other ways. In oncology, drugs can be given that are taken up specifically by malignant cells. Exposure to laser light of a particular wavelength causes these drugs to break down into toxic products, which cause death of the tissue. This is known as the photochemical effect. Photoablation is another use of lasers commonly utilized during eye surgery. It causes the destruction of tissues without the generation of significant amounts of localized heat.

Table 10.3.1 gives some examples of surgical lasers and their properties.

Table 10.3.1: Some lasers used in surgery with their wavelengths/colours and uses.

Laser	Type	Wavelength (nm)	Colour
Nd:YAG	Solid	1064	Infrared
CO_2	Gas	10600	Infrared
Argon	Gas	480–515	Blue–green
Helium–neon	Gas	633	Red
Ruby	Solid	694	Red
Chemical dye (e.g. rhodamine)	Liquid	570–640	Yellow–red
Excimer laser (e.g. XeCl)	Gas	353	Ultraviolet

How it works

Generating a laser beam

Energy from a source such as an intense flash of light or an electric current is passed through a substance called the lasing medium. This can be a solid, liquid or gas and gives the type of laser its name (e.g. CO_2 laser, argon laser, etc.). The lasing medium also dictates the specific wavelength of light the laser produces.

At rest, electrons in the molecules and atoms that make up the lasing medium are in a stable low energy state. When energy from the light flash or electric current (known as the pump) is applied to the lasing medium, many electrons are excited into an unstable higher energy level. When more than half of the molecules in the lasing medium have an electron in an excited state, this is known as population inversion and is fundamental to creation of a laser beam. Some of these excited electrons spontaneously decay back to their resting state, emitting a photon in a random direction as they do so. This is known as *spontaneous* emission. If this photon happens to hit another excited electron, it will cause it also to decay back to its resting state, in the process releasing another photon of radiation that is parallel to, in phase with and of the same wavelength as the first. This is known as *stimulated* emission.

As more photons are emitted, they collide with more excited electrons which in turn emit more photons. This process is known as amplification.

The lasing medium is housed in a 'resonator', a chamber with a mirror at either end. One mirror is fully reflective, while the other is partially reflective (i.e. some of the light that hits it passes through it – perhaps 5% – while the rest is reflected). Most light is therefore reflected back into the lasing medium and stimulates the emission of more photons. Some light that is parallel with the axis of the laser apparatus will pass through the partially reflective mirror and form the laser beam.

In some lasers the resonator may also house a Brewster's window, through which the laser light passes before leaving the resonator. These windows are made from a variety of materials such as germanium or compounds of zinc and are positioned at an angle to the incident light so that only p-polarized photons can get through while s-polarized photons are reflected. The resulting laser beam is therefore composed of p-polarized light only. CO_2 lasers, in particular, often use Brewster's windows and are therefore polarized lasers. In contrast, Nd:YAG lasers are not polarized.

The laser beam can be aimed directly at a target, or passed into a fibreoptic cable or mirrored tubing.

Continuous wave versus pulse wave lasers

There are several refinements to the method outlined above.

The first produces a continuous wave (CW) laser. When the lasing medium is continuously pumped by the power source, an equilibrium develops between the number of atoms that have an excited electron and the number of photons emitted. The result is a continuous, uninterrupted beam. Continuous wave lasers are used less frequently in modern surgery because the continuous output can lead to excessive heating of tissues adjacent to the target, and unsatisfactory surgical results.

In contrast, in pulsed wave (PW) lasers, the beam output is split into short pulses. The duration of each pulse may range from milliseconds to femtoseconds (10^{-15} seconds) depending on the laser and the method of generating the pulses. Methods include Q-switching, mode locking and pulsed pumping, although the details of how these differ is beyond the scope of this book. The result is that the heating effect is confined to a smaller area, and collateral damage is easier to avoid.

Laser output and classification
The laser beam that leaves the resonating chamber is often too diffuse to be used for surgery, therefore, a lens may be used to focus the beam. The irradiance (or power density) is the power of the laser divided by the diameter of the beam. It is therefore measured in watts per m^2.

The actual effect of a laser on a tissue depends on both the irradiance of the laser and the amount of time that the tissue is exposed to it. The fluence (or energy density) is a measure of the amount of energy delivered to the tissue and it is equal to the irradiance multiplied by the exposure time. Power multiplied by time equals energy, and therefore fluence is measured in joules per m^2.

Lasers are classified into seven groups by the International Electrotechnical Commission (IEC) depending on how hazardous they are considered to be, which in turn will depend on the irradiance, fluence, wavelength, and pulse characteristics. *Table 10.3.2* describes this classification in more detail. Surgical lasers are almost always class 4 devices.

Applications
The application of a particular laser depends on its wavelength (dictated by its lasing medium), its depth of penetration into tissues, and which substances absorb its wavelength most efficiently. The CO_2 laser (wavelength of 10.6 μm) penetrates tissues by approximately 0.2 mm and is absorbed by water. It is therefore good for superficial cutting. On the other hand, the Nd:YAG (neodymium: yttrium-aluminium-garnet, wavelength 1064 nm) laser is also absorbed by water but vaporizes tissues to a depth of up to 6 mm. The Argon laser (wavelength 480 nm) is absorbed very efficiently by haemoglobin (and to a slightly lesser extent by melanin) but not by water. It therefore passes through the water in tissues with little effect, but is useful for blood coagulation and some surgery in dermatology. *Figure 10.3.1* shows how different laser light is absorbed by different tissues.

⊕ Advantages
- An excellent bloodless field is possible during surgery.
- Permits surgery in very small or confined areas.

⊖ Disadvantages
- Considerable safety risks accompany laser surgery (see below and *Table 10.3.2*).

Table 10.3.3: The IEC classification of laser devices.

Class	Description
1	No risk to the eyes or skin and safe for accidental viewing in all circumstances (including use with lensed viewing instruments such as microscopes).
	Not safe for prolonged deliberate viewing.
1M	No risk to the eyes or skin and safe for accidental viewing as long as this does not occur via lensed viewing instruments.
2	Lasers in this class must produce a beam with a wavelength in the visible spectrum.
	No risk to the naked eye in time frames less than that needed to initiate the blink reflex (approximately 0.25 seconds), even if this occurs with lensed viewing instruments. Deliberate prolonged viewing is likely to result in eye damage.
	No risk to the skin.
2M	Lasers in this class must produce a beam with a wavelength in the visible spectrum.
	No risk to the naked eye in time frames less than that needed to initiate the blink reflex, as long as this does not occur via lensed viewing instruments.
	No risk to the skin.
3R	Lasers with a wavelength greater than 302.5 nm producing between 1 and 5 mW belong in this class.
	Low risk of eye injuries from exposure to beam.
	No risk to the skin.
3B	Intentional or accidental exposure of the eye to laser beam will result in injury, even if of very short duration.
	Low risk of skin burns.
4	Highly dangerous lasers. Continuous wave power over 0.5 watts with no upper limit to this laser class.
	Eye and skin injury will result if exposed to the beam.
	Exposure to diffuse reflections of laser light is also likely to cause injuries.
	Combustion of materials exposed to the beam is likely.

⚠ Safety

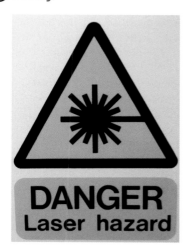

Fig. 10.3.2: Warning sign.

- Safety aspects of laser surgery depend on the type of surgery being performed. Some safety precautions should be taken in all theatres where a laser is being used, while others are only required if the laser is being used in the airway.
- Safety considerations for all theatres where a laser is in operation.
  - A designated laser safety officer should be present.
  - Eye protection (specific to the wavelength of the laser being used) must be worn by the patient and all staff in theatre. Laser beams can cause serious eye damage, even if they have been reflected, because the cornea and lens refocus the light onto the retina. Permanent blindness may result.
  - Warning signs should be clearly displayed outside theatre (*Fig. 10.3.2*) and doors should be locked to prevent people walking in.

- ○ Equipment should have a matt finish to help prevent reflection of the laser beam.
- ○ The patient should be covered in non-combustible drapes, and wet gauze should be used to protect exposed tissue adjacent to the area where surgery is being performed.
- ○ Ideally, the laser will have a low-power targeting laser to show where the laser is pointing.
- Safety considerations for laser airway surgery include all the above, plus the following.
  - ○ Laser beams may cause ignition of tissues and equipment in the presence of combustible gases such as oxygen and nitrous oxide. The use of the latter should be avoided altogether during laser airway surgery, and the FiO_2 kept as low as safely possible. Modern volatile agents are not flammable or explosive and most authorities regard them as safe to use with lasers. Theoretically, they may undergo pyrolysis during an airway fire and yield toxic compounds. However, because they are used in small concentrations, this problem is not usually considered significant.
  - ○ Nitrogen does not support combustion, and so reducing FiO_2 using air is appropriate. However, some authorities suggest the use of heliox instead. Helium has a higher thermal conductivity than nitrogen and therefore conducts heat away from its source faster. Airway fires may be less likely if heliox is used instead of air. However, routine surgery using this gas may become expensive.
  - ○ Most standard ETTs are made of PVC, and will ignite shortly after exposure to some lasers. This is a major hazard, and there are ETTs made of stainless steel or aluminium for use during laser airway surgery to avoid this.
  - ○ Procedures should be in place for the immediate management of an airway fire, should it occur. All staff in the theatre should know the agreed drill (see *Fig. 10.3.3*).

Action by surgeon	Action by anaesthetist
Stop using laser	Immediately cease ventilation
Remove source of fire and extinguish in water	Disconnect breathing system
Inform anaesthetist	Remove ETT if still present
Flood area with 0.9% saline	
Suggested action following extinction of fire	
Ventilate with 100% oxygen by mask	
Maintain anaesthesia	
Rigid laryngoscopy and bronchoscopy to assess damage and remove debris	
Consider bronchoalveolar lavage	
Re-intubate, or if damage is severe perform tracheostomy	
Arterial blood gas, chest X-ray	
Consider ITU management and short course of steroids	

Figure 10.3.3: Possible procedure for early management of an airway fire in theatre.

Other notes

Surgical lasers can be highly hazardous if used incorrectly and their power output can be up to approximately 200 watts (continuous wave lasers), placing them firmly in class 4.

In comparison, the most powerful laser beam ever recorded at the time of writing was produced by the National Ignition Facility (NIF) in the USA in 2012, where lasers are used experimentally in an attempt to provoke the nuclear fusion of hydrogen atoms. This laser can produce pulses of over 500 trillion (5×10^{14}) watts!

10.4 Arterial tourniquet

Overview

Arterial tourniquets are high pressure cuffs for use on a limb in order to prevent blood flow. They are applied in much the same way as a blood pressure cuff, although extra padding is required to help prevent pressure damage to nerves and other structures.

Uses

Arterial tourniquets are used after exsanguination of a limb to prevent blood reaching the surgical site and therefore allow surgeons to operate in a bloodless field. They are commonly used in orthopaedic surgery, particularly during total knee replacement.

Intravenous regional anaesthesia (Bier's block) also requires the use of an arterial tourniquet to prevent the local anaesthetic reaching the systemic circulation. They may also be used in isolated limb perfusion techniques in the management of local malignancy.

How it works

The limb is exsanguinated by raising it above the level of the heart and often by using an Esmarch bandage or a Rhys–Davies exsanguinator (an elongated rubber doughnut which compresses the limb as it is rolled along it). The tourniquet is then inflated to a pressure 50–100 mmHg above systolic pressure preventing arterial flow past the cuff. Typical maximum inflation pressure is approximately 250 mmHg.

⊕ Advantages

- Easy to apply, provides the surgeon with a bloodless field in which to operate.

⊖ Disadvantages

- The time that the tourniquet can be used for is limited to approximately 120 minutes, because permanent ischaemic damage may occur after this.
- Alcoholic skin preparations used for asepsis during surgery can be absorbed by the padding under the tourniquet and be held against the skin for significant time periods. Chemical burns can be the result.
- Temporary nerve damage (neuropraxia) may occur, leading to weakness or paraesthesia in the limb after surgery. This is often incorrectly attributed to regional anaesthetic techniques that have been used.
- Muscle damage has been known to occur, even to the extent of rhabdomyolysis on very rare occasions. Stiffness, swelling and weakness in a muscle that was under the tourniquet may be observed.
- Tourniquet pain develops soon after inflation of the cuff, and is difficult to treat. It is a severe dull ache at the site of compression, and may be felt in awake patients even if a regional nerve block has been performed. In patients under general anaesthesia, tourniquet pain manifests as slowly rising pulse and blood pressure that is unresponsive to the usual treatment.
- Haemodynamic compromise when the tourniquet is released may be severe, especially in the elderly, in hypovolaemic patients, or in those with impaired cardiac function.

⚠ Safety

There are no absolute contraindications, but careful consideration should be given to the risks versus benefits before arterial tourniquets are used in:

- people with sickle cell disease, because the oxygen supply to the affected limb is minimal; red cells that remain in the limb may sickle and result in a crisis, as limb exsanguination prior to inflation of the tourniquet is unlikely to be 100% complete
- those with peripheral vascular disease
- limbs known to have deep vein thrombosis, because a pulmonary embolus could result if the clot was dislodged during compression
- patients with local infection or tumour underlying the exsanguinator or tourniquet.

Chapter 11
Radiological equipment

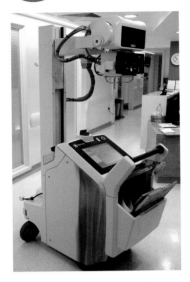

Fig. 11.1.1: A portable X-ray machine.

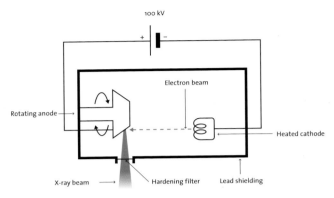

Fig. 11.1.2: Diagram of an X-ray tube.

Overview

Imaging using X-rays is ubiquitous in modern medicine. Anaesthetists may be required to provide anaesthesia or sedation during imaging, or may carry out X-ray guided procedures themselves (most commonly during the management of chronic pain). It is therefore necessary for anaesthetists to have a general understanding of what X-rays are and, in particular, knowledge of how to work around them safely.

Uses

X-rays have numerous uses, including diagnostic imaging (plain films, contrast studies and computed tomography, CT) and real-time imaging of interventions using fluoroscopy.

X-rays may also be used therapeutically in radiotherapy.

How it works

X-rays lie between gamma and ultraviolet radiation in the electromagnetic spectrum. Those used for medical imaging have photon energies of around 10–100 keV (wavelengths of approximately 0.01–0.1 nm).

In an X-ray tube the negatively charged cathode, which is a heated filament, releases electrons from its surface. The anode, usually made of a rotating tungsten disc, is placed at the other end of a vacuum-filled tube. A large voltage is placed across the tube, causing electrons to accelerate rapidly from cathode to anode. When the electrons collide with the anode, around 1% of their energy is released as X-rays, with the rest converted to heat. This heat must be dissipated, hence the rotating disc which allows cooling.

The tube is lead-shielded so that the X-ray beam only escapes in the desired direction. Low energy, 'soft' X-rays with energies <10 keV, would be fully absorbed in the body, increasing the dose but not producing an image. The beam is therefore 'hardened' by passing through an aluminium filter on leaving the tube. The soft X-rays are absorbed, leaving the hardened rays as the beam. These are at the correct energy so that some will pass through the patient and be detected, whilst others are absorbed (e.g. by bone).

⊕ Advantages

- Plain films, CT and fluoroscopy are cheap and widely available.
- Many images can be interpreted by non-radiologists.

⊖ Disadvantages

- Radiation exposure to both patient and staff are significant risks.
- Intravenous iodinated contrast may be nephrotoxic.

⚠ Safety

Anaesthetists are regularly exposed to X-rays. It follows that knowledge of the risks they pose, and methods used to minimize those risks, is essential.

Radiation doses

The sievert (Sv) is the SI unit of dose equivalent radiation. It attempts to quantitatively evaluate the biological effects of ionizing radiation (as opposed to the gray (Gy), which defines an absorbed amount of energy). Background radiation in the UK is on average $0.007\,mSv.day^{-1}$.

Table 11.1.1: Radiation dose to the patient of common imaging modalities

Intervention	Dose equivalent (mSv)	Equivalent background radiation
Chest/dental X-ray	0.07	10 days
CT head	2.5	1 year
CT chest/abdo/pelvis	10	4 years
Coronary angiogram	10	4 years

Risks from radiation exposure are hard to quantify. The available figures are largely based on populations exposed to relatively high levels of ionizing radiation for short periods, mainly Japanese atomic bomb survivors. The effect of longer term, low level exposure is harder to establish. Healthcare professionals in developed countries are not believed to have an increased risk of developing cancer. Nevertheless, in the absence of good evidence of a safe level, radiation protection specialists advise minimizing dose as far as possible.

Minimizing dose

Radiation dose in a healthcare setting may be reduced in the following ways.

- *Shielding.* Lead aprons reduce dose equivalent by up to 80%. Lead glass, solid walls, thyroid shields and glasses also offer protection.
- *Increasing the distance from the X-ray tube.* Radiation obeys the inverse square law, so dose falls with the square of the distance. Moving away from the source is therefore one of the most effective ways to minimize the dose.
- *Decreasing exposure time.*

The ALARP principle

There are radiation dose limits set in the UK; however, it is not legally sufficient to keep dosage below a set limit, so doses must be kept **A**s **L**ow **A**s **R**easonably **P**racticable.

11.2 Ultrasound

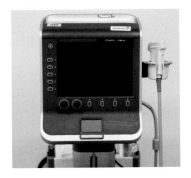

Fig. 11.2.1: The Sonosite S-Nerve ultrasound machine is specifically designed for anaesthetics and has settings for nerve blocks and vascular access.

Overview

The term ultrasound is used to describe a sound wave at a higher frequency (and therefore pitch) than the upper limit of human hearing. This is around 20 kHz, though the frequencies used in medicine are from 2 to 20 MHz.

Uses

Medical ultrasound has imaging and therapeutic uses; it is also used in humidifiers and to clean medical instruments.

Imaging takes place in real time and may be used for diagnostic purposes (echocardiography, soft-tissue imaging and fetal scanning) or to aid placement of invasive devices (for venous access, chest drains and nerve blocks).

The direct therapeutic uses of ultrasound will be less familiar to anaesthetists, but include tumour ablation and treatment of renal stones.

How it works

Creating and detecting ultrasound waves

An ultrasound probe may be used for surface or invasive use and its design will depend on the site to be imaged, taking into account the depth, tissue type and the acoustic window available. An acoustic window is a gap through which the ultrasound beam can pass, for instance between ribs.

The probe contains a piezoelectric transducer that vibrates when an electric current flows, producing a sound wave. Sound waves are mechanical waves transmitted by vibrating particles, and are therefore not part of the electromagnetic spectrum; they are non-ionizing.

The focused wave is transmitted to the patient. Refraction and reflection of sound can occur as it passes from air into tissue because of the sudden change in the density of the medium through which it is travelling. This effect is reduced by applying a water-based gel between the probe and the skin. The step change in density between the water-based gel and body tissue is significantly less than between air and tissue, therefore the sound waves are refracted and reflected far less.

Within the patient, reflections occur at boundaries between tissue layers. Some of these reflections return to the probe, the piezoelectric transducer then operates in reverse, and the sound energy is converted to an electric current. Microprocessors are used to convert information in this current into the image. In order to allow time for the reflection to return and be transduced, a brief pause follows each ultrasound pulse.

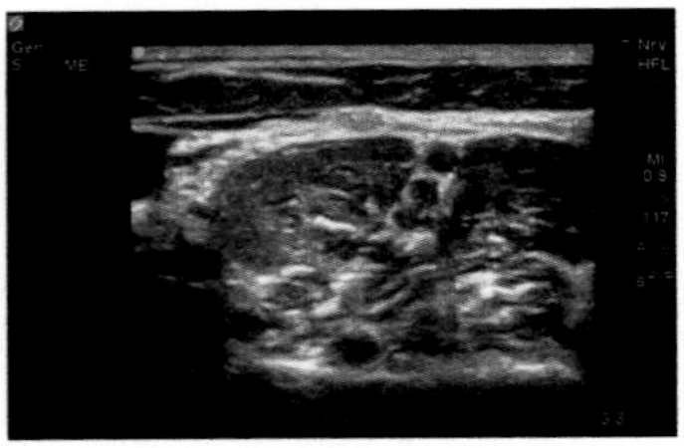

Fig. 11.2.2: A B-mode scan of the brachial plexus at an interscalene level (from Sonosite website www.sonosite.com).

Displaying the image

Most anaesthetists will be familiar with a scan based on a moving B-mode (brightness-mode) image. In B-mode, the time taken for the reflection to reach the transducer is used to calculate the depth of the tissue. Pixel brightness depends on the strength of the reflection and the final image is a 2D plane through the body. Sequential B-mode pulses are used to produce the real-time moving image.

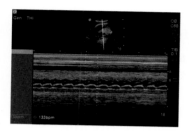

M-mode (motion mode) is also used in medical imaging, particularly in cardiac scans, because the higher sampling rate and format in which the information is displayed allow more accurate measurements to be taken.

Three-dimensional ultrasound is also becoming available and digitally combines scans from multiple 2D transducers to produce a moving 3D image.

Fig. 11.2.3: An M-mode scan of the fetal heart (from Sonosite website www.sonosite.com.)

Effect of frequency

High frequencies (therefore short wavelengths) produce images of high resolution. Unfortunately, attenuation of ultrasound in tissues is greatest at high frequencies and therefore the depth that can be scanned is limited. In order to image deeper tissues, resolution must be sacrificed.

Doppler ultrasound

The Doppler effect is the change in frequency that occurs when a wave is reflected off an object that is moving relative to the observer. This change of frequency is called the Doppler shift. When the object is moving towards the observer there is an increase in frequency; conversely, when it is moving away, there is a decrease in frequency. It is the Doppler effect that causes the change of pitch in a siren as an ambulance passes. More usefully, however, it can be employed to measure velocity, particularly of blood, during an ultrasound scan. Since the Doppler effect relies on movement towards or away from the probe, flow perpendicular to the probe is not detected.

Continuous wave (CW) Doppler is used to display velocity as a graph against time, or to produce the familiar audible signal of arterial flow. It is also employed by transoesophageal cardiac output monitors. A CW Doppler signal is an amalgamation of the velocities of all the objects that the beam has encountered. This makes the measurement of specific intra-cardiac flows, such as those across valves, difficult.

Pulsed wave (PW) Doppler is used to overcome the deficiencies of CW Doppler. The transducer alternates transmission and reception of ultrasound in a similar way to an M-mode transducer. This allows the transducer to measure the signal from a particular depth along the beam by waiting the appropriate time for the signal to return from that location.

Colour Doppler overlays Doppler information relating to direction of movement on a standard 2D image.

Using basic ultrasound controls to optimize the image

In general a 6-13 MHz linear transducer will produce an adequate view of blood vessels and superficial nerves without much adjustment of the machine settings. There are, however some simple steps that can improve the image.

Depth – as the depth is increased, the object being scanned becomes smaller, therefore reducing the depth improves the accuracy with which an object can be targeted. If the depth is too shallow, important structures may be missed off the bottom or sides of the field of view.

Gain – increasing gain increases the brightness of the image, but may introduce noise. Gain may be adjusted for the whole image, or for near or far fields.

Focus – the highest resolution will be found in the focal zone, which is set by many machines in the centre of the image. It is often also possible to adjust the focal zone to ensure it includes the object of interest and thus optimize the image.

Advantages

- Relatively simple to use, cheap and widely available.
- Non-ionizing.
- Real-time imaging – in anaesthetics this facilitates placement of lines and nerve blocks.
- Ability to overlay a Doppler image.

Disadvantages

- Bone represents a barrier to ultrasound and obscured tissues cannot effectively be imaged.
- Air also represents a barrier and may impair scans in the chest or if air is injected subcutaneously during the course of a procedure.
- Because deep tissues are poorly imaged, obesity may result in an inadequate scan.
- It can be difficult to interpret a stored image so the report is usually made by the sonographer who performed the scan. However, if more expert advice is required, that expert must usually scan again.
- Ultrasound scans are notoriously operator-dependent.

Safety

Diagnostic ultrasound is essentially safe; however, infection is a potential hazard if probes are not properly decontaminated between patients.

11.3 MRI and compatible equipment

Random magnetic moments

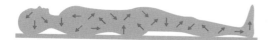

Fig. 11.3.1: The magnetic moments of protons within the body are normally aligned randomly.

Aligned magnetic moments

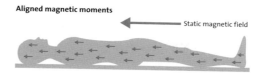

Static magnetic field

Fig. 11.3.2: When the patient lies in the scanner, the magnetic moments align with the static magnetic field.

Overview

Magnetic resonance imaging (MRI) uses strong magnetic fields to create images by determining the distribution of protons within the subject. It is a highly complex process which requires sophisticated mathematics and quantum mechanics to explain fully. We have instead briefly described the 'classical model' of MRI, which allows non-mathematicians some insight into what is happening.

More important to the anaesthetist than an understanding of MRI physics, is knowledge of the safety aspects and the equipment required when anaesthetizing a patient in the MRI suite. These elements are therefore covered in more detail.

Uses

MRI may be used to image any body part. It is, however, particularly useful for imaging soft tissues, including the CNS. From an anaesthetic standpoint, MRI is the modality of choice for diagnosis of epidural haematoma and abscess.

How it works

The static magnetic field
A superconducting electromagnet with a field strength of around 1.5–3 tesla (T) forms the largest component of the scanner (1 T is equal to 10 000 gauss, or approximately 20 000 times the strength of the earth's magnetic field). The field produced by the electromagnet is known as the static magnetic field because it does not vary.

In order to remain superconducting, the electromagnet's coils must be kept at a few degrees above absolute zero and are therefore surrounded by liquid helium contained within vacuum-insulated walls.

Alignment of magnetic moments
All charged particles possess a quantity known as a magnetic moment, which determines their interaction with a magnetic field. This can be thought of as the particle's own very small magnetic field and the magnetic moment therefore tends to align with the external field. The more powerful the external field, the more alignment takes place.

Protons (hydrogen nuclei) are the charged particle targeted in MRI because, as a component of water, they are widespread throughout the body. When the patient is placed in the bore of the scanner, the magnetic moments of the protons tend to align with the strong field (*Fig. 11.3.2*).

Radiofrequency pulses
During a scan, pulses of radiofrequency energy are used to flip the protons' magnetic moments out of alignment. As the magnetic moments relax back to their original positions, energy is released.

This energy is detected by the scanner and used to form the image. Multiple pulses in a particular sequence are used depending on the image required.

Gradient fields

During the scan, secondary 'gradient' magnetic fields are also applied to vary the field strength slightly from one position in the patient to the other. This process allows the scanner to localize signals it receives in three dimensions, in other words, to identify where in the patient a particular signal has originated. It is the rapidly changing gradient fields that cause the loud knocking noises during an MRI scan, because the coils that produce them vibrate on their mountings.

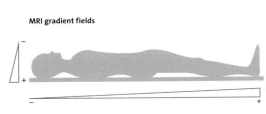

MRI gradient fields

Fig. 11.3.3: The arrangement of gradient magnetic fields during a scan.

Contrast

Most MRI contrast agents are paramagnetic compounds of gadolinium, a rare metal. Side-effects are rare and, unlike CT contrast, contrast does not need to be administered under pressure, so any available IV access may be used. Gadolinium is also much less nephrotoxic than iodinated CT contrast.

Advantages

- MRI has excellent soft tissue resolution.
- There is no ionizing radiation involved.

Disadvantages

- Most equipment cannot be taken into the scan room (see below).
- Many patients find the narrow bore of the scanner claustrophobic; it also impedes access.
- MRI is contraindicated in many patients who have medical implants.
- Scan times are far slower than CT and may take several hours.

Safety

Safety considerations when anaesthetizing a patient in an MRI scanner are frequently examined. Hazards may either harm the patient directly, or may interfere with the normal operation of equipment.

Problems caused by the static magnetic field

- *Projectiles.* There have been fatalities caused by oxygen cylinders or sharp ferromagnetic objects being accelerated into the bore of the scanner. Staff working in MRI must be fully trained and alert to the risk. Alarms are available to detect ferromagnetic objects before they enter the scan room.
- *Indwelling metal.* Individuals with ferromagnetic material within their bodies are not permitted in the scan room. Care must be taken with medical implants including intracranial clips and heart valves (though some are safe), as well as individuals with shrapnel injuries and metal workers who may have metal splinters in their eyes.
- *Electronic devices.* Implanted devices, such as pacemakers, and external equipment, such as monitors and infusion pumps, are likely to malfunction in the presence of the static field.

The static magnetic field extends beyond the scan room and shielding is used to minimize the extent of this 'fringe field'. Passive shielding consists of a large mass of steel, in the walls, ceiling and floor of the scan room. Active shielding may also be used, consisting of a second electromagnet surrounding the scanner with an opposing magnetic field.

The area contained within the fringe field's 0.5 mT (5 gauss) contour is controlled and off-limits to those with implanted devices. It is marked by a line known as the 5 gauss line. A second line, much closer to the scanner, is the 50 gauss line, beyond which most electronic equipment will malfunction.

Problems caused by radiofrequency pulses
- Radiofrequency energy causes currents to be induced within monitoring cables, particularly if coiled. This causes heating and may lead to burns.

Acoustic noise
- The rapidly changing gradient magnetic fields give rise to acoustic noise levels in excess of 100 dB. Patients, whether anaesthetized or not, and staff who remain in the scan room, must be protected with ear plugs.

Location and patient access
- The MRI suite is an isolated site and is for many anaesthetists an unfamiliar environment with unfamiliar equipment.
- The patient is positioned largely out of sight and the airway and IV access may be difficult.

Quench
- A quench refers to the events that occur when the liquid helium cooling the electromagnet rapidly boils and is vented from the scanner.
- Quenching may occur spontaneously due to a fault, or may be activated in order to turn off the magnetic field in a life-threatening emergency. Quenching may cause permanent damage to the scanner.
- Whilst the scan room design should vent the helium gas externally, there is a risk of a hypoxic environment if systems do not function appropriately.

Anaesthetic equipment for use in MRI

There are two possible options when giving an anaesthetic within an MRI scanner: the use of standard equipment, located outside the scan room via extensions and waveguides, or the use of specialized equipment which is MR compatible. In either case, patients are anaesthetized outside the scan room before being transferred in, allowing standard anaesthesia and resuscitation equipment to be used.

Table 11.3.1: Classification of MRI equipment

MR safe – an item that poses no known hazards in all MRI environments.	MR
MR conditional – an item that poses no known hazard in a specified MRI environment within specified conditions of use (i.e. may be conditional on field strength, scan sequence, routing of cables, etc.).	⚠ MR
MR unsafe – poses hazards in all MRI environments.	Ⓜ̸R

Wave guides (and their use with unsafe equipment)

Wave guides are brass conduits which pass through the wall of the scan room without breaking the magnetic shielding. A standard anaesthetic machine, infusion pumps, or monitoring may then be located outside the 5 gauss line, usually in the control room. Long extensions are then attached to the breathing circuit, gas monitoring and infusion lines and passed through the waveguides.

Advantages

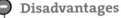

- Familiar, cheaper equipment can be used.
- The machine is situated with the anaesthetist outside the scan room.

Disadvantages

- It is inconvenient to set up, requiring disconnections in infusion lines.
- A significant delay in capnography is introduced.
- The high breathing system volume causes delay following alteration of inspired gas concentrations.
- The machine is not next to the patient which is challenging in an emergency.

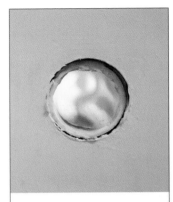

Fig. 11.3.4: A wave guide is simply a brass conduit through the scan room wall.

Anaesthetic delivery

MR-conditional anaesthetic machines and infusion pumps are available from the major manufacturers which function up to several hundred gauss.

A wide range of non-ferromagnetic airway equipment is also available. It should be noted that ETTs have a small metal clip in the pilot balloon that should be taped away from the area to be scanned because it impairs the image.

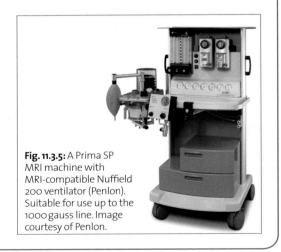

Fig. 11.3.5: A Prima SP MRI machine with MRI-compatible Nuffield 200 ventilator (Penlon). Suitable for use up to the 1000 gauss line. Image courtesy of Penlon.

Monitoring

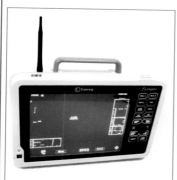

Fig. 11.3.6: An Expression MRI telemetric monitor (Invivo).

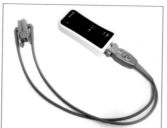

Fig. 11.3.7: A telemetric MRI conditional pulse oximeter (Invivo). Light is transmitted to the oximeter using fibreoptics to prevent induction of currents.

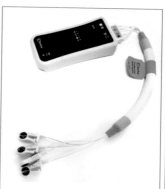

Fig. 11.3.8: A telemetric ECG module (Invivo) which attaches to 4 electrodes placed centrally on the chest. The short insulated cable ends in a wireless transmitter.

Monitors are usually telemetric in order to avoid long cables. An ideal set-up has a monitor in the scan room and linked monitor in the control room.

Non-invasive blood pressure: nylon connectors are used in place of metal.

Pulse oximeter: fibreoptic cabling and telemetry prevent induced currents and burns.

ECG: carbon electrodes are used and are placed a few centimetres apart on the chest so that short cables can be used, lessening induced currents. Cables must not be coiled and must be padded away from the skin. The ECG, particularly the ST-segment, is distorted by currents induced in the aortic blood during a scan.

Unsafe equipment

Anything not known to be MR safe or conditional must be assumed to be unsafe. This may include oxygen cylinders, airway equipment, patient trolleys, drip stands, defibrillators, surgical instruments and personal items.

In an emergency, it is usually safest to take the patient out of the scan room so that a full range of familiar equipment can be used.

Chapter 12
Miscellaneous

12.1 Electricity and electrical safety

Introduction

Throughout this book, pieces of equipment used in anaesthesia have been described that use electrical power. Many of these are found in theatre, in close proximity to the patient, the surgeon, the anaesthetist and other theatre staff. It is important that the anaesthetist has a good understanding of the electrical principles and what measures can be taken to render electrical equipment as safe as possible.

Charge and Ohm's law

Charge (Q) is the property of some subatomic particles that causes them to experience a force when in proximity to other charged particles. It is measured in coulombs (C). Electrons are particles that have a negative charge, and are able to move about in some materials. The freedom of the electrons to move within the material varies. Those that allow electrons to move easily are known as conductors and those that do not are known as insulators. Resistance is a measure of the difficulty electrons have moving in a particular material, and is measured in ohms (Ω).

The charge on a single electron is -1.602×10^{-19} C. If a conductor is arranged in such a way that there is a deficit of electrons in one place and a surplus in another, the electrons experience a force that will move them from where there is surplus to where there is a deficit. The areas of surplus and deficit are known as poles. The number of electrons (or amount of charge) that moves past a fixed point per unit time is the current (I), which is measured in amperes (amps or A). One amp is the movement of one coulomb of charge (or 6.24×10^{18} electrons) per second.

The magnitude of the force that causes the movement of the electrons between poles is known as the potential difference (or voltage), and is measured in volts (V). One volt is the potential difference between two poles in a conductor that causes the flow of one amp of current when the resistance is one ohm. The ohm is therefore similarly defined as the resistance that allows a current of one amp to flow when there is a potential difference of one volt. This is Ohm's law:

Potential difference (V) = Current (I) × Resistance (R)

Power

Electrical energy in joules (J) is equal to the product of charge and voltage. The power generated in watts (W) is the energy dissipated per unit time (i.e. joules per second). As stated above, charge per unit time is current. Therefore, power is equal to voltage multiplied by current. This is Joules' law:

Power (P) = Voltage (V) × Current (I)

By substitution of Ohm's law into Joules' law, it can be seen that power is also equal to the square of the current multiplied by the resistance:

$P = VI$

Therefore, $P = I(IR) = I^2R$

Earth

Earth (or 'ground') is the reference potential from which voltage is measured, i.e. voltages are quoted as a potential difference relative to earth. Current will flow from a potential difference to earth by taking the route of least resistance. In order to experience an electric shock, a person must be somewhere in the pathway connecting the potential difference to earth.

Mains electricity

Electrons are induced to move when a conducting material is in motion within a magnetic field. This is known as induction. Power stations utilize fossil fuels or nuclear energy to heat water and produce steam that turns a turbine. The turbine causes rotation of a magnet within an arrangement of conductor coils and this generates electricity.

Due to the rotation of the magnet the polarity of the potential difference rapidly changes back and forth, and electricity generated in this way produces an alternating current (AC) – a current whose direction changes backwards and forwards. This is in contrast to electricity from a battery whose current constantly flows in one direction, known as direct current (DC). The number of times the AC changes direction per second (its frequency) is measured in hertz (Hz). Impedance (Z) is usually used in place of resistance when discussing AC because it includes resistance and two other mechanisms affecting current flow in AC, induction and capacitance (see below). Impedance is also measured in ohms but is dependent on the frequency.

The electricity generated in UK power stations is at the relatively low frequency of 50 Hz because low frequencies are more economical to transmit over long distances.

A graph of potential difference against time or current against time will both produce a sine wave for AC electricity. Because the potential difference is constantly changing, it is difficult to quote a voltage for the system. A way around this problem is to quote the root mean square (RMS) voltage. One of the simplest ways of deriving this value is to rapidly sample the voltage. Each sample is squared, which gives each value a positive number. The sum of the squares divided by the number of samples gives the mean square. The square root of this is the RMS voltage.

Electricity is transmitted through power wires from the power station to the substation at the hospital with a very high voltage (many thousands of volts), where a transformer reduces it to the UK mains supply voltage of 240 V RMS. The peak voltage of mains electricity in the UK is approximately 340 V.

A high transmission voltage over the fixed electrical resistance offered by the cabling means that the current can remain low. As mentioned above, power dissipated is equal to the square of the current multiplied by the resistance. Therefore, the higher the current the more power is lost in heat energy. Electricity is therefore transmitted with a high voltage and low current in order to minimize power loss.

Current flows from the substation into the hospital via the live wire (coloured brown in the UK), where it powers equipment, and then back to the substation via the neutral wire (coloured blue in the UK) to complete the circuit. The neutral wire in the substation is then connected to earth. If the current is able to find a path to earth that has a lower impedance than the neutral wire, it will take it. If this new path includes a human body, that person may experience an electric shock.

Inductance

As described above, inductance is the production of an electrical current when a conductor is in motion within a magnetic field. Similarly, when an AC electrical current flows a magnetic field is generated. A current flowing in a wire can therefore induce a current in an adjacent wire to which it is not physically connected.

Capacitance

A capacitor is a system that consists of two electrical conductors separated by an insulator known as the dielectric. Direct current flows from a power source and electrons collect on one of the conductor plates, causing it to become negatively charged. At the same time, electrons move from the opposite plate back towards the power source, causing this plate to become positively charged. A potential difference therefore exists between the two capacitor plates. This potential difference increases with time until its voltage is equal to that of the power source. At this point the current flow ceases. The capacitor can be discharged when the circuit is altered, e.g. in a defibrillator (see Section 9.18).

Capacitance is the ability to store charge and it is measured in farads (F). One farad is when a potential difference of one volt is applied across the capacitor and causes the storage of one coulomb of charge. Therefore:

$$\text{Potential difference } (V) = \frac{\text{Charge } (Q)}{\text{Capacitance } (C)}$$

The stored charge can also be expressed as energy in joules. As mentioned above, the expression relating electrical energy to charge and potential difference is:

Energy (E) = Charge (Q) × Potential difference (V)

However, in the case of the energy on a capacitor this expression is modified. Due to the fact that like charges repel, it becomes more difficult to add electrons to the negative capacitor plate as it charges, and a higher amount of energy is required to charge the capacitor by a given amount. The energy needed to add charge to a capacitor given a particular potential difference becomes:

$\Delta E = \Delta Q.V$

However, as the capacitor is charged, the potential difference across it increases. Therefore the change in potential difference that occurs when charging occurs is given by:

$$\Delta V = \frac{\Delta Q}{C}$$

Which means:

$\Delta Q = C \Delta V$

Substitution of ΔQ into the energy expression gives:

$\Delta E = C \Delta V.V$

The change in energy in the capacitor over the whole process of charging can be obtained by integration:

$\int dE = C \int V \, dV$

Which gives the result:

Energy (E) = ½ × Capacitance (C) × Potential difference squared (V^2)

Substituting charge for capacitance gives:

Energy (E) = ½ × Charge (Q) × Potential difference (V)

This result shows that although the energy supplied by the power source is $Q.V$, only half of this is actually transferred onto the capacitor. The rest is dissipated as heat due to the resistance of the circuit.

If AC is applied to a capacitor, the capacitor rapidly charges and discharges at the same frequency as the current. This property of AC therefore allows current flow through the circuit despite the presence of the insulating dielectric.

Capacitive coupling is a reason a patient may become part of an electrical circuit. A patient lying on an operating table is a conductor, as is the operating lamp above the table. The air between the patient and the lamp is an insulator and acts as a dielectric in a capacitor. As the lamp is supplied by mains AC, a circuit may be set up between the lamp and the patient. Wires and cables in contact with the patient may also become part of the circuit and current may also flow in them in this situation.

Effects of electricity on the human body

The effect of electricity on the human body depends on the magnitude of the current and its frequency, as well as where in the body the electricity is applied.

The mains frequency of 50 Hz is, unfortunately, the most dangerous and has the highest probability of inducing cell membrane dysfunction in excitable cells such as skeletal muscle and cardiac myocytes. Equipment such as is used in diathermy is able to pass large currents through patients without the risk of electrocution because it uses very high frequencies. *Table 12.1.1* shows the effects of varying amplitudes of 50 Hz current on the human body.

Table 12.1.1: The effects of different amplitudes of 50 Hz electric current on the human body.

Current (mA)	Effect on human body
<1	Imperceptible
1	A tingling feeling can be felt where current is applied
5	Painful
8	Likely to cause burns
15	Skeletal muscle tetany, the 'can't let go' phenomenon
50	Skeletal muscle paralysis and respiratory arrest
100	Ventricular fibrillation and cardiac arrest

In theory, an adult wearing high impedance footwear on a dry anti-static floor should have an impedance of approximately 240 kΩ. Therefore, with a mains RMS voltage of 240 V, only 1 mA of current should flow. However, this may vary if incorrect footwear is worn or the impedance is reduced in another way, perhaps by the spillage of an electrolyte-rich solution on the floor. The impedance may also be lowered significantly if the person is touching an object that provides a low electrical resistance route to ground, such as a drip stand. In these situations, a much higher current will flow.

Microshock and leakage currents

Current density is the current divided by the area or volume through which it passes. When a current of 100 mA passes from one hand to the other only a fraction (less than 1%) actually passes through the heart, because the rest of the current passes through other tissues. However, the current density is still sufficient to induce VF.

If a device such as a cardiac catheter or a pulmonary artery catheter is inserted into the heart, a small current may flow directly to the myocardium. This current may be many times smaller than that which caused VF as it passed from one hand to the other, but because it only flows through a small area, the current density may be the same and therefore it is still sufficient to induce VF. This is known as microshock, and currents are of the order of 50–100 μA.

No piece of equipment is insulated so well that absolutely no current will flow if the equipment gains a slightly higher potential than earth. This may be due to static charge build-up, inductance or capacitive coupling. The small currents that flow from equipment to earth are called leakage currents, and although they are small they may sometimes cause microshocks if they flow through the patient. Classification systems exist that rank equipment depending on the maximum leakage currents they will allow (see below).

Classification of equipment
Modification of electrical equipment can make it safer. Different classification systems are used depending on whether the modifications are designed to prevent macroshock or microshock.

Macroshock
Equipment is classified into three groups depending on the technique used to prevent it from delivering an electric shock to a user in the event of a fault.

- Class I equipment requires that any part that can come into contact with the user (e.g. the casing) is connected to an earth wire. This forms the third wire at the plug and it is coloured yellow and green in the UK. While the neutral wire runs back to the substation and is earthed there, this third wire in the plug allows another low resistance local connection to earth. If a fault occurs so that the casing of the equipment becomes live, a large current will flow to earth. In the process, the fuse in the plug will melt and break the circuit disconnecting the power. If the earth wire was not present, the fault could cause a large current to flow to earth via a user touching the unearthed casing, thus resulting in electrocution.
- Class II equipment does not require an earth wire, although it may still be present. All accessible parts are either double-insulated or have a single reinforced insulation layer. This insulation acts as an extra barrier against the possibility of these parts becoming live.
- Class III equipment requires no more than 24 V to power. This is achieved using a transformer that reduces the mains supply voltage, or using a battery; this system is called safety extra low voltage (SELV). It does not necessarily prevent a shock from being received, but the shock will be less severe than one received directly from the mains. Microshock is still possible.

Microshock
Equipment that is made to be inserted into the body is classified into a further three groups, depending on the maximum amount of leakage current that could flow in the presence of a single electrical fault.

- Type B ('body') equipment has a maximum leakage current of 500 µA if used with a Class I safety technique, or 100 µA if used with a Class II technique. Equipment may be considered IB or IIB respectively.
- Type BF ('body floating') leakage current standards are the same as Type B. However, Type BF equipment also incorporates an isolating transformer. Current that flows into the transformer coils from the mains causes induction in an adjacent circuit, called the floating circuit. The floating circuit can then be connected to equipment to be used with the patient. The presence of the transformer means that the patient circuit is not physically connected to the mains circuit and therefore is not earthed. This means that current from another source cannot find its way to earth via this circuit and therefore the likelihood of a shock is reduced.
- Type CF ('cardiac floating') equipment has a maximum leakage current of 50 µA if used with a Class I safety technique (ICF), or 10 µA if used with a Class II technique (IICF). Type CF equipment is the only equipment considered safe for direct contact with the heart.

Electrical symbols

Type B equipment

Maximum leakage current of 500 μA if Class I equipment, or 100 μA if Class II.

Fig. 12.2.1: Type B equipment symbol.

Type BF equipment

Maximum leakage currents are same as Type B equipment, but Type BF also has a floating patient circuit.

Fig. 12.2.2: Type BF equipment symbol.

Type CF equipment

Maximum leakage current of 50 μA if found in Class I equipment, or 10 μA if found in Class II equipment. Also has a floating patient circuit. Type CF is the only equipment type considered safe for insertion into the heart.

Fig. 12.2.3: Type CF equipment symbol.

Class II equipment

Class II equipment may or may not have a fused earth wire, but it has double insulation or a single layer of reinforced insulation. Class I and Class III equipment do not have a symbol.

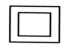

Fig. 12.2.4: Class II equipment symbol.

Battery

A battery consists of one or more electrochemical cells and produces a potential difference, causing DC to flow if a circuit is completed between its terminals.

Fig. 12.2.5: Battery.

Earth

Earth (or 'ground') is the reference potential from which other voltages are measured.

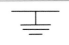

Fig. 12.2.6: Earth.

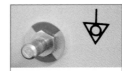

Fig. 12.2.7: The equipotential earth symbol found on the back of an anaesthetic machine.

Resistor

The resistance of a component is equal to the potential difference across it in volts divided by the current flowing in amps. This is Ohm's law. Many pieces of equipment (e.g. invasive blood pressure monitors) rely on resistors arranged as a Wheatstone bridge.

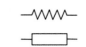

Fig. 12.2.8: Symbols used for a standard resistor.

Variable resistor

The resistance of these components is not fixed and can be altered depending on need. They are also used in the Wheatstone bridge.

Fig. 12.2.9: Symbols used for a variable resistor.

Capacitor

A capacitor can be charged by DC and then discharged at a later time. AC is unable to charge capacitors due to its continually changing polarity.

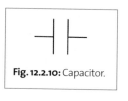

Fig. 12.2.10: Capacitor.

Inductor

An inductor consists of coils of wire through which a current flows. The current generates a magnetic field, and may induce a current to flow in adjacent wires.

Fig. 12.2.11: Inductor.

Transformer

A transformer uses an inductor to transfer current from one circuit to another. It contains two sets of coils, one connected to each circuit. If the number of coils is different on the two sides of the transformer, the voltage will be stepped up or down in proportion to the number of coils present.

Fig. 12.2.12: Transformer.

Switch

A switch is a reversible interruption in a circuit and it must be closed to allow current to flow.

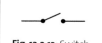

Fig. 12.2.13: Switch.

Diode

This component allows current to flow in one direction only. A theoretically ideal diode has zero resistance to current flow in one direction (forward) and infinite resistance in the opposite direction (reverse).

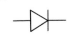

Fig. 12.2.14: Diode.

Therefore, AC will be converted to direct current because only the forward component can pass the diode. This is known as rectification.

Amplifier

An amplifier uses external electrical power to increase the amplitude of an input signal.

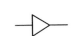

Fig. 12.2.15: Amplifier.

12.3 Cardiac pacemakers

Overview

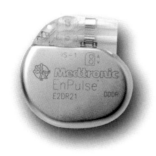

Fig. 12.3.1: The EnPulse permanent pacemaker. Image reproduced with permission from Medtronic.

Cardiac pacemakers can be temporary or permanent.

Permanent pacemakers are implanted subcutaneously, usually inferior to the left clavicle, and are connected to wires (also commonly called leads) that pace the heart at the endocardial surface. These wires are usually inserted via the subclavian vein, passing through the superior vena cava to terminate in either the right atrium or right ventricle. Modern pacemakers commonly have two wires, with one terminating in each chamber, and are known as dual chamber pacemakers. A biventricular pacemaker may have two or three wires: the first paces the right ventricle and septum as normal; the second is inserted through the right atrium, into the coronary sinus, passing along a cardiac vein in order to pace the lateral wall of the left ventricle; a third wire may be present to pace the atria.

Temporary pacemakers are much larger external devices. They are connected to wires that pace the heart at either the endocardial surface or the epicardial surface. The former are inserted into the heart via a central vein (transvenous pacing), while the latter are often inserted during cardiac surgery.

Transcutaneous pacing is also a form of temporary pacing. Many defibrillator machines have a function which allows pacing via standard chest pads as long as the ECG is also connected.

Uses

Permanent pacemakers are used to treat patients with bradycardia caused by sick sinus syndrome, atrioventricular (AV) conduction blocks, slow atrial fibrillation (AF) and other conditions. Biventricular pacemakers are used to resynchronize ventricular contraction in patients with bundle branch block and cardiac failure, and have been shown to increase life expectancy in this condition.

Temporary pacing wires are used during emergency situations, or as a short term solution while the patient is waiting for a permanent pacemaker to be fitted, or in the hours to days after cardiac surgery when arrhythmias are relatively common.

Transcutaneous pacing is used in emergencies when there is severe bradycardia and haemodynamic compromise. It is usually a very short-term solution that can be used while a temporary transvenous wire is arranged. It is painful while conscious, and so the patient should be sedated.

How it works

Pacemakers stimulate cardiac depolarization by delivering a small electrical current or voltage via the pacing wire. When the stimulus is sufficient that a cardiac depolarization follows every pacing impulse, this is known as electrical capture. The smallest current or voltage needed to cause capture is known as the threshold. Electrical capture can sometimes occur without the heart contracting in response. It is therefore important to check that mechanical capture has also occurred by checking the patient's pulse.

Pacemakers can be programmed to sense the intrinsic electrical activity in the heart caused by spontaneous depolarizations. The magnitude of the voltage (which is in the order of millivolts) that the pacemaker is able to detect can be set, and is known as the sensitivity. If the sensitivity is set high (i.e. the voltage it is able to detect is low), the pacemaker will detect most intrinsic activity but may also detect a lot of interference. If the sensitivity is set low then the interference may be ignored but some cardiac activity may be missed.

Note that pacemaker output may be set in current (mA) or voltage (V), depending on the model, but that sensitivity is always set as a voltage (mV).

Pacemakers can be set in different modes depending on the patient's underlying rhythm and pathology. In 2001 the North American Society of Pacing and Electrophysiology (NASPE) and the British Pacing and Electrophysiology Group (BPEG) revised a code of up to five letters that describes the mode of a pacemaker (see *Table 12.3.1*).

Table 12.3.1: Permanent pacemaker codes agreed by NASPE and BPEG.

Code letter	Meaning	Possible settings
1st	Chamber being paced	O = none, A = atrium
		V = ventricle, D = dual (both)
2nd	Chamber being sensed	O = none, A = atrium
		V = ventricle, D = dual (both)
3rd	What action should be taken if electrical activity is sensed?	O = sensing switched off
		I = inhibition (do not pace)
		T = trigger (pace)
		D = dual (T&I)
4th	Programmability settings	O = none
		R = rate modulation
5th	Multisite pacing	O = none, A = atria
		V = ventricles, D = dual

If the 4th and 5th letters are set to 'O', they are usually not quoted. Therefore, the simplest pacemaker is therefore VOO (or AOO). This will pace the heart via the single specified chamber at the set rate, regardless of the intrinsic cardiac activity. In VOO there is a risk of delivering the pacing stimulus at the same time as the ventricle is repolarizing from an intrinsic beat. This is known as R-on-T and can cause ventricular fibrillation (VF).

It is therefore safer to sense as well as pace. When a chamber is sensed, the pacemaker needs to know what action to take if intrinsic activity is detected. For example, VVI will pace and sense the ventricle. If an intrinsic depolarization is detected, the pacemaker will inhibit itself and not pace over the heart's spontaneous activity, thereby preventing R-on-T. Similarly, in VAT ventricular pacing would be triggered if an atrial depolarization was detected. In theory, this could be used to pace in the presence of complete AV block. In practice, DDD mode is usually used.

In DDD pacing, both chambers are paced, both are sensed, and the pacemaker can be triggered or inhibited in response to a sensed depolarization. If the pacemaker is in DDD mode and the heart is in normal sinus rhythm, then the P-wave will be sensed in the atria, which will inhibit any output from the atrial wire. As the P-wave is conducted, the ventricle responds with a QRS complex. This is sensed by the ventricular wire and further output is inhibited. However, if there is sick sinus syndrome with a DDD pacemaker the situation changes. There is no P-wave sensed in the atrium, so an atrial pacing stimulus is triggered. This is then conducted normally through the AV node causing ventricular depolarization which is sensed and therefore ventricular pacing is inhibited. Similarly, if there is AV conduction block with DDD mode, the atrium depolarizes spontaneously and this is sensed so atrial pacing is inhibited. The depolarization of the atria is then not conducted to the ventricles. The lack of ventricular activity is sensed and a ventricular pacing stimulus is triggered.

Some pacemakers can be rate modulated. This is indicated in the 4th letter of the code and means that the pacemaker can spontaneously change the pacing rate. These pacemakers are able to detect an increased respiratory rate, movement, increased temperature or other variables that may indicate the requirement for a faster heart rate.

The 5th letter indicates the presence of multisite pacing, showing that the pacemaker can pace more than one site in the specified type of chamber. For example, a biventricular pacemaker in DDD mode with rate modulation would be noted as DDDRV because both ventricles are being paced rather than just one (which would be DDDRO).

Interrogation and reprogramming
Permanent pacemaker boxes are implanted subcutaneously and can be interrogated and reprogrammed non-invasively by placing a wand over the skin. The wand wirelessly communicates with the pacemaker and is connected to a computer.

Different brands use different equipment and so the make of the pacemaker must be known in order to programme it. Patients are given a card with these details which they should bring with them to medical appointments. The devices can also be identified by markings visible on a chest X-ray.

⊕ Advantages

- Provides definitive treatment for bradyarrhythmias.
- Long battery life (usually 5–10 years).

⊖ Disadvantages

- Risk of infection, which may result in endocarditis.
- Susceptible to interference and subsequent pacemaker malfunction, especially in theatre.
- Diathermy:
  - Interference from diathermy in particular may be interpreted by the pacemaker as intrinsic cardiac activity and cause inhibition or triggering of pacing.
  - Interference may also cause the pacemaker to revert to a back-up mode (perhaps VOO) which runs the risk of VF as described above.
  - The pacemaker is susceptible to damage from diathermy currents, and microshock can also occur resulting in VF. Ideally diathermy should be avoided altogether in patients with pacemakers. If it must be used, bipolar diathermy is preferential to unipolar, and if unipolar diathermy must be used then the ground plate should be placed as far from the pacemaker as possible and diathermy only used in short controlled episodes.
- If DC cardioversion using an external defibrillator is required for any reason, the pads must be placed a minimum of 10 cm from the pacemaker. The pacemaker should be interrogated and settings checked afterwards.
- The communication between pacemakers and the computer wands that interrogate them is not encrypted. It is has been shown that it is possible to interrogate, reprogramme and switch off pacemakers from some distance. This problem has only recently been recognized, and plans are being made to tackle it.

ⓘ Safety

- If a patient with a pacemaker requires elective surgery, the pacemaker should have been checked within the preceding 3 months to ensure normal function. The cardiology centre that inserted the pacemaker should be contacted to take advice such as whether a cardiac physiologist should be present during surgery.
- If emergency surgery is required, the above steps should still be followed as far as is possible.
- If central venous catheters are to be used, care must be taken not to dislodge the pacing wires, especially if they are new and more mobile. A femoral approach may sometimes be considered safer.
- The use of a magnet as a solution for pacemaker problems, either in theatre or otherwise is not recommended. The application of a magnet to the pacemaker can have unpredictable results, from causing it to change to a back-up mode such as VOO, to reverting to factory settings, to performing various self-tests, to switching off entirely.
- People with pacemakers cannot go into MRI scanners.

Other notes

Temporary pacemakers are often encountered in critical care, especially in patients who have recently had cardiac surgery. These pacemakers work in the same way as the permanent ones described above, except that they are more easily reprogrammed, because the pacemaker electronics are external. Many different models of temporary pacemaker are available, but they will all allow the pacing rate, the pacing mode, output current, sensitivity voltage and other variables to be changed easily. They also often have a button that can be pressed in an emergency that switches the pacemaker to an asynchronous mode such as DOO or VOO and forces it to use the highest current output available. These modes will not sense any intrinsic activity, but simply give the best possible chance of adequate cardiac pacing in an emergency situation.

Table 12.3.2 provides a list of other possible problems that may be encountered with temporary (or permanent) pacemakers, and a list of simple solutions.

Table 12.3.2: Trouble-shooting temporary pacemaker problems.

What's the problem?	What does it look like?	Why is it a problem?	What might have caused it?	How can it be fixed?
No atrial capture	Atrial pacing spikes not followed by P-waves	Poor cardiac output / complete heart block / ventricular standstill	Pacing current set too low Low pacemaker battery Drugs (e.g. sodium / calcium channel blockers) Displacement or fracture of leads (possibly inside patient)	Increase pacemaker output in milliamps Reverse polarity of leads Replace battery
No ventricular capture	Ventricular pacing spikes not followed by QRS complexes			
No atrial sensing	P-waves are present, but atrial pacing spikes are still present (seen just after the P-wave)		Sensitivity on pacemaker is set too low Low pacemaker battery Displacement or fracture of leads (possibly inside patient)	Increase sensitivity by reducing mV threshold
No ventricular sensing	Normal QRS complexes are present but a ventricular pacing spike is present during the complex	Risk of R-on-T and ventricular fibrillation		
Over-sensing	Patient's rate / rhythm is insufficient, but no pacing occurs	Poor cardiac output / complete heart block / ventricular standstill	Sensitivity on pacemaker is set too high	Reduce sensitivity by increasing mV threshold
Cross-talk. Ventricular wire senses atrial spike and interprets it as ventricular QRS	Atrial pacing spike followed by P-wave, but then ventricular spike is absent		Ventricular sensitivity or atrial current set too high	Reduce sensitivity of ventricular channel or reduce pacemaker output from atrial channel in milliamps or volts

In all cases, check cables, electrodes and pacemaker battery. Replace if necessary. Try viewing ECG in different lead to reassess problem. Correct metabolic imbalances such as electrolyte abnormalities and acid–base disturbance. In acute cases, prepare for transcutaneous pacing and draw up chronotropic drugs. Be ready to begin cardiopulmonary resuscitation.

12.4 Implantable cardiovertor defibrillators

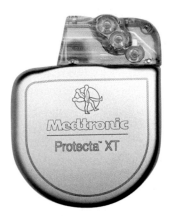

Fig. 12.4.1: The Protecta XT internal cardioverter defibrillator. Image reproduced with permission from Medtronic.

Overview

Implantable cardiovertor defibrillators (ICDs) are similar devices to permanent pacemakers and are implanted under the skin, with wires passing through central veins into the heart. Modern ICDs almost always have pacing functions, but they are also able to deliver a DC shock to the heart to treat tachyarrhythmias such as VF or VT.

Uses

ICDs are used instead of standard permanent pacemakers to treat people who are known to be at high risk of developing a ventricular tachyarrhythmia. This includes those who have previously had sustained VT or VF, those with significantly impaired left ventricular function (except in the initial 40 days post-myocardial infarction), and patients with specific types of hypertrophic obstructive cardiomyopathy or long QT syndrome. Several other indications also exist.

In addition to DC cardioversion and defibrillation, ICDs often also have other functions such as overdrive pacing which enable them to treat tachycardias without delivering a shock.

How it works

Detection of abnormal rhythms occurs in the same way as sensing via a standard permanent pacemaker, although a specific rhythm recognition algorithm is used. If the microprocessor decides that cardioversion is required, then a shock is delivered. The effect is the same as that which occurs with an external defibrillator although less energy is required (in the region of 10 to 30 joules).

The ICD may later be interrogated to determine the cause of the arrhythmia because it records a snapshot of the rhythm leading up to arrest. Its settings, or the patient's medication, may then be altered to try to prevent this in the future.

Overdrive pacing works by attempting to pace faster than a prevailing tachycardic arrhythmia and then subsequently reducing the rate once control is achieved.

The North American Society of Pacing and Electrophysiology (NASPE) and the British Pacing and Electrophysiology Group (BPEG) have produced a coding system similar to the one they use for permanent pacemakers (see *Table 12.4.1*).

Table 12.4.1: ICD codes.

Code letter	Meaning	Possible settings
1st	Chamber to be shocked	O = none, A = atrium
		V = ventricle, D = dual (both)
2nd	Anti-tachycardia pacing chamber	O = none, A = atrium
		V = ventricle, D = dual (both)
3rd	Anti-tachycardia detection	E = ECG, V = ventricle
		H = haemodynamic
4th	Pacing chamber	O = none, A = atrium
		D = dual (both)

⊕ Advantages

- Provides definitive treatment of bradyarrhythmias as well as being able to treat tachyarrhythmias.
- Long battery life, depending how many shocks are delivered. One shock will reduce the battery life by approximately 2 weeks.

⊖ Disadvantages

- Disadvantages of permanent pacemakers also apply to ICDs.

ⓘ Safety

- If a patient who has an ICD requires surgery, the same precautions should be taken as with a normal pacemaker. In addition, a cardiac electrophysiologist should disable the shock and anti-tachycardia function. An external defibrillator should be readily available.
- A patient with an ICD who collapses should be treated according to the ALS algorithm. A tingling may be felt in the hands of the individual performing chest compressions, but this will not be dangerous. VT or VF that is refractory to internal cardioversion should be treated with DC cardioversion via external paddles placed at least 10 cm from the ICD.
- Other safety issues of ICDs are the same as those for permanent pacemakers.

Other notes

On a chest X-ray, it is often possible to tell the difference between a normal permanent pacemaker and an ICD by looking at the wires. At least one of the ICD wires will have a thickening along several centimetres of its length, which is the electrode used to deliver a shock. Non-ICD pacemakers will not have this.

In the past, inadequate decontamination of anaesthetic equipment has led to the transmission of pathogenic organisms such as *Pseudomonas aeruginosa* and *Staphylococcus aureus*.*Mycobacterium tuberculosis* and the hepatitis C virus have also been found in breathing systems and filters after use. More recently concerns have been raised over the possible spread of prion diseases such as variant Creutzfeldt–Jakob disease (vCJD) by medical equipment. It is therefore important that if equipment is reusable, it is properly decontaminated between patients.

Equipment can be classified depending on its likelihood of transmitting an infectious organism.

- *Critical equipment* is equipment that penetrates the skin or mucous membrane to enter a normally sterile space or vascular space. Examples include surgical tools, intravascular cannulae, urinary catheters. Endotracheal tubes are also considered critical equipment despite not normally penetrating mucous membranes.
- *Semi-critical equipment* is equipment that comes into contact with skin or mucous membranes but does not enter a normally sterile or vascular space. Examples include laryngoscopes and temperature probes.
- *Non-critical equipment* is that which only comes into contact with intact skin, or is not in contact with the patient at all. Examples include non-invasive blood pressure cuffs, ECG electrodes, ultrasound probes and pulse oximeters.

Decontamination
Decontamination is the process of rendering a piece of equipment ready for use by the removal of macroscopic and microscopic contaminants in quantities sufficient to prevent a harmful reaction.

Different degrees of decontamination are required, depending on how critical the equipment is. Most decontamination in hospitals is done in the Sterile Services Department, although non-critical equipment can be decontaminated in the anaesthetic room.

Cleaning
Cleaning refers to the initial stage of decontamination. It is the only stage for non-critical equipment, but other classes of equipment will go on to be disinfected or sterilized after cleaning. Macroscopic material is removed as are many micro-organisms; however, infectious agents may survive the cleaning process.

Cleaning is performed by washing at a low temperature with a detergent to remove macroscopic debris. The low temperature is important, as high temperatures may cause proteins to condense and coagulate, leaving a film under which micro-organisms can escape removal.

Debris can be removed manually, by automated machines, or by ultrasonic cleaning. In the latter, the equipment is placed in water and ultrasound is used at a frequency of 50–400 kHz to produce longitudinal pressure waves. The areas of rarefaction in the sound waves have a very low pressure compared to the areas of compression. Billions of microscopic bubbles form at these low pressure areas, but they are short lived and collapse in on themselves in a process known as cavitation. The formation and collapse of these bubbles dislodges debris from the equipment.

It is important that equipment is disassembled as far as possible to allow thorough cleaning to occur.

Disinfection
Disinfection is a decontamination process that is intermediate between cleaning and sterilization. It will remove almost all microbial pathogens, including most viruses, but will not remove bacterial spores. Mycobacteria may also survive. Most semi-critical equipment is disinfected (*Fig. 12.5.1*).

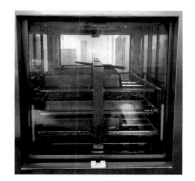

Fig. 12.5.1: Disinfection of surgical instruments.

Chemical disinfectants include gluteraldehyde (which can also be used for sterilization under different conditions), peracetic acid and chlorine-releasing substances that may be corrosive.

Pasteurization is a disinfection process that involves heating the equipment to 70–80°C for half an hour. The advantage of this is that there are no toxic chemicals used.

Sterilization

Sterilization is the most thorough stage of decontamination, and is defined as the complete removal of all forms of microbial life, including bacterial spores. In practice, the level of sterilization is expressed as the probability that any microbial life survived the sterilization process. This probability is known as the sterility assurance level and, for most pieces of equipment, a probability of 1 in a million (1 in 10^6) is sufficient. Critical equipment should be sterilized prior to use.

Equipment can be sterilized by exposure to chemicals, high temperatures, radiation or a combination of these.

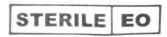

Fig. 12.5.2: A product bearing this symbol has been sterilized using ethylene oxide.

Chemicals used for sterilization include ethylene oxide, gluteraldehyde and hydrogen peroxide. They are used for equipment that cannot tolerate heating. Ethylene oxide is an explosive and flammable gas that is a highly effective sterilizing agent due to its toxicity, but requires up to 12 hours at temperatures of up to 65°C to work. *Figure 12.5.2* shows the symbol for a piece of equipment that has been sterilized using ethylene oxide. Gluteraldehyde is a liquid into which equipment must be submerged for over 10 hours to achieve good sterilization – time periods of less than this will achieve disinfection. Another chemical used is hydrogen peroxide which has the advantage of needing just a short time – some machines are able to sterilize in under half an hour. However, high concentrations are needed which are very toxic and penetration of equipment is not as good as with some other methods. Other chemicals that can be used in sterilization processes are ozone, chlorine bleach, and silver.

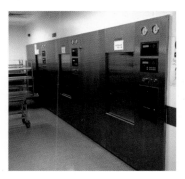

Fig. 12.5.3: Hospital autoclaves.

Autoclaves are the most common method of sterilization in the UK because they are efficient, safe, fast and reliable (*Fig. 12.5.3*). Equipment is cleaned, disinfected, rinsed and dried and then packaged and placed in the autoclave. The air in the autoclave is replaced with high pressure saturated steam at a temperature of either 121°C or 134°C for 15 minutes or 3 minutes, respectively. The fibres of the packaging initially allow steam to enter and come into contact with the enclosed instruments. By the end of the process, the fibres within the packaging swell and produce an airtight seal around the sterile instruments.

Irradiation of equipment with gamma rays, electron beams, high energy X-rays, or ultraviolet light may also be used, primarily industrially by manufacturers. This is not a method commonly used in hospitals.

Decontamination of fibreoptic bronchoscopes

Bronchoscopes must be cleaned immediately following use and should then be sent for disinfection. They are discussed separately here, because they are a rare example of a reusable piece of equipment that is cleaned by the anaesthetist.

Cleaning is the most important part of the process. The external surfaces of the scope are thoroughly wiped with an enzymatic detergent which breaks down tissue residues. At least 50 ml of this solution are then aspirated through the suction channel of the scope and in some cases a flexible brush may also be pulled through the channel. Following this, sterile water is aspirated to remove the remaining detergent.

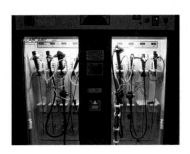

Fig. 12.5.4: Storage of endoscopes with air circulation.

The scope is then placed in a tray with an indication that it has been used and has not yet been disinfected (often a red cover). It is then transported to the hospital sterilizing services unit. Here it is disinfected using a liquid immersion method, such as with peracetic acid. This liquid may also be automatically pumped through the endoscope channels. The scope is dried and stored in a cabinet with dry, filtered air pumped through it to prevent the growth of micro-organisms (*Fig. 12.5.4*).

A note about prions

A group of rare diseases, including vCJD, are caused by infectious agents known as prions. These are proteins with an abnormal tertiary structure that are able to induce existing, normally folded proteins into adopting the same abnormal structure. A chain reaction occurs that results in accumulation of the abnormal protein and ultimately cell death. No treatments have been identified to date.

Prions have been shown to be highly resistant and difficult to remove from equipment. Only total denaturation of the protein is sufficient to render the prion inactive. In some circumstances, partially denatured prion proteins have been observed to reactivate under laboratory conditions.

Neither standard high pressure autoclaving at 134°C for 3 minutes, nor exposure to proteases or radiation or many of the chemicals described above, is sufficient to denature prion proteins.

One possible removal method suggested by the World Health Organization is to immerse the equipment with the prion into 1 M sodium hydroxide solution for 1 hour and then transfer to an autoclave and heat to 134°C for another hour. After this, the equipment should be cleaned again and the subjected to a standard sterilization process.

If feasible, single use disposable equipment should be used when prion disease is a possibility.

12.6 The Wheatstone bridge

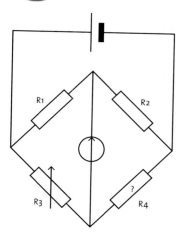

Fig. 12.6.1: The Wheatstone bridge circuit diagram.

Overview

The Wheatstone bridge was made popular by Sir Charles Wheatstone in 1843, 10 years after it was first invented by Samuel Christie for use in the telegraph machine.

Several pieces of anaesthetic equipment rely on the precise measurement of electrical resistance and the Wheatstone bridge is an electrical circuit that makes this possible. It is a null deflection device and so it is very accurate.

Uses

Examples of equipment incorporating a Wheatstone bridge include pressure transducers and electrical thermometers such as thermistors.

How it works

The Wheatstone bridge is a circuit containing four resistors. Two are of a fixed value (designated R1 and R2), one is variable (R3), and one is the unknown resistance being measured (R4). The resistors are arranged on opposite sides of a circuit so that R1 and R2 are in parallel with R3 and R4. A potential difference is placed across the two sides and a galvanometer compares the current flow between them.

If the current on one side of the circuit is greater, the resistance through that side must be less. The resistance in R3 is then altered until the galvanometer indicates no difference in the current between the two sides of the circuit, i.e. until R1/R2 = R3/R4. At this point, R4 can be calculated by using the equation R4 = (R2/R1)·R3.

Continuous electronic alteration of R3 so that no deflection occurs in the galvanometer as R4 varies, means that R4 can be calculated very accurately with a rapid response time. This is known as 'null deflection'. The resistance in R4 can then be displayed (as a waveform in the case of invasive blood pressure monitoring, for example).

The MHRA

Until the mid 1990s, medical devices and equipment were not formally regulated, although the UK Department of Health and the Scientific and Technical Branch (STB) worked to try to ensure the quality and safety of new medical products that appeared on the market. Following the incorporation of the STB with the NHS in the 1980s, a new agency was established, the Medical Devices Directorate (MDD). This subsequently became the Medical Devices Agency (MDA) in 1994 and was merged with the equivalent regulator of medicines, the Medicines Control Agency (MCA) in 2003. This result of this merger was the Medicines and Healthcare products Regulatory Agency (MHRA).

The MHRA is a UK government body responsible for ensuring that the medicines, blood products and equipment used in healthcare are acceptably safe. All equipment, from that described in this book to breast implants, wound dressings and PET scanners must be granted a licence by the MHRA before it can be used in the UK. The agency is able to force the withdrawal of a product from the market and can also prosecute manufacturers if it deems that regulatory laws have been broken. It works closely with NICE, the European Medicines Agency (EMEA), and the US Food and Drug Administration (FDA).

In order that a new piece of medical equipment is granted a licence, it must first have a CE mark (see below). Manufacturers need to be able to substantiate their claims about their product before a licence is granted, and these data come from clinical or laboratory trials. In cases where the device is so new that no clinical trials have yet been performed, a licence from the MHRA must be obtained to start one in the UK. Approximately 20% of such applications are refused on the grounds of patient safety concerns or health policy restrictions.

Although all new medicines are required to undergo clinical trials before a licence is granted, not all new medical devices are, because it is considered impractical or unnecessary to test some new equipment on patients when laboratory testing can suffice. The decision regarding whether a clinical trial is required depends on the type of device, how novel it is, its intended use and the potential it has to cause harm.

As well as granting licences, the MHRA is also responsible for monitoring the safety and quality of devices that are already in use. Effective monitoring and vigilance is achieved by regular inspections of manufacturing facilities, routine annual sampling and testing of equipment, the receipt of reports about design faults in equipment by healthcare professionals, gathering intelligence regarding counterfeit or illegal devices and enforcing laws that concern medical equipment.

If manufacturers become aware of a fault with their product, they must report it to the MHRA by law. The MHRA may also obtain information regarding a fault with a piece of equipment via their own testing programmes, reports from healthcare professionals, or other routes. Warnings and alerts are published by the MHRA regarding problems with equipment that is currently in use so that healthcare professionals may easily become aware of them. Approximately 8000 device reports are received every year, and the number is rising. This reflects the rising number of new pieces of equipment that are appearing on the market each year, rather than a fall in standards.

The CE mark

Strict rules and regulations set out by European Union (EU) legislation govern the way in which medical devices (and many other products) must be manufactured if they are to be marketed in the European Economic Area (EEA). It is a legal requirement that all medical devices sold in the UK have a CE mark.

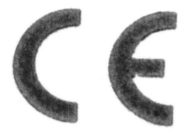

Fig. 12.7.1: The CE mark. A product bearing this symbol has been manufactured to standards that conform with European Union legislation.

In order to show that a manufacturer has complied with the regulations, their product is stamped with the CE (Conformité Européenne) mark, and this allows free trade on the European market. The mark does not indicate that that the product was made in the EU.

It is the manufacturer's responsibility to carry out the assessment of conformity with EU rules and to affix the CE mark to the product. However, for all but the simplest devices, this assessment is verified by an independent certification organization known as a Notified Body (NB). Another of the responsibilities of the MHRA is to appoint NBs in the UK and it is therefore known as the Competent Authority for the UK. Other European countries have their own Competent Authorities that appoint their own NBs. All NBs are regularly audited in order to ensure continuous high standards.

The British Standards Institute and the Kitemark

The British Standards Institute (BSI) was established in 1901 and began suggesting standards for steel and iron sections for use in civil engineering projects. It was therefore the world's first

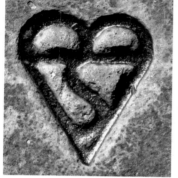

Fig. 12.7.2: The Kitemark symbol of the BSI.

standards body. In 1903, the Kitemark began to be applied to goods to inform consumers that they were 'up to standard' and complied with the BSI's recommendations. Since then, the BSI has expanded considerably. It operates in approximately 150 countries and has suggested standards for a wide range of products, from military equipment to office furniture.

The BSI played a considerable role in the establishment of the International Organization for Standardization (ISO) in 1947 and its European equivalent, the Comité Européen de Normalisation (CEN) in 1964.

One of the many current roles of the BSI is as a British NB. It therefore verifies that products that have been given the CE mark actually comply with European manufacturing legislation.

International standardization

The ISO is based in Geneva and has 163 member countries. It issues standards that have been agreed upon through worldwide consensus by bodies such as the BSI and CEN. These standards can be voluntarily applied by manufacturers to their products. In order to ensure that ISO itself is standardized and is not altered around the world because of the local language, the name ISO is said to be derived from the Greek *isos*, meaning equal. ISO standards are applied to a diverse range of products and systems, and some take their name directly from the standard. For example, the light sensitivity of camera film and of digital camera sensors is referred to as the ISO number.

The Global Harmonization Task Force (GHTF) was a body concerned with the international standardization of medical equipment in particular. In 2012, its role was taken over by the International Medical Device Regulators Forum (IMDRF), which had been established in 2011. The IMDRF is a voluntary group of regulators from around the world and is made up of representatives from Europe, Australia, Brazil, Canada, Japan and the United States. The World Health Organization (WHO) is an official observer. It is hoped that the IMDRF will help accelerate international agreement regarding manufacturing standards of medical equipment.

12.8 Intraosseous needles

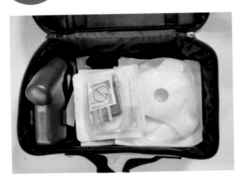

Fig. 12.8.1: An EZ-IO (Vidacare) grab bag. The bag contains all the items required for rapid intraosseous access, including the drill, needle, extension and fixation device.

Overview

Intraosseous (IO) needles provide an alternative means of accessing the circulation in situations where IV access is difficult or impossible to obtain. Their use may allow rapid, life-saving infusion of drugs, fluid or blood.

Needles may be inserted manually, via spring-loaded introducers, or using drill devices such as the widely available EZ-IO (Vidacare).

Uses

Intraosseous devices provide reliable access to the circulation. They are of particular use where intravenous access is difficult to obtain rapidly, such as in:

- peri-arrest and cardiac arrest situations
- trauma
- paediatrics
- obstetrics.

How it works

The marrow of long bones contains a non-collapsible network of vessels, held open by the structure of the bone itself even in profoundly shocked patients. Drugs and fluids administered into the marrow therefore can be rapidly flushed into the circulation.

Manual insertion of an intraosseous needle

The most common site for insertion is the flat section of the antero-medial tibia, around 2 cm below the tibial tuberosity. Ensuring this distance from the tibial tuberosity means that the needle avoids the growth plate in children. Flexing the knee and externally rotating the hip optimizes positioning.

- Use aseptic technique.
- In the awake patient, inject local anaesthetic from the skin down to the periosteum.
- Insert the needle directly through the skin, down to the bone.
- To enter the bony cortex, grip the needle between finger and thumb, holding it near the skin for stability. Use the palm to exert pressure on the needle hub. Use a back and forth twisting motion to advance through the cortex.
- As the needle enters the marrow space a loss of resistance is felt. At this point, stop inserting further. The needle should now be gripped firmly by the bone.
- Remove the inner trochar and use a syringe to aspirate marrow. The marrow may be used for a group and save if necessary. Note that aspiration is not always possible, even in correctly placed needles.
- The needle should flush easily and there should be no sign of extravasation.
- Secure the needle with tape. Fashioning a support, for instance using gauze may be helpful.
- When using the EZ-IO, the needle attaches to the drill magnetically. The drill is then used instead of manual rotation to advance the needle through the skin and into the bony cortex.

A similar loss of resistance is felt as the needle advances into the marrow at which point the drill is removed, and the needle used as in the steps above.

Alternative access points include the antero-lateral aspect of the distal femur (3 cm above the lateral condyle), the distal tibia and the proximal humerus.

Using intraosseous access
- *Fluids:* Marrow affords a relatively high resistance to flow when compared with IV access devices. Fluids must therefore usually be infused under pressure using a syringe, pressure bag or pump.
- *Blood products:* all blood products may be administered.
- *Drugs:* all emergency drugs may be used; they must be flushed into the circulation.

Advantages
- Insertion is usually straightforward.
- All resuscitation fluids, emergency drugs and blood products may be administered.
- Marrow aspirate may be used for a group and save.

Disadvantages
- Insertion may be painful.
- Complications include:
  - incorrect placement leading to extravasation of drugs (relatively common) and compartment syndrome (rare)
  - injury to the growth plate
  - fracture
  - infection.

Safety
There are few contraindications, but they include:

- existing fracture of the bone to be used
- osteogenesis imperfecta.

12.9 Cell salvage

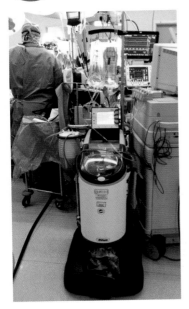

Fig. 12.9.1: Cell salvage apparatus.

Overview

Cell salvage allows blood collected from the surgical field to be washed, filtered, reconstituted and transfused back into the same patient. Cell salvage can be continuous or intermittent. It can be performed intra-operatively, by collecting blood directly from the surgical site, or post-operatively by collecting blood directly from surgical drains.

Uses

It is used in cases where significant blood loss is expected, such as in cardiothoracic or vascular surgery. It is also useful in patients who have rare blood groups and auto-antibodies, where finding a suitable donor is difficult. It may also be acceptable to some religious groups who might otherwise refuse an allogenic blood transfusion. There is also an economic benefit because the use of cell salvage can reduce demand on dwindling blood bank stocks.

How it works

There are six steps involved in cell salvage.

Step 1 – *Suction:* of blood from the surgical field, through low pressure, wide bore, double lumen tubing. The low pressure and wide bore of the tubing reduces red cell damage during collection. A second internal tube within the body of the suction tubing delivers an anticoagulant such as citrate directly to its distal end. Therefore blood is mixed with the anticoagulant as soon as it is collected, which reduces the risk of it clotting within the length of the suction tubing.

Step 2 – *Filtration:* microaggregates and other debris from the operative site are filtered using a filter whose pore size ranges from 40 to 150 µm.

Step 3 – *Separation:* a centrifuge is used to separate out the red cells.

Step 4 – *Washing and resuspension:* in isotonic saline.

Step 5 – *Disposal:* waste products such as white blood cells, platelets, plasma, fat and free haemoglobin are collected in a waste bag.

Step 6 – *Cell salvage and reinfusion:* the resuspended, washed red cells are collected in a bag at room temperature. The cell salvaged blood must be reinfused within 4 hours of processing.

Note that the blood remains citrated, so calcium may need to be administered to neutralize the citrate, especially if there is any liver dysfunction. The quality of the cell salvaged blood depends on the volume of wash required, the quality of the blood before washing, the type of surgery and any residual contamination within it.

⊕ Advantages

- Reduces demand for allogenic (donated) blood.
- Reduces risk of transmitting allogenic transfusion related infections (e.g. HIV).
- No risk of ABO incompatibility.
- May be acceptable to some religious groups who would otherwise refuse allogenic blood transfusion.

- Cells are infused at room temperature.
- Cell saved blood contains near normal levels of 2,3-diphosphoglycerate (2,3-DPG), which improves oxygen delivery.

Disadvantages

- High initial capital outlay.
- High cost of disposables.
- Staff training required.
- Risk of red cell damage during collection and processing (skimming).
- Risk of bacterial contamination.
- Risk of fat and amniotic fluid emboli.
- Citrate within resuspended blood can contribute to a systemic coagulopathy.

Safety

There are some circumstances where the transfusion of cell salvaged blood remains controversial. These include cancer surgery, obstetrics and non-sterile surgery (e.g. bowel perforation), where there is a risk of transfusing cancer cells, amniotic fluid or bacteria systemically. The risk can be mitigated by using a second suction system to remove undesirable substances before using the cell salvage suction.

Chapter 13
Sample FRCA questions

1 Medical gases

Multiple choice questions

For each of these questions, mark every answer either true (T) and false (F)

(1) The vacuum insulated evaporator:
    a) Stores oxygen at below its critical temperature.
    b) Contains oxygen as liquid and vapour.
    c) May be mounted on a weighing scale.
    d) Actively cools its contents to −160°C.
    e) Has a pressure-releasing valve set to around 700 kPa.
(2) Concerning the delivery of supplemental oxygen:
    a) The Hudson mask acts as a variable performance device.
    b) The nasopharynx acts as an oxygen reservoir.
    c) The Venturi mask may act as a variable performance device.
    d) Nasal high flow generates PEEP.
    e) The Venturi principle states that a fluid will increase its velocity as it flows through a constriction.
(3) With regard to a medical gas cylinder:
    a) It is usually made of chromium molybdenum (chromoly) or aluminium.
    b) A size E cylinder will yield 340 litres of oxygen when full.
    c) Its valve block is engraved with its testing pressure.
    d) The filling ratio for nitrous oxide cylinders in the UK is 0.67.
    e) Air cylinders have a blue body and white shoulders in the UK.

Short answer questions

(1) Describe how medical gases are stored for use in anaesthetics. Include in your answer:
    a) The vacuum insulated evaporator.
    b) Cylinders and cylinder banks.

Viva questions

(1) Describe the scavenging system in use at your hospital. What are its main components? What are its safety features?
(2) What are the safety features of the medical gas supply to your anaesthetic machine?

2 Airway equipment

Multiple choice questions

For each of these questions, mark every answer either true (T) or false (F).

(1) Regarding fibreoptic intubation:
    a) A glass fibre is approximately 20 μm in diameter.
    b) The light source is usually at the tip of the scope.
    c) The tip may be manoeuvred in four directions using the control knobs.
    d) Awake fibreoptic intubation is indicated in a child with epiglottitis.
    e) Total internal reflection occurs at angles of incidence below the critical angle.

(2) A patient requires a cricothyroidotomy:
    a) The 4th National Audit Project (NAP 4) suggests that needle cricothyroidotomy is more effective than surgical techniques.
    b) The cricothyroid membrane connects the cricoid cartilage to the thyroid gland.
    c) In needle cricothyroidotomy, a patent upper airway is required for expiration.
    d) Devices smaller than 4 mm ID are considered 'small cannula' devices.
    e) Surgical cricothyroidotomies should be performed by experienced surgeons only.

(3) Regarding the LMA:
    a) It may be useful in a 'can't intubate, can't ventilate' scenario.
    b) Aperture bars may prevent the epiglottis blocking the airway.
    c) It is a definitive airway.
    d) A size 2 LMA is suitable for children weighing 10–20 kg.
    e) The classic LMA seals to a relatively low airway pressure of less than 20 cmH$_2$O.

Short answer questions

(1) Describe an airway device for delivering high pressure (jet) ventilation via each of the following routes. Include the benefits and disadvantages of each route.
    a) Supraglottic.
    b) Transglottic.
    c) Trans-tracheal.

(2) Describe how you would perform an awake fibreoptic intubation on a patient presenting for elective surgery, with a known difficult airway.

Viva questions

(1) What are the indications for the use of a double lumen endotracheal tube? How is it inserted? How might it be incorrectly placed and how would you detect this?

(2) Describe the indications for tracheostomy. What types of tracheostomy tubes are available? What are the key points in giving an anaesthetic for a tracheostomy insertion?

3 Breathing systems

Multiple choice questions

For each of these questions, mark every answer either true (T) or false (F).

(1) Regarding the Bain breathing system:
    a) It is a co-axial variant of the Lack system.
    b) Fresh gas flows through the inner tubing.
    c) It is more efficient for controlled ventilation than a circle system.
    d) It may be used in conjunction with a ventilator.
    e) Fresh gas flow should not be lower than alveolar minute ventilation.

(2) Soda lime:
    a) Is located after the APL valve in a circle system.
    b) Is part of the original Waters circuit.
    c) Usually comprises sodium hydroxide, calcium hydroxide and potassium hydroxide.
    d) Undergoes an exothermic reaction.
    e) Produces compound A in a reaction with sevoflurane.

(3) Regarding the Humphrey ADE block:
   a) It is less efficient than conventional Mapleson breathing systems.
   b) When in the Mapleson A configuration, it allows fresh gas flows as low as $50\,ml.kg^{-1}.min^{-1}$, before carbon dioxide is rebreathed.
   c) 15 mm externally corrugated smooth bore tubing is used with it to reduce resistance.
   d) It can only be used in adults.
   e) It comprises an integrated pressure relief valve that opens at pressures exceeding $60\,cmH_2O$.

Short answer questions

(1) Describe the circle system. Include in your answer:
   a) A diagram showing the location of the constituent parts, with a description of each of their functions.
   b) The advantages of the system.
   c) The disadvantages of the system.

Viva questions

(1) Draw the breathing circuits in the Mapleson system. Explain why some are in common clinical use whereas others are not.
(2) What are the advantages of the reservoir bag? What is the law of Laplace? How does it reduce barotrauma?

4 Ventilators

Multiple choice questions

For each of these questions, mark every answer either true (T) or false (F).

(1) When ventilating a patient using pressure control mode:
   a) The flow during inspiration is constant.
   b) Flow is high at the beginning of inspiration.
   c) The tidal volume delivered is fixed.
   d) The ventilator triggers each breath.
   e) Barotrauma is less likely than when volume control is used.
(2) The Penlon Nuffield 200 ventilator:
   a) Is a pneumatically driven and controlled, time cycled, constant flow generator.
   b) With a standard adult patient valve attached, the lowest tidal volume that can be achieved is 250 ml.
   c) Three dials allow adjustment of the inspiratory time, expiratory time and tidal volume.
   d) The standard adult patient valve incorporates a pressure relief valve that opens at pressures in excess of $60\,cmH_2O$.
   e) The Newton valve, used in conjunction with a Penlon Nuffield 200 ventilator, can deliver tidal volumes of 10–300 ml.
(3) Concerning high frequency oscillatory ventilation (HFOV):
   a) Both inspiration and expiration are active.
   b) Relies on the Venturi principle to entrain surrounding air.
   c) The diaphragm oscillates at 3–15 Hz.
   d) Bias flow is the constant flow of gas through the ventilator.

e) Two recent multicentre randomized controlled trials, OSCAR and OSCILLATE, have suggested that there is no mortality benefit associated with HFOV.

Short answer questions

(1) List the indications for high frequency *jet* ventilation. How does it differ from high frequency *oscillatory* ventilation? What are the main disadvantages and risks associated with high frequency *jet* ventilation?

(2) What criteria should be met before a patient can be weaned from an ITU ventilator? Describe two ventilator modes you might use during this process; what are their relative advantages and disadvantages?

Viva questions

(1) What is PEEP and how does it affect gas exchange? Is there a difference between PEEP and CPAP during positive pressure ventilation? In what ways might a ventilator generate PEEP? What are the physiological risks associated with excessive PEEP?

(2) How might you classify ventilators used in clinical practice? Describe your ideal ventilator.

5 Anaesthetic delivery

Multiple choice questions

For each of these questions, mark every answer either true (T) or false (F).

(1) Plenum vaporizers:
  a) Have a low internal resistance.
  b) Require a pressurized fresh gas flow.
  c) Fully saturate fresh gas that pass through their vaporization chambers.
  d) Include the Oxford Miniature Vaporizer.
  e) Such as the Tec 5 series are accurate to +/− 1% of the dial setting at flows of 15–200 ml.min^{-1} at 21°C.

(2) Concerning the delivery of desflurane via a Tec6 vaporizer:
  a) Desflurane has a boiling point close to room temperature.
  b) Desflurane is pressurized to 2 atmospheres.
  c) Requires an electrical supply.
  d) A differential pressure transducer compensates for changes in the fresh gas flow.
  e) The output is unaffected by ambient temperature.

(3) Regarding target controlled infusions of propofol:
  a) The induction dose required can be calculated by multiplying the initial volume of distribution by the desired plasma or effect site concentration.
  b) Targeting the effect site concentration (Ce) leads to a quicker induction than targeting the plasma concentration of propofol (Cp).
  c) Targeting the effect site concentration (Ce) leads to temporary overshooting of the plasma concentration during induction.
  d) The Marsh and Schneider pharmokinetic models for target controlled infusions tend to over-dose children.
  e) Remifentanil target controlled infusions use the Schneider model for plasma or effect-site targeting.

Short answer questions

(1) What are the advantages and disadvantages of total intravenous anaesthesia (TIA) compared to volatile anaesthesia? How might you reduce the risk of awareness whilst delivering a total intravenous anaesthetic?

(2) Describe how and why a vaporizer delivering desflurane is different from one delivering isoflurane.

Viva questions

(1) What is latent heat of vaporization and specific heat? What relevance do these have during vaporization?

(2) How does the function of a Tec5 sevoflurane vaporizer change at altitude?

(3) Classify vaporizers.

6 Monitoring equipment

Multiple choice questions

For each of these questions, mark every answer either true (T) or false (F).

(1) The fuel cell:
   a) Is also known as the polarographic electrode.
   b) Has a potassium hydroxide electrolyte solution.
   c) Requires an external power source.
   d) Has a positive anode made from gold and a negative cathode made from lead.
   e) Requires gas to be dried before it is analysed, because water vapour interferes with the signal.

(2) Regarding gas analysis:
   a) The paramagnetic analyser gives an acceptable estimation of oxygen partial pressure in a gas mixture, but is not completely accurate.
   b) The wavelength of a laser beam will be reduced as it passes through a mixture of gases.
   c) N_2, O_2, helium, hydrogen and ozone are all gases that cannot be detected by infrared analysis.
   d) Side-stream capnographs utilize a 1.2 mm diameter Teflon tube to carry gas from the breathing system to the analyser.
   e) The Severinghaus CO_2 electrode needs to be calibrated regularly.

(3) Concerning rotameters:
   a) They are variable orifice fixed pressure flowmeters.
   b) Bobbins must not be swapped between rotameter tubes.
   c) At equilibrium, the pressure drop across the bobbin when gas is flowing around it is equal to the weight of the bobbin divided by the cross-sectional area of its base.
   d) The rotameter tube is cylindrical.
   e) The rotameter will function completely normally at high temperatures and at high altitudes.

Short answer questions

(1) What are the minimum standards for monitoring patients under general anaesthesia as recommended by the AAGBI? What extra monitoring would you consider using for patients undergoing a major laparotomy and why?

(2) Discuss the different methods of measuring the concentration of oxygen in a gas mixture.

Viva questions

(1) How can blood pressure be measured?
(2) What measurements does a thromboelastograph make? What do they mean?

7 Filters and humidifiers

Multiple choice questions

For each of these questions, mark every answer either true (T) or false (F).

(1) A heat and moisture exchanger (HME):
   a) Is an active humidification device.
   b) Produces 100% relative humidification of inspired gases.
   c) May be impregnated with hygroscopic salts.
   d) Has an internal resistance which increases with use.
   e) Efficiency falls as tidal volumes and inspiratory flow rates increase.
(2) With regard to active humidification of gases:
   a) Gases that are fully saturated with water at body temperature (37°C) have an absolute humidity of $17\,g.m^{-3}$.
   b) It is an energy dependent process.
   c) There is a risk of bacterial contamination in a bubble humidifier reservoir.
   d) Ultrasonic nebulized humidifiers are more efficient than HMEs.
   e) Surface bath humidifiers may be heated to 40–60°C.
(3) Filters:
   a) The relative contribution of inertial impaction to filtration efficiency increases as the density of a given particle decreases.
   b) A nominal filter rating of 99% at $0.5\,\mu m$ means that 99% of contaminants equal to or greater than $0.5\,\mu m$ in diameter have been successfully removed by the filter.
   c) An epidural filter is able to filter particles as small as $0.2\,\mu m$.
   d) Packed red cells must be given through an in-line mesh filter with a pore size of $20–40\,\mu m$.
   e) Both inertial and diffusional impaction work best when filtering solid particles from a gas rather than a liquid.

Short answer questions

(1) How is whole blood converted to various blood products? What filtration processes are required pre-storage and at the time of delivery?

Viva questions

(1) What is the difference between absolute and relative humidity? What is the dew point? What is the absolute humidity of fully saturated air at room temperature and at body temperature?
(2) Through what mechanisms does a filter remove particles from a flow of liquid or gas?

8 Regional anaesthesia

Multiple choice questions

For each of these questions, mark every answer either true (T) or false (F).

(1) With respect to a sub-Tenon's block:
   a) Hyaluronidase is an enzyme which breaks down connective tissue and therefore improves the spread of the local anaesthetic.
   b) Proxymetacaine is used to disinfect the eye.
   c) The patient is typically asked to look inferio-medially whilst the block is performed.
   d) Moorfield's forceps are used to grasp the conjunctiva and the underlying Tenon's capsule together around 2 mm from the inferonasal limbus.
   e) The block has been administered safely in patients on warfarin, aspirin and clopidogrel.

(2) With regards to electrical nerve stimulation:
   a) A supramaximal stimulus should be applied.
   b) For a given current amplitude, shorter impulse durations will preferentially stimulate smaller nerve fibres.
   c) Less energy is needed to stimulate a nerve that is adjacent to the anode than one adjacent to the cathode.
   d) Rheobase is the minimum current amplitude of indefinite duration that results in an action potential.
   e) The energy required to depolarize a neuron and the distance between the neuron and electrode is related by the inverse square law.

(3) With respect to central neuraxial blockage:
   a) Use of a Quincke spinal needle is associated with a higher incidence of post-dural puncture headache, compared to the use of a Whitacre needle.
   b) The Sprotte spinal needle has a diamond-shaped cutting tip.
   c) A Luer connection comprises a male connector with a 6% taper and a matching female receptor.
   d) Commonly used epidural needles are 8 cm long and 20G or 22G in size.
   e) Adult epidural catheters range from 18 to 20G in diameter and up to 915 mm in length.

Short answer questions

(1) List the indications for a performing a sub-Tenon's block. What are its relative strengths and weaknesses compared to a peribulbar block? Describe how you would perform a sub-Tenon's block.

(2) Describe how you would manage an inadvertent dural puncture with an 18G Tuohy needle, whilst performing an epidural for labour.

Viva questions

(1) How would you perform a femoral nerve block using a nerve stimulator? What initial settings would you use on the stimulator? Why?

(2) How can we measure the depth of neuromuscular blockade?

9 Critical care

Multiple choice questions

For each of these questions, mark every answer either true (T) or false (F).

(1) Pulmonary artery catheters:
   a) Utilize the Fick principle to estimate cardiac output.
   b) Are known to improve outcome in patients treated in intensive care.
   c) Are associated with pulmonary artery rupture that has a mortality rate of approximately 30%.
   d) Typically have four to five lumens.
   e) Have a balloon at the tip that should be inflated with 1–5 ml of air.

(2) Regarding defibrillators:
   a) They have an inductor in the charging circuit.
   b) They include an inductor in the discharge circuit in order to increase the speed of energy delivery.
   c) The discharge waveform can be monophasic or biphasic.
   d) They should only be used by highly trained members of medical staff.
   e) Have a capacitor that discharges according to the equation $V = V_{max} \cdot (1 - e^{-t/RC})$.

(3) Regarding intracranial pressure measurement:
   a) Normal ICP is 15–20 mmHg.
   b) The tip of an external ventricular drain (EVD) is surgically placed in the lateral ventricle.
   c) Intraparenchymal monitors may be extradural, subdural or subarachnoid.
   d) EVDs can be used to treat raised intracranial pressure as well as measure it.
   e) EVDs have a lower rate of infection when compared with other ICP monitors.

Short answer questions

(1) Outline the different modes of renal replacement therapy and describe how they differ. What are the possible complications of this therapy?

(2) Describe the principles of the intra-aortic balloon pump and how it may benefit a patient with cardiac failure. What are the possible complications of using this piece of equipment?

Viva questions

(1) Draw a cardiopulmonary bypass circuit. Which different types of blood pump are available and what are the advantages and disadvantages of these? How does 'mini-bypass' differ from normal bypass?

(2) Can you outline the different methods of measuring cardiac output in the intensive care unit? Which do you prefer to use and why?

10 Surgical equipment relevant to anaesthetists

Multiple choice questions

For each of these questions, mark every answer either true (T) or false (F).

(1) Regarding chest drains:
   a) These should be inserted using a trocar in an emergency situation.
   b) Underwater seals should be primed with a volume of water equal to the patient's tidal volume.

c)   They should never be clamped.
d)   They should only have suction applied if advised by a respiratory physician or thoracic surgeon.
e)   The use of live ultrasound is advised by the British Thoracic Society (BTS) when inserting drains for the removal of fluid.

(2) Surgical diathermy:
a)   Uses alternating current.
b)   Has a frequency of approximately 50 Hz.
c)   Produces a heat energy that is proportional to the square of the current multiplied by the resistance.
d)   Does not produce significant heat at the diathermy plate due to the low current density.
e)   Produces diathermy smoke that is harmless.

(3) Regarding lasers:
a)   The photothermal effect describes a laser's ability to vaporize water by generating heat.
b)   Photoablation is the destruction of tissues due to the generation of heat.
c)   The lasing medium may be a solid, liquid or gas.
d)   The carbon dioxide laser beam is infrared.
e)   The Nd:YAG laser has a liquid lasing medium.

Short answer questions

(1) What are the properties of laser light? How is a laser beam produced? What are the safety considerations of laser surgery?

(2) List the indications and contraindications to using an arterial tourniquet during surgery. What are some of the complications of using this piece of equipment?

Viva questions

(1) Why are patients not electrocuted by diathermy? What is the difference between monopolar and bipolar diathermy? How do diathermy modes differ (e.g. cut, coag, blend)?

(2) Pretend I am a patient who requires a chest drain for a pleural effusion. Explain to me why I need it, how you will insert it and what complications are possible.

11 Radiology equipment

Multiple choice questions

For each of these questions, mark every answer either true (T) or false (F).

(1) When giving an anaesthetic in the interventional radiology suite:
a)   Radiation exposure is reliably minimized by wearing a lead apron.
b)   Beam softening improves safety.
c)   The radiation dose should be kept inside legal limits.
d)   The radiation dose 3 m from the source is 9 times lower than that at 1 m.
e)   The dose during an angiogram may be equivalent to over 100 chest X-rays.

(2) Regarding magnetic resonance imaging:
a)   Most current scanners have a magnetic strength of over 3 tesla.
b)   An electromagnet cooled by liquid nitrogen is used.
c)   MRI is superior to CT in imaging the spinal cord.
d)   A standard anaesthetic machine must be kept outside the 50 gauss line.
e)   MRI conditional equipment poses no known hazard under specified conditions.

(3) Regarding medical ultrasound:
- a) It uses sound waves between 2 and 20 kHz.
- b) Piezoelectric crystals produce and detect reflected sound waves.
- c) B-mode produces a 2-dimensional image.
- d) M-mode is used in cardiac scans because it is more accurate.
- e) The Doppler effect is the change in amplitude of a sound wave that occurs when a wave is reflected off an object that is moving relative to the observer.

Short answer questions

(1) When giving an anaesthetic in an MRI scanner:
- a) What are the safety concerns relating to anaesthetic and monitoring equipment?
- b) How may these safety concerns be addressed?

Viva questions

(1) What are the broad categories of ultrasound use in medicine? What specific uses does ultrasound have in anaesthetics? What settings might you adjust on an ultrasound scanner when inserting a CVP line? What effect would this have on the image?

(2) What is ionizing radiation? Under what circumstances may an anaesthetist be exposed? What features of an X-ray machine reduce unnecessary radiation exposure? How may staff and patients be further protected?

12 Miscellaneous

Multiple choice questions

For each of these questions, mark every answer either true (T) or false (F).

(1) Concerning electrical safety:
- a) In type BF equipment all accessible parts are shielded from live parts by two layers of insulation.
- b) Two concentric squares is the symbol for type III equipment.
- c) Only type CF equipment is safe to be inserted into the heart.
- d) A floating circuit is one where the part connected to the patient is electrically isolated from the mains circuit.
- e) The maximum accepted leakage current from type CF equipment is 50 mA.

(2) Regarding the regulation of medical devices:
- a) The Medicines and Healthcare products Regulatory Agency (MHRA) is responsible for ensuring that the medicines, blood products and equipment used in healthcare are acceptably safe.
- b) In order that a new piece of medical equipment is granted a licence, it must first have a CE mark.
- c) If manufacturers become aware of a fault with their product, they must report it to the MHRA by law.
- d) The CE mark (Conformité Européenne) indicates that a product was manufactured in Europe.
- e) All new medical equipment must undergo clinical trials on patients before they are approved for sale.

(3) Regarding permanent pacemakers:
   a)   They have wires that are usually inserted through the subclavian artery.
   b)   A biventricular pacemaker may have 3 wires.
   c)   The first code letter of the five letters that are used to describe a pacemaker refers to the chamber being paced.
   d)   VVI mode is less likely to trigger VF than VOO mode.
   e)   Rate modulation allows the pacemaker to automatically change its rate when it detects increased activity, which might require an increased cardiac output.

Short answer questions

(1) Discuss the precautions that are taken in theatre to prevent staff and patients from suffering electric shocks from equipment.
(2) Draw a simple Wheatstone bridge circuit. Describe how it is used during the measurement of arterial blood pressure.

Viva questions

(1) How are cardiac pacemakers classified? How may the presence of a permanent pacemaker alter your anaesthetic plan for a patient?
(2) What do you understand by the term 'decontamination'? How is anaesthetic equipment classified in terms of the risk it poses to patients from infection? How is equipment decontaminated?

ANSWERS TO MCQs

Chapter 1 – Medical gases

(1)	The VIE	TTTFT	(Section 1.1)
(2)	Supplemental oxygen	TTTTF	(Sections 1.9–1.13)
(3)	Cylinders	TFTFF	(Section 1.3)

Chapter 2 – Airway equipment

(1)	Fibreoptic intubation	TFFFF	(Section 2.10)
(2)	Cricothyroidotomy	FFTTF	(Section 2.16)
(3)	LMA	TTFTT	(Section 2.6)

Chapter 3 – Breathing systems

(1)	The Bain system	FTFTT	(Section 3.5)
(2)	Soda lime	TTTTT	(Section 3.7)
(3)	Humphrey ADE	FTTFT	(Section 3.6)

Chapter 4 – Ventilators

(1)	Pressure control ventilation	FTFTT	(Section 4.1)
(2)	Penlon Nuffield 200	TFFTT	(Section 4.5)
(3)	HFOV	TFTTT	(Section 4.10)

Chapter 5 – Anaesthetic delivery

(1)	Plenum vaporizers	FTTFF	(Section 5.5)
(2)	Desflurane Tec6	TTTTT	(Section 5.6)
(3)	TCI of propofol	TTTFF	(Section 5.12)

Chapter 6 – Monitoring equipment

(1)	The fuel cell	FTFFF	(Section 6.3)
(2)	Regarding gas analysis	FTTTT	(Sections 6.4–6.6, 6.12, 6.22)
(3)	Concerning rotameters	TTTFF	(Section 6.2)

Chapter 7 – Filters and humidifiers

(1)	HME	FFTTT	(Section 7.1)
(2)	Active humidification	FTTTT	(Section 7.2)
(3)	Filters	FTTFT	(Section 7.3)

Chapter 8 – Regional anaesthesia

(1)	Sub-Tenon's block	TFFFT	(Section 8.8)
(2)	Electrical nerve stimulation	TFFTT	(Section 8.1)
(3)	Central neuraxial blockade	TFTFT	(Sections 8.3 & 8.4)

Chapter 9 – Critical care

(1)	Pulmonary artery catheters	FFTTF	(Section 9.8)
(2)	Defibrillators	FFTFF	(Section 9.20)
(3)	Regarding intracranial pressure	FTFTF	(Section 9.11)

Chapter 10 – Surgical equipment relevant to anaesthetists

(1)	Chest drains	FFFTT	(Section 10.2)
(2)	Surgical diathermy	TFTTF	(Section 10.1)
(3)	Regarding lasers	TFTTF	(Section 10.4)

Chapter 11 – Radiological equipment

(1)	Radiation safety	FFFTT	(Section 11.1)
(2)	MRI	FFTFT	(Section 11.3)
(3)	Medical ultrasound	FTTTF	(Section 11.2)

Chapter 12 – Miscellaneous

(1)	Concerning electrical safety	FFTTF	(Sections 12.1 & 12.2)
(2)	Regulation of equipment	TTTFF	(Section 12.7)
(3)	Permanent pacemakers˙	FTTTT	(Section 12.3)

Index